Pediatric Surgery

Editor

JOHN D. HORTON

SURGICAL CLINICS
OF NORTH AMERICA

www.surgical.theclinics.com

Consulting Editor
RONALD F. MARTIN

October 2022 • Volume 102 • Number 5

ELSEVIER

1600 John F. Kennedy Boulevard • Suite 1800 • Philadelphia, Pennsylvania, 19103-2899

http://www.surgical.theclinics.com

SURGICAL CLINICS OF NORTH AMERICA Volume 102, Number 5
October 2022 ISSN 0039–6109, ISBN-13: 978-0-323-98651-9

Editor: John Vassallo, j.vassallo@elsevier.com
Developmental Editor: Arlene Campos

Surgical Clinics of North America (ISSN 0039–6109) is published bimonthly by Elsevier Inc., 360 Park Avenue South, New York, NY 10010-1710. Months of publication are February, April, June, August, October, and December. Business and Editorial Offices: 1600 John F. Kennedy Blvd., Suite 1800, Philadelphia, PA 19103-2899. Periodicals postage paid at New York, NY and additional mailing offices. Subscription prices are $456.00 per year for US individuals, $1240.00 per year for US institutions, $100.00 per year for US & Canadian students and residents, $547.00 per year for Canadian individuals, $1283.00 per year for Canadian institutions, $552.00 for international individuals, $1283.00 per year for international institutions and $250.00 per year for foreign students/residents. To receive student/resident rate, orders must be accompanied by name of affiliated institution, date of term, and the *signature* of program/residency coordinator on institution letterhead. Orders will be billed at individual rate until proof of status is received. Foreign air speed delivery is included in all *Clinics* subscription prices. All prices are subject to change without notice. POSTMASTER: Send address changes to *Surgical Clinics*, Elsevier Health Sciences Division, Subscription Customer Service, 3251 Riverport Lane, Maryland Heights, MO 63043. **Customer Service (orders, claims, online, change of address): Telephone: 1-800-654-2452 (U.S. and Canada); 314-447-8871 (outside U.S. and Canada). Fax: 314-447-8029. E-mail: journalscustomerservice-usa@elsevier.com (for print support); journalsonlinesupport-usa@elsevier.com (for online support).**

Reprints. For copies of 100 or more, of articles in this publication, please contact the Commercial Reprints Department, Elsevier Inc., 360 Park Avenue South, New York, New York 10010-1710. Tel. 212-633-3874, Fax: 212-633-3820, E-mail: reprints@elsevier.com.

Surgical Clinics of North America is also published in Spanish by McGraw-Hill Interamericana Editores S.A., P.O. Box 5-237 06500 Mexico D.F. Mexico; and in Portuguese by Interlivros Edicoes Ltda., Rua Comandante Coelho 1085, CEP 21250, Rio de Janeiro, Brazil; and in Greek by Paschalidis Medical Publications, Athens Greece.

Surgical Clinics of North America is covered in *MEDLINE/PubMed (Index Medicus), EMBASE/Excerpta Medica, Current Contents/Clinical Medicine, Current Contents/Life Sciences, Science Citation Index,* and *ISI/BIOMED.*

Contributors

CONSULTING EDITOR

RONALD F. MARTIN, MD, FACS
Colonel (Retired), United States Army Reserve, Department of General Surgery, Pullman
Regional Hospital and Clinic Network, Pullman, Washington

GUEST EDITOR

JOHN D. HORTON, MD
Department of Surgery, Madigan Army Medical Center, Tacoma, Washington

AUTHORS

MEADE BARLOW, MD, FACS, FAAP
Pediatric Surgery and Pediatric Trauma, Mary Bridge Children's Hospital and Health
Network, Tacoma, Washington

ERICA BRENNER, MD, MSCR
Assistant Professor, Department of Pediatrics, Division of Gastroenterology, University of
North Carolina School of Medicine, Chapel Hill, North Carolina

MARILYN W. BUTLER, MD, MPH, MPhil
Professor, Department of Surgery, Division of Pediatric Surgery, Oregon Health & Science
University, Portland, Oregon

JENNIFER T. CASTLE, MD
Department of Surgery, University of Kentucky College of Medicine, Lexington, Kentucky

SARAH CHOKSI, MD
PGY-3, General Surgery, Albany Medical Center, Albany, New York

WOO S. DO, MD
Clinical Fellow, Pediatric Surgery, Boston Children's Hospital, Boston, Massachusetts

J. DUNCAN PHILLIPS, MD, FACS, FAAP
Surgeon-in-Chief, WakeMed Children's Hospital, Co-Director, WakeMed Chest Wall
Deformity Center, Raleigh, North Carolina; Clinical Associate Professor of Surgery, The
University of North Carolina at Chapel Hill, Chapel Hill, North Carolina

MARY J. EDWARDS, MD
Professor, Pediatric Surgery, Albany Medical Center, Albany, New York

MAURICIO A. ESCOBAR Jr, MD, FACS, FAAP
Pediatric Surgery and Pediatric Trauma, Mary Bridge Children's Hospital and Health
Network, Tacoma, Washington

ELIZABETH FIALKOWSKI, MD
Associate Professor, Pediatric General Surgery, Oregon Health & Science University, Portland, Oregon

JACE FRANKO, MD
General Surgery, Madigan Army Medical Center, Tacoma, Washington

COLIN D. GAUSE, MD
Department of Surgery, Division of Pediatric Surgery, Providence Health & Services, Portland, Oregon

AJAY S. GULATI, MD
Professor, Department of Pediatrics, Division of Gastroenterology, University of North Carolina School of Medicine, Chapel Hill, North Carolina

XIAO-YUE HAN, BS, MD
Department of Surgery, Oregon Health & Science University, Portland, Oregon

TORBJORG HOLTESTAUL, MD
General Surgery, Madigan Army Medical Center, Tacoma, Washington

JOHN DAVID HOOVER, MD, FACS, FAAP
Co-Director, WakeMed Chest Wall Deformity Center, Raleigh, North Carolina

PATRICK J. JAVID, MD
Professor of Surgery, University of Washington School of Medicine, Seattle Children's Hospital, Seattle, Washington

ALFRED KENNEDY Jr, MD
Chair, Department of Pediatric Surgery, Geisinger Health System, Danville, Pennsylvania

SANJAY KRISHNASWAMI, MD
Professor of Surgery, Division of Pediatric Surgery, School of Medicine, Surgeon-in-Chief, Doernbecher Children's Hospital, Oregon Health & Science University, Portland, Oregon

BRITTANY E. LEVY, MD
Department of Surgery, University of Kentucky College of Medicine, Lexington, Kentucky

CRAIG W. LILLEHEI, MD
Senior Associate in Surgery, Pediatric Surgery, Boston Children's Hospital, Associate Professor of Surgery, Harvard Medical School, Boston, Massachusetts

LAUREN MALONEY, BS
Oregon Health & Science University, Portland, Oregon

GRANT MORRIS, MD, MPH
Department of Pediatric Gastroenterology, Geisinger Health System, Danville, Pennsylvania

PATRICK N. NGUYEN, MD
PGY-4, General Surgery, Albany Medical Center, Albany, New York

EDWARD PENN, MD
Greenville ENT Allergy and Associates, Prisma Upstate, Greenville Memorial Hospital, Greenville, South Carolina

ADAM PETCHERS, MD
PGY-4, General Surgery, Albany Medical Center, Albany, New York

MICHAEL R. PHILLIPS, MD
Assistant Professor, Departments of Surgery and Pediatrics, University of North Carolina School of Medicine, Chapel Hill, North Carolina

LAURA N. PURCELL, MD, MPH
Department of Surgery, University of North Carolina School of Medicine, Chapel Hill, North Carolina

ROBERT L. RICCA, MD
Associate Professor of Surgery, Division of Pediatric Surgery, University of South Carolina, Prisma Health Upstate, Greenville Memorial Hospital, Greenville, South Carolina

DAVID A. RODEBERG, MD, FACS
Division of Pediatric Surgery, University of Kentucky College of Medicine, University of Kentucky, Lexington, Kentucky

LEIGH TARYN SELESNER, BA, MD
Department of Surgery, Oregon Health & Science University, Portland, Oregon

VICTORIYA STAAB, MD, FAAP, FACS
Jersey Shore University Medical Center, Hackensack Meridian Health, Farmingdale, New Jersey

MCKINNA TILLOTSON, BS
Oregon Health & Science University, Portland, Oregon

JOSEPH TOBIAS, MD
Oregon Health & Science University, Portland, Oregon

LTC RYAN M. WALK, MD, FACS
Assistant Professor of Surgery and Pediatrics, Uniformed Services University of the Health Sciences, Walter Reed National Military Medical Center, Bethesda, Maryland

DANIELLE WENDEL, MD
Associate Professor of Pediatrics, University of Washington School of Medicine, Seattle Children's Hospital, Seattle, Washington

Contents

Esophageal atresia (EA) with tracheoesophageal fistula (TEF) is among the most common congenital anomalies requiring surgical intervention in infancy. General surgeons practicing in rural or austere environments may encounter emergency situations requiring their involvement. Respiratory emergencies can arise in the neonatal period; the recommended approaches are the ligation of the fistula through the chest or occlusion of the distal esophagus through the abdomen. As survivors of the condition reach late adulthood, general surgeons can anticipate encountering these patients. An understanding of risk factors, common symptoms, associated anomalies, and the appropriate diagnostic evaluation will facilitate care.

Pediatric ingestions encompass a wide range of diseases, including foreign body ingestions, caustic ingestions, and aspiration. Specific topics of interest in the pediatric age group for adult general surgeons are button batteries and magnets, which have significant morbidity and mortality and require a high index of suspicion to provide timely care. Evaluation and management of these cases should be tailored to the offending agent and managed at an appropriate pediatric center.

Perforated appendicitis continues to be a significant cause of morbidity for children. In most centers, ultrasound has replaced computed tomography as the initial imaging modality for this condition. Controversies surrounding optimal medical and surgical management of appendicitis are discussed. Management of intussusception begins with clinical assessment and ultrasound, followed by image-guided air or saline reduction enema. When surgery is required, laparoscopy is typically utilized unless bowel resection is required. The differential diagnosis for pediatric gastrointestinal bleeding is broad but often made with age, history, and physical examination. Endoscopy or laparoscopy is sometimes needed to confirm a diagnosis or for treatment.

Congenital abdominal wall defects vary from abdominal wall hernias to severe congenital structural anomalies that include gastroschisis, omphalocele, and prune belly syndrome. The conditions often carry various associated anomalies and require multidisciplinary treatment approaches. Complex surgical reconstructive techniques are frequently required and prenatal, perioperative, and long-term follow-up is critical to ensuring the best possible outcomes.

The small intestine is a complex organ system that is vital to the life of the individual. There are several congenital anomalies that occur and present most commonly in infancy; however, some may not present until adulthood. Most congenital anomalies of the small intestine will present with obstructive symptoms, whereas some may present with vomiting, abdominal pain, and/or gastrointestinal bleeding. Various radiologic procedures can aid in the diagnosis of these lesions that vary depending on the particular anomaly. The congenital anomalies of the small intestine discussed include Meckel diverticulum, duodenal web, duodenal atresia, jejunoileal atresia, and intestinal duplications.

In this article, we aim to provide the general surgeon with a clinical blueprint to navigate disorders of gut rotation. We emphasize that bilious emesis in a newborn is malrotation with volvulus until proven otherwise. Although an upper GI series can establish the diagnosis, surgical intervention should not be delayed until the child is ill-appearing. Following detorsion, the key steps are to broaden the mesentery, fully Kocherize the duodenum, and mobilize the cecum. If nonviable bowel is encountered, the principles of damage control can be applied to children. Every effort should be made to preserve bowel length.

Children with underlying neurologic conditions or developmental delay may have undergone prior surgical therapy to improve quality of life. These patients may present to the emergency room with complications associated with these procedures or present requiring emergent or urgent surgical management of a new diagnosis. An understanding of the anatomic variation and known long-term complications of these devices is important for any surgeon who may be called to care for these patients. The goal of this article was to provide recommendations that will assist the general surgeon in the surgical management of children with neurologic impairment or developmental delay.

Medical and surgical care for children with intestinal failure has evolved so that long-term life expectancy is common even in the setting of the shortest bowel lengths. The long-term administration of parenteral nutrition has become safe with alterations in lipid formulation, and the risk of liver injury has been dramatically reduced. Well-established techniques for bowel lengthening and tapering exist to increase the absorptive capacity of the remnant bowel. These advances allow for ongoing intestinal rehabilitation in the child with the ultimate goal of enteral autonomy while the use of intestinal transplantation in this population has declined in recent years.

Cystic fibrosis is an autosomal-recessive defect in the cystic fibrosis transmembrane conductance regulator (CFTR) gene located on chromosome 7
that affects 1 in 2500 live White births. Defects in the gene lead to abnormally thick secretions causing chronic obstruction in the respiratory and
gastrointestinal tracts. Common gastrointestinal pathology in children
with cystic fibrosis includes meconium ileus in infancy and distal intestinal
obstruction syndrome in childhood and exocrine pancreatic insufficiency,
constipation, and rectal prolapse. This article describes the presentation,
diagnosis, and management of these conditions in patients with cystic
fibrosis, from birth to adulthood.

Pectus excavatum, carinatum, and arcuatum are 3 developmental chest
wall deformities that may evolve during childhood and cause cardiac
and/or pulmonary compression. Evaluation may include nonsurgical subspecialty consultations and imaging studies. Treatment may be nonoperative or surgical. Long-term follow-up studies have identified rare
complications of traditional open repair. Routine in utero ultrasonography
has led to increasing identification of congenital lung anomalies, including
congenital cystic adenomatoid malformations, pulmonary sequestrations,
and bronchogenic cysts. Short-term follow-up studies have suggested
that some lesions may regress spontaneously. Minimally invasive techniques, including thoracoscopy, may allow for early surgical resection
with less morbidity than traditional open surgery.

Key differences exist in pediatric and adult inflammatory bowel disease
(IBD), and a multidisciplinary approach focused on meeting these needs
should be implemented. In an emergency situation, surgical management
of pediatric IBD should focus on patient stabilization with an eye toward
future intestinal function.

SURGICAL CLINICS
OF NORTH AMERICA

THE CLINICS ARE AVAILABLE ONLINE!
Access your subscription at:
www.theclinics.com

Foreword

Pediatric Surgery

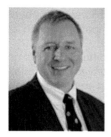

Ronald F. Martin, MD, FACS
Consulting Editor

Right patient, right clinical team, right facility, and right time: the Holy Grail of medical care and particularly true of surgery. I might throw in "right diagnosis" as well, as that should not always be considered a given. This basic premise of having patients cared for in the most optimal environment would be the backbone as well as the measuring stick of any worthwhile health care system that anyone might want to construct in an ideal world. Yet, it is not how we function here in the United States, and we are not alone in this dilemma.

If we take away malice and greed as the reasons for failing to achieve an "idealized" system (and let us only do that in theory for the moment), then what is it that prevents us from having an idealized system? Is it too few doctors? Too few nurses? Too few dollars? Too few devices? Too little imagination? In many cases, some or all the above are deeply ingrained in the problem. For resources-poor areas—whether locally poor or poor on a country-wide basis—lacking resources is probably the prime driver of system weakness. In areas where net resource availability is not the prime driver of system weakness, the remaining significant contributors to suboptimal systems are resource distribution, network (formal or informal) malalignment, and lack of agreement between the providers of health care and the consumers of health care as to what is needed. One may note that all the factors that are not associated with "too little stuff" are fundamentally sociopolitical issues. To which we must then reenter into our analysis the potential for malice and greed.

I would submit that the two populations of patients who best exemplify our need for strong systems arrangements and keen attention to resource distribution are the pediatric population and those who require organ transplantation services. For the latter, we have a very well-developed regional/national clinical system in place and a very well-described method of handling the financial requirements of it. The former group, our children, are not quite so organized, especially the fiscal pieces.

Surg Clin N Am 102 (2022) xiii–xv
https://doi.org/10.1016/j.suc.2022.08.010
0039-6109/22/© 2022 Published by Elsevier Inc.

surgical.theclinics.com

The genesis of the variance between the pediatric group and the transplant group is easy to understand on some levels. Children are largely healthy on a day-to-day basis until they aren't. Someone on an organ transplant list knows she/he is sick all the time and is waiting for a literal lifeline. There is usually time to establish clinical relationships over large distances and prepare for what may be required. For the more general pediatric population, children mostly live wherever their parents/guardians live—which is pretty much everywhere. Unless something comes up, most children don't need to develop a relationship with providers of complex or even inpatient health care. However, things come up with great routine that alter that need.

This conundrum of services that are required sometimes in some places but not at all times in all places brings us back to the main concern that drives our work at the *Surgical Clinics*—how do we divide work and responsibility between the generalist and specialist? Spoiler alert: in the grand scheme, there is no right answer. To make matters more challenging, I would submit that the dilemma is much more complicated for pediatric care. Even within the range of "pediatric care," there are further subdivisions that may alter our analysis. Subgroups could be constructed by factors such as children with single system disease, children who weigh more than our average health care provider, children who can receive care and go directly home with capable support. Of course, all these factors are routinely considered at some level.

There are many facets of the surgical care of children that can be offered in many kinds of environments with excellent results and patient/family satisfaction. There are some other types of care that it matters greatly which environment is being utilized, bringing us back to right patient, team, facility, time, and diagnosis.

The "right diagnosis" part of the equation becomes much more challenging in the pediatric population, especially in facilities that are not pediatric centered. Being a good clinical diagnostician is essential to providing good patient care. That said, being a good clinical diagnostician in this era means having a good working relationship with our diagnostic imaging colleagues as well. Having people who are good at both skill sets for the care of children in facilities that do not specialize in pediatric care is rare.

A friend of mine who was a US Marine officer once told me that he always had two plans so that if one didn't work, he had another. That made me think that Marines are geniuses because, in my time in the Army, I needed many more backup plans than that whenever possible. The concept of fallback plans also formidably has affected my thinking on patient care: whether it has been overseas in hostile, austere environments or here in the United States with a full complement of subspecialty help or little to no help from any other specialist, or even generalist, depending on time of day. Add to that the resource availability outside of the operating room from nursing care, family support, pharmacy, and so forth, and the pediatric patient group can become quite a logistical and dispositional challenge. When one who does not usually provide surgical care for children does engage in this care, she/he had best be prepared for what to do should the situation that is encountered be markedly different from that which was expected.

As with so many other aspects of life, self-education about solid fundamentals will go a long way to securing the tools required to avoid rushing in where angels fear to tread. Our Guest Editor for this issue, Dr John Horton, is an excellent pediatric surgeon who not only serves our children but also serves our country in the US Army. I had the privilege of working with him directly during my time working for the Department of Defense after I had retired from military service. He is an excellent clinician, an excellent teacher of surgery, and a tremendous colleague. He and his fellow contributors have generated an excellent collection of articles that will inform all of us well. They have taken great care to not only focus on the issues that children face but also help address how those issues track to the adult phase of these patients' lives.

Still, no matter how well informed you may be, the main consideration in the surgical care of children is whether one has the totality of resources required to address all the likely issues and perhaps many of the unlikely ones as well. All families want to stay as close to home as possible, but very few want to stay close to home if that would adversely affect their child—and those that would consciously do so give us one more thing to consider.

I realize that we surgeons alone cannot solve all the problems, stagnations, inertia, and other woes that affect our health care system easily or maybe not at all. Yet, I would like to think that if there were some areas that a divided people might gather around, it would be the care of our children. Most children are not possessed of the tools to fend for themselves, and they must rely on adults until they can. Being well versed in what one can do to help in the moment and how we can educate others to do the right things to build a better overall system is an essential for all of us who wish to be leaders in the betterment of our society.

Ronald F. Martin, FACS
Colonel (retired), United States Army Reserve
Department of General Surgery
Pullman Surgical Associates
Pullman Regional Hospital and Clinic Network
825 SE Bishop Boulevard, Suite 130
Pullman, WA 99163, USA

E-mail address:
rfmcescna@gmail.com

Management of Anorectal Malformations and Hirschsprung Disease

Colin D. Gause, MD[a],*, Sanjay Krishnaswami, MD[b]

KEYWORDS

- Anorectal malformations • Hirschsprung disease • Adult • General surgeon
- Continence • Bowel management • Long-term

KEY POINTS

- Surgical management of anorectal malformations (ARM) and Hirschsprung disease (HD) requires placement of normal intestine with the center of the anal sphincter complex.
- The predominant contributor to impaired quality of life in ARM and HD patient is related to bowel continence.
- All patients with ARM and many with HD will require long-term bowel management in order to achieve social continence.

INTRODUCTION

Anorectal malformations (ARM) and Hirschsprung disease (HD) are hindgut anomalies in which the rectum is either abnormally located or abnormal in function, respectively. Management of these disease processes centers on isolation of normal colon or rectum and placement within the anal sphincter complex. Although these diseases are addressed in infancy by pediatric surgeons, even appropriate surgical repair requires ongoing, lifelong management in regard to continence, sexual satisfaction, fertility, and quality of life by general surgeons, urologists, and gynecologists.

BACKGROUND
Anorectal Malformations

In patients with an ARM, the rectum is either blind ending (imperforate anus, 5%), stenotic or atretic (1%), drains onto the perineum (perineal fistula) (10%–18%), empties

[a] Department of Surgery, Division of Pediatric Surgery, Providence Health & Services, 9427 Southwest Barnes Road, Clinic Office Suite 395, Portland, OR 97225, USA; [b] Department of Surgery, Division of Pediatric Surgery, Oregon Health & Science University, Mail Code CDW7, 3181 Southwest Sam Jackson Park Road, Portland, OR 97239, USA
* Corresponding author.
E-mail address: cdgause@gmail.com
Twitter: @Nirazila (C.D.G.); @JayKrishnas (S.K.)

Surg Clin N Am 102 (2022) 695–714
https://doi.org/10.1016/j.suc.2022.07.005
0039-6109/22/© 2022 Elsevier Inc. All rights reserved.

surgical.theclinics.com

Abbreviations	
ARM	Anorectal malformation
ART	Assisted reproductive technologies
HAEC	Hirschsprung-associated enterocolitis
HD	Hirschsprung disease
IND	Intestinal neuronal dysplasia
ISA	Internal sphincter achalasia
ROOF	Remnant of original fistula
UTI	Urinary tract infection

into an organ space (rectourethral fistula and rectovesical fistula in men, rectovestibular fistula in women; 70%–80%), rectovaginal fistula (<1%), or represents a cloacal anomaly (5% of females). Cloaca is a complex ARM found in girls wherein the gastrointestinal, reproductive, and urinary tracts join as a common channel before emptying onto the perineum as a single perineal orifice (**Figs. 1** and **2**, **Table 1**). Approximately 50% to 60% of patients with ARM will have an associated anomaly of another organ

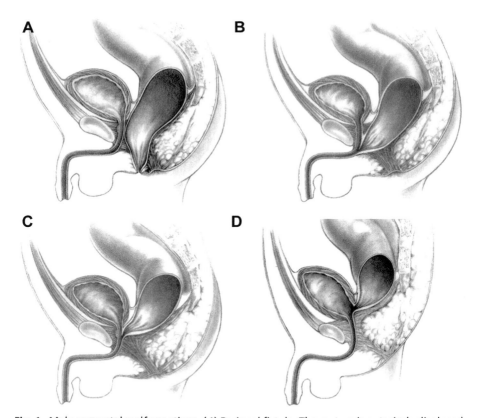

Fig. 1. Male anorectal malformations. (*A*) Perineal fistula. The rectum is anteriorly displaced, outside of the anal sphincter complex (*gray*, striated), (*B*) rectobulbar urethral fistula, (*C*) rectoprostatic urethra fistula, and (*D*) rectovesical fistula. (*Adapted from* Ashcraft's Pediatric Surgery, 6th Edition, Elsevier Saunders, March 10, 2014.)

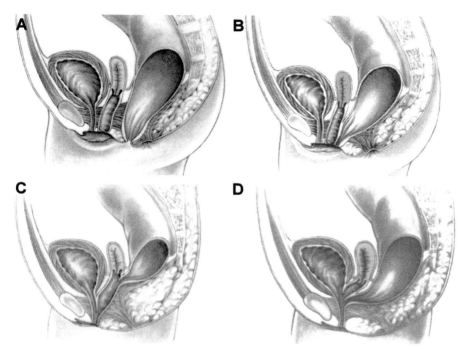

Fig. 2. Female anorectal malformations. (*A*) Perineal fistula. (*B*) Rectovestibular fistula. The rectum empties into the vestibule of the vagina, between the labia minora and distal to the vaginal opening, (*C*) rectovaginal fistula, and (*D*) cloacal anomaly. (*Adapted from* Ashcraft's Pediatric Surgery, 6th Edition, Elsevier Saunders, March 10, 2014.)

system, and surgeons need to be aware of the potential need for assistance in management from other specialists, particularly urology and neurosurgery, when applicable. Genitourinary anomalies are common (30%–54%), most often seen in patients with sacral deformities,[1] and include vesicoureteral reflux, renal agenesis and dysplasia, cryptorchidism, and hypospadias.[1-6] Spine anomalies (30%–50%) include tethered cord, myelomeningocele, vertebral, and sacral defects. Cardiac anomalies (30%) include Tetralogy of Fallot and endocardial cushion defects, such as atrial and ventricular septal defects. Gynecologic anomalies may occur, and

Table 1	
Classification of anorectal malformations	
Male	Rectobulbar urethra fistula
	Rectoprostatic urethra fistula
	Rectovesical fistula
Female	Rectovestibular fistula
	Rectovaginal fistula
	Cloaca
Both	Rectal atresia/ARM without fistula
	Anorectal stenosis
	Rectoperineal fistula

include uterine malformations, vaginal anomalies (septa, atresia), and Mullerian anomalies.[7,8]

Diagnosis of ARM is largely clinical but may be supplemented with radiography and, in the case of cloaca, endoscopy. Patients with higher malformations are most often initially managed with a colostomy proximal to the fistula, with definitive surgical management delayed until the patient reaches a few months of age. Lower malformations typically undergo complete reconstruction at the time of diagnosis. In all cases, definitive management requires identification of the distal rectum, separation of the abnormal communication between the rectum and any involved organs, and placement of the rectum within the center of the anal sphincter complex. This involves a perineal approach with the degree of dissection dependent on the location of the rectum or fistula (**Fig. 3**). Combined approaches through both the perineum and the abdomen, using minimally invasive techniques, are becoming increasingly more common,[9] particularly for higher malformations, with some avoiding a posterior sagittal incision entirely.[10]

Hirschsprung Disease

The rectum of patients with HD is properly positioned within the anal sphincter complex but is abnormal in function. In HD, intestinal ganglion progenitor cells, which regulate effective relaxation and peristalsis, fail to completely migrate caudally in utero. The absence of ganglion cells in the submucosal (Meissner's) and myenteric (Auerbach) plexuses of the intestine thus results in a colon that is tonically contracted. This clinically presents as a large bowel obstruction at the terminal migratory site of ganglion cells. Approximately 50% to 60% of patients have at least one abnormality of another organ system, including congenital heart disease, intestinal malrotation, genitourinary anomalies, limb anomalies, hearing loss, and intellectual developmental disorder.[11] A chromosomal abnormality is present in 12% of cases, with trisomy 21 as the most frequent.

Initial management of HD varies based on surgeon preference. Many manage the functional obstruction with scheduled home colonic irrigations while allowing the patient to grow for a period of several months, whereas others proceed to immediate resection and reconstruction. Rarely, these patients are managed with colostomy creation just proximal to the aganglionic segment in an area of normal colon (leveling

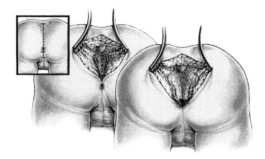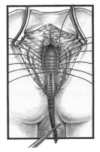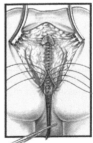

Fig. 3. Posterior sagittal approach for ARM. A posterior sagittal incision is made from the coccyx to perineal body in the midline. The parasagittal fibers run parallel to the incision and divided and retracted. The rectum is identified, separated from attachments to the genitourinary system, where applicable, and placed in the center of the anal sphincter complex. (*Adapted from* Ashcraft's Pediatric Surgery, 6th Edition, Elsevier Saunders, March 10, 2014.)

colostomy) at the time of diagnosis. This is particularly useful in cases of Hirschsprung enterocolitis. Definitive management requires resection of the abnormal, aganglionic distal bowel, with anastomosis of normal, ganglionated bowel to the distal anal canal within the center of the anal sphincter complex. This is most often accomplished via the Swenson, Duhamel, or Soave procedures (**Fig. 4**).

Although ARM and HD are fundamentally different disease processes, they have an identical treatment goal, which is a functioning gastrointestinal tract with associated continence. This is accomplished by placement of normal, functioning intestine within the center of the anal sphincter complex on the perineum, with postoperative bowel management strategies tailored to the patient's symptoms as related to constipation and incontinence. It is therefore not surprising that ARM and HD overlap in many aspects of long-term management.

IMMEDIATE COMPLICATIONS

Patients who undergo surgical management of ARM and HD are at risk for specific complications related to a perineal dissection in proximity to the genitourinary tract with an associated coloanal anastomosis. These complications can result in long-term issues that the general surgeon needs to be aware of. Wound infection and separation of the perineal anastomosis may occur even with meticulous operative technique and wound care. In the event of wound separation comprising a large portion of the anastomosis or significant retraction of the rectum, the anastomosis may need to be surgically revised, which increases the risk of anastomotic stricture and issues with urinary or gastrointestinal continence in the future. Bladder or urethral injury can result in urine leak, stricture, or fistula, requiring operative repair or dilations.

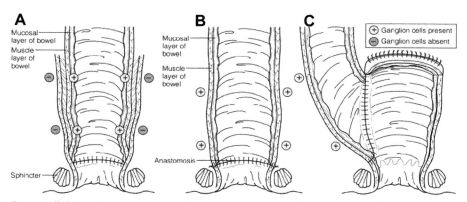

Fig. 4. Pull-through Procedures for Hirschsprung disease. (*A*) Soave: In an effort to avoid pelvic nerve injury, aganglionic colon and rectum are resected in an endorectal fashion, leaving an aganglionic seromuscular "cuff" through which ganglionated bowel is pulled through and anastomosed to the anal canal. The muscular cuff is then split posteriorly to prevent recurrent obstruction. (*B*) Swenson: All aganglionic colon and rectum is resected with end-to-end anastomosis of ganglionated bowel to the anal canal, (*C*) Duhamel: Aganglionic bowel is resected up to the rectum, which is left intact. A presacral dissection is performed, and ganglionated bowel is then pulled through and anastomosed to the native rectum via a posterior, distal transverse enterotomy in the native rectum. After anastomosis, the anterior portion of the neorectum is native and the posterior portion is the ganglionated pull-through segment. This creates a larger reservoir and avoids an anterior dissection and potential injury to autonomic nerves of the bladder. All methods have shown equivalent outcomes. (*Adapted from* Coran's Pediatric Surgery, 7th Edition, Mosby, February 28, 2012.)

Neurogenic bladder can be seen after an extensive bladder dissection, which can cause recurrent urinary tract infections due to stasis and abnormal bladder emptying. The patient may require intermittent catheterization or even cystostomy. Rectal injury or devascularization can cause a stricture. A twisted pull-through can cause a bowel obstruction requiring revisional surgery. Pelvic nerve injury can cause chronic pain, paresthesias, loss of sensation, or weakness. Many minor complications may not be evident until they cause chronic symptoms later in life.

LONG-TERM COMPLICATIONS—DISEASE SPECIFIC
Anorectal Malformations

Remnant of original fistula
In the ARM patient with a fistulous connection to the genitourinary tract, if the rectum is not separated close to the wall of the vagina, urethra, or bladder, a remnant may remain. This remnant or pseudodiverticulum of tissue is an area of flow stasis, which, when occurs on the bladder or urethra, may result in recurrent urinary tract infections, passage of mucous, urinary dribbling, incontinence, and, in rare cases, degeneration to adenocarcinoma.[12] Practitioners should have a high index of suspicion for patients with repaired ARM who present with the above symptoms. Diagnosis includes pelvic MRI, voiding cystourethrogram, with confirmation via examination under anesthesia with cystoscopy.[13] Repair is individualized and can include a combination of open and minimally invasive techniques.

Recurrent fistula
Patients with an ARM and associated fistula are at risk for fistula recurrence. Fortunately, this complication is rare, occurring in 0.5% to 1% of cases.[14] Patients with a long common wall are at highest risk, and this can occur at any point in life. Recurrent fistulae should be treated with fistula takedown with placement of an interposition tissue flap in order to minimize recurrence. Buccal mucosal flap[15,16] and gracilis muscle interposition[17] have been used with excellent results. General surgeons should not hesitate to enlist the aid of their urology colleagues for both vaginal and urologic fistulae takedown and repair.

Genitourinary
Patients with ARM and associated recto-urinary tract fistula or cloaca are associated with anomalies of genitourinary function, even after repair. Urinary incontinence is seen in 16%, more common in women, and more frequent in high severity anomalies.[18] Vesicoureteral reflux can result in recurrent urinary tract infections, pyelonephritis, and chronic renal insufficiency (CRI). Indeed, CRI is the biggest contributor to decreased life expectancy in these patients.[19] Patients with repaired cloaca are at highest risk, with 50% suffering chronic renal failure by around age 11[20] and may require intermittent catheterization or bladder augmentation.[21] Urology involvement for assessment, evaluation of reflux, and ongoing care is often necessary.

Neurogenic bladder is present in approximately 22% to 36% of patients[18] and is more often seen in severe sacral or spine anomalies. Medical management, botulinum toxin injection, intermittent catheterization, pelvic floor physical therapy, biofeedback therapy, or in severe cases, suprapubic cystostomy may be needed.

Cryptorchidism is seen in 19% to 33% of patients,[6,22,23] and is more common in those with more severe malformations[24] and vertebral anomalies.[6] General surgeons and primary care physicians should perform a focused examination on testicular position, characteristics, and size and be aware of the need for urologic referral for any abnormalities.

Gynecologic

Patients with ARM have a spectrum of gynecologic anomalies. Dysmenorrhea may occur due to partial or complete obstruction of menstrual flow, with patients presenting with severe menstrual cramps. Obstruction may require removal of old blood, or resection of hemiuteri, fallopian tubes, blind vaginas, or hemivaginas.[25] Dyspareunia and difficulty with tampon application may result from a vaginal septum. Infertility may be the result of uterine didelphys (double uterus), unicornuate or bicornuate uterus, cervical atresia, or even absent uterus.[25,26] Female patients with ARM should undergo screening for gynecologic anomalies at birth. However, if not done previously, or if new or chronic symptoms are present, surgeons should engage with their gynecology colleagues for assistance and possible vaginoscopy, hysteroscopy, and/or pelvic MRI.

Patients with repaired cloacal malformations will often have undergone vaginal reconstruction in order to facilitate menstruation or sexual activity.[27] This is most often performed with small or large bowel,[28,29] whereas vaginal stenosis can be treated with buccal mucosal graft.[16] An obstructed uterus requires operative intervention and may require hysterectomy.[26] Reconstruction is often required.

Hirschsprung Disease

Hirschsprung-associated enterocolitis

Hirschsprung-associated enterocolitis (HAEC) is a complication of HD in which patients develop enterocolitis of varying degrees of severity. HAEC manifests with one or more signs and symptoms including fever, emesis, feeding intolerance, abdominal distention, foul-smelling stools, and potentially sepsis. The cause is poorly defined but is likely due to a combination of an abnormal enteric nervous system, abnormal mucin production, insufficient immunoglobulin production, and abnormal intestinal flora.[30] Treatment includes resuscitation, antibiotics, and colonic decompression and irrigations. Lack of improvement may require urgent stoma creation. Although HAEC is most often seen in neonates, older children and adults can develop HAEC even after a technically sound pull-through and at any point in life. Most studies show that the incidence of HAEC is similar no matter what type of pull-through was previously performed.[31–33] Regardless, recognition is critical because these patients can decompensate rapidly and repeated bouts of enterocolitis have long-term effects on bowel function and continence.

Aganglionosis

Acquired aganglionosis occurs following a properly performed pull-through in which normal, ganglionated colon is used for the anastomosis but ganglion cells are progressively lost over time.[34] The cause is unknown but may be due to ischemia of the pull-through or as a result of bouts of enterocolitis. Patients present with symptoms of progressive obstruction.[35] Acquired aganglionosis is diagnosed via biopsy just proximal to the anastomosis. In infants, an endorectal biopsy of mucosa and submucosa is sufficient as the pathologic findings in the submucosal plexus correlate well with those of the myenteric plexus. However, older children and adults should undergo posterior, full-thickness, operative biopsy in order to obtain a sufficient sample containing mucosa, submucosa, and muscle. Biopsies should be taken in a near circumferential fashion as the transition zone from normal to abnormal intestine may by asymmetrically oriented. When acquired aganglionosis is confirmed, the treatment is a repeat pull-through.

Persistent aganglionosis occurs when a segment of abnormally ganglionated intestine was used in the initial pull-through. This typically occurs when the transition zone (segment immediately proximal to the aganglionic colon where ganglion cells are present but not completely normal in size, function, and distribution) is anastomosed to the anal canal.[36] This condition should be uncommon in adults because it usually leads to symptoms early in the postoperative course. Persistent aganglionosis is treated identically to acquired aganglionosis.

Intestinal neuronal dysplasia

Intestinal neuronal dysplasia (IND) is a poorly understood disease, which affects the submucosal nerve plexus. Patients present with constipation and associated continence issues. X-ray and barium enema reveal a variable segment of dilated bowel. Diagnosis should be performed with a combination of radionuclide transit study,[37] manometry,[38] and full thickness biopsies throughout the abnormal segment(s).[39] Pathologic evaluation requires sophisticated special staining and thick sections,[40] and the surgeon should be in close discussion with the pathologist throughout the process. Although the cause is unclear, some think IND is a result of chronic obstruction, further emphasizing the importance of lifelong bowel management on outcomes. If the segment of IND is isolated, treatment is a resection or repeat pull-through. If diffuse IND is seen, bowel management strategies are used.

Internal sphincter achalasia

All patients with HD lack a normal/proper recto-anal inhibitory reflex (RAIR).[41] Internal sphincter achalasia (ISA) occurs when there is incomplete full relaxation of the internal anal sphincter because of this abnormal reflex pathway. Patients may present similarly to the initial diagnosis of HD, although the neorectum itself is normal in ganglion cell size and distribution. Diagnosis is made with anorectal manometry, which will reveal elevated internal anal sphincter resting pressure. Internal anal sphincter botulinum toxin injection is a useful diagnostic and therapeutic test[42] and can be repeated as needed. Topical alternatives include nitroglycerine and nifedipine. Operative treatment options include internal sphincterotomy and myectomy.[43–45] However, one must be aware that these patients are already at risk of incontinence after surgical management of HD, and muscle-splitting procedures can contribute to worsening incontinence.[46,47] Fortunately, ISA usually resolves by age 5 but if persists to adulthood, one will need to consider the above treatment strategies.

LONG-TERM COMPLICATIONS: ANORECTAL MALFORMATIONS AND HIRSCHSPRUNG DISEASE
Mechanical Obstruction

Although uncommon, patients with a properly positioned but partially twisted pull-through may present with symptoms later in life, including recurrent bowel obstructions, "stenosis" and, in the case of HD, recurrent enterocolitis. A patient with an ARM or HD and coloanal anastomosis with recurrent bowel obstructions thus cannot be presumed to simply have adhesive disease. Workup should include lower endoscopy and barium enema to delineate anatomy. Treatment requires revision of the coloanal anastomosis.

Stricture

Strictures are not uncommon in the management of both ARM and HD. First-line management includes serial dilations, which can be performed as an outpatient procedure or at home, with patients self-administering home dilations using disposable plastic Hegar dilators. Intralesional steroid, injected within the lesion, when combined with dilations, seems to decrease the risk of recurrence.[48,49] Topical mitomycin C has been used as an adjunct to dilations and can decrease the need for repeat interventions in children.[50] Recalcitrant strictures may require surgical therapy, including Heineke-Mikulicz strictureplasty or anoplasty revision. Skin level strictures may benefit from diamond flap anoplasty.[51,52]

Prolapse

Prolapse may occur if the rectum is not adequately secured to the anal muscle complex, or if the muscle is inadequate, and is exacerbated by constipation, which is common in both ARM and HD. Prolapse is more common after repair of ARM, and varies widely, ranging from 3.8% to 60%.[53,54] The rate of prolapse is higher in patients with more severe ARM, tethered cord, and vertebral anomalies.[55] First-line treatment of prolapse includes management of constipation. Refractory cases should be treated only if symptomatic, and management depends on the degree of prolapse. Circumferential prolapse is most often approached transanally, using rectal mucosectomy and muscular plication.[54] Traditional techniques including Delorme procedure and Altemeier perineal rectosigmoidectomy. Minimally invasive rectopexy techniques may also be used. Partial circumference prolapse can be managed with hemicircumference resection of redundant rectum.

Sexual Dysfunction

Difficulties with sexual arousal, intercourse, and sexual relationships are not uncommon in patients with both ARM and HD. Men are at risk of erectile dysfunction, present in 8.8% to 16% of those with ARM and 8.8% to 11% with HD.[18,56] Men with a history of repaired ARM and rectourethral fistula can have absent, incomplete, or retrograde ejaculation,[18,22,57] with the incidence related to the severity of the anomaly. Women report sexual distress in 20% to 45% of cases and sexual dysfunction in 30% to 53%,[18,56,58,59] with urinary continence predicting sexual functioning.[60]

Patients with ARM have been found to delay coitus when compared with controls.[61] Many patients with ARM are not sexually active, ranging from 53% to 56%,[26,62] either due to difficulties with relationships or physical discomfort with sexual activity.[26] Fortunately, women with ARM and sexual dysfunction related to vaginal stenosis or short vagina can be treated with augmentation vaginoplasty, which improves vaginal capacity and the ability to engage in penetrative intercourse.[63] Adults of both genders with HD report limitation of sexual relationships,[64] and women with HD have been noted to be in less stable relationships when compared with controls.[65] Importantly, approximately 60% of patients with both ARM and HD report insufficient attention is paid to addressing sexuality by health-care providers.[58]

Fertility

Conception and live birth can be challenging but attainable in both ARM and HD. These patients, in particular those with ARM, require more assistance from reproductive technologies (ART) than controls.[66] Patients with ARM should be referred to an experienced gynecologist to assess the patency of the reproductive tract,[67] which may require vaginal dilations or reconstruction to allow for vaginal intercourse,[67,68] needed in up to 56% of patients with cloaca.[27] The vaginal introitus should be sufficient to accommodate a 24 or 26 Hegar dilator for comfortable penetrative intercourse.[67] Men with ARM have both lower testicular volume and ejaculatory difficulties, and should be promptly evaluated for testicular function if there is concern for infertility.[22]

Women with ARM or HD can safely become pregnant and have a live birth. Although women with ARM have a lower childbirth rate, this is specific to the more severe anomalies, with minor anomalies having similar rates to controls.[69] Despite using ART more often, most pregnancies in women with ARM are spontaneous and do not require in vitro fertilization.[8] Despite the fact that most babies born to a mother with ARM are born premature due to preterm premature rupture of membranes,[8,27] there is no reported difference in mortality related to prematurity.[8] Although cesarean section is often required, and in many cases recommended,[70] particularly for cloacal anomalies,[68] patients can be candidates for vaginal delivery if followed closely.[71,72]

The primary pregnancy-associated morbidity is related to urinary tract infection and worsening CRI in the mother, and renal function should be followed closely.[8,68] An important note when caring for these patients as they try to conceive, is that women with a bladder augmentation have a 57% false-positive pregnancy test and require a serum confirmation.[73] This is thought to be due to mucus production in enterocytoplasties interfering with urine pregnancy tests.

Bowel Continence

ARM patients are at high risk of developing difficulties with continence throughout life,[57,61,74,75] with fecal soiling, constipation, and obstipation being common. Constipation is the most common functional disorder (approximately 32%)[76] and is more closely associated with minor/low anomalies, whereas true incontinence is more associated with severe/high anomalies. Not surprisingly, patients with more minor anomalies are similar to controls in regard to continence.[77]

Most ARM patients have an intrinsic functional disorder related to their disease.[78–81] Normal continence depends on the interaction of voluntary pelvic floor musculature, anorectal sensation, and motility. The pelvic floor voluntary skeletal muscles (levators, muscle complex, external sphincter) in these patients are underdeveloped to varying degrees. Sensation may be impaired due to the absence of a true anal canal, which is instead replaced with the neorectum at the time of surgical repair, which does not provide the same degree of precise sensation. Rectal distention can be felt by these patients but primarily with solid stool. Soft and liquid stools are difficult to appreciate and thus keep under voluntary control. Motility is also altered in these patients because of the above. When bowel movements are not properly managed over time, patients can develop a megarectum, which becomes functionally hypomotile. Abnormal motility is most notable with "low" defects, where the megarectum results in constipation and overflow incontinence. Patients with "high" defects, in which the rectosigmoid reservoir is absent, may instead have loose stools, exacerbated by the aforementioned poorly developed pelvic floor muscles.[82]

The 2 most important aspects of the initial workup for both constipation and incontinence are evaluating for the presence of a stricture, which can be treated with dilations, and assessing the location of the neoanus in relation to the anal sphincter muscles. A normal anus is of adequate size, lined with mucosa, has a dentate line, and is located with the anal sphincter complex.[80] The appearance or location otherwise is irrelevant. This is critical because attempts to relocate or manipulate an otherwise normal anus that simply seems off-center, or abnormal in appearance, are unnecessary and potentially dangerous because they will not improve on the function of the normal anorectal complex. The position of the anus in relation to the sphincters is diagnosed by examination under anesthesia and electrical stimulation of the sphincters using a nerve stimulator, of which there is a variety available.[83] The anal opening should be directly in the center of the sphincter complex. A malpositioned anus, if affecting quality of life or causing obstructive symptoms, should be treated with a repeat pull-through. If the malposition is minor and the patient's stooling can be controlled with a bowel management regimen, a redo pull-through can be avoided.

Patients with HD have historically been thought to have favorable continence outcomes in the absence of an improperly performed pull-through. However, recent studies suggest that these patients have varying degrees of impaired bowel control when compared with age-matched controls, with anywhere from 5% to 48% of patients suffering from constipation or impaired continence,[84–87] with effects on social activity and quality of life. In many patients, incontinence results from a functional megacolon caused by stool holding behaviors and overflow incontinence, in which liquid stool leaks around impacted stool, which appears similar to true incontinence. Patients with HD who present in adulthood with incontinence should undergo a digital rectal examination to evaluate for the presence of stricture and hard stool within the rectal vault, and a barium enema should be performed. If a stricture is present, dilations can be performed. If stricture is absent and barium enema or abdominal radiography is consistent with constipation, a reasonable next step is to treat constipation empirically with a combination of stool softeners and/or motility agents and enemas. If this is unsuccessful during a period of weeks to months with adjustments, one must consider the rare scenario of acquired aganglionosis or a transition zone pull-through, and circumferential biopsies should be performed. If stricture is absent and ganglion cells are present and normal in appearance and distribution, a motility workup should be performed using a radionuclide study.[37] If motility is abnormal but isolated to one location, focal resection is an option. Diffuse abnormal motility requires bowel management strategies. If motility is normal, anorectal manometry can be used to diagnose internal sphincter achalasia, for which botulinum toxin injections are therapeutic. Proceeding to internal sphincterotomy and myectomy should be done with an abundance of caution, for the reasons mentioned previously. If soiling is present in the absence of any objecting findings in the testing above, one needs to consider that the sphincter may have been damaged during the initial operation or a prior muscle-splitting treatment of internal sphincter achalasia. Sphincter and muscle damage can result in abnormal sensation and inability to differentiate gas and stool, which cannot be treated with surgery and requires bowel management programs or a permanent colostomy in refractory cases. Management of constipation and incontinence in patients with ARM and HD requires a systematic approach in order to appropriately categorize the type of dysfunction present and treat it appropriately (**Fig. 5**).

Quality of Life

The quality of life of patients with ARM and HD is negatively affected by their disease, and most of the impact revolves around urinary and bowel continence, and sexual dysfunction.[57,59,61,88]

Children and young adults with ARM report shame, feeling "different," and more psychosocial and psychological problems than their peers, with women more affected than men.[89] Fecal continence seems to the primary contributor, which results in emotional distress, mental health issues, and impairment in general well-being.[74,90–92] Poor functional outcome is reported in 30% to 46% of patients requiring protective aids, frequent underwear changing,[59,75] or the need for retrograde or antegrade enemas.[93] Functional outcome seems to be directly related to disease severity[88] and anorectal function, with manometric findings correlating resting pressure, squeeze pressures, and absent RAIR with poor outcomes.[94] Importantly, social difficulties during childhood may affect the quality of life later in life despite improvements in bowel function,[88,95] with adults reporting ongoing difficulties with schooling, employment, and mental health.[96,97] Patients with cloaca seem to have similar quality of life as other women with ARM.[98]

Patients with HD face similar difficulties related to bowel function and continence, with soiling present in 4% to 7.5%, which affects their social life due to dependence

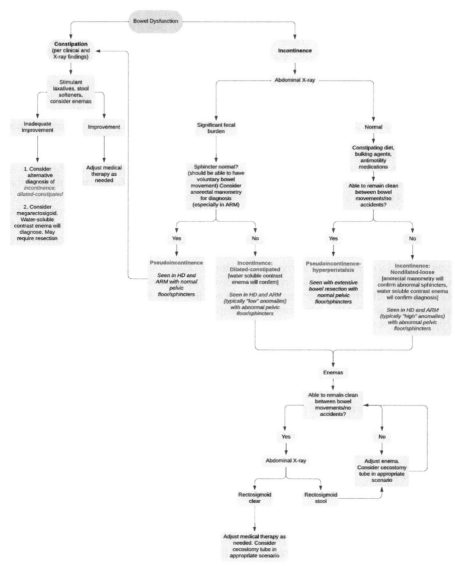

Fig. 5. Bowel management.

on diapers.[99] Patients report unhappiness and anxiety, straining, diarrhea, and incomplete evacuation.[100–102] Although some report symptom improvement over time,[64,103,104] others do not,[105] and regardless, continence remains abnormal when compared with controls,[103] and continues to negatively affect the quality of life.[91,103] Fortunately, these effects on quality of life seem to decrease with age,[99,106] with many reporting similar scores as their peers by late teens or early 20s.[107,108] Despite this, overall quality of life scores are lower when compared with the general population,[108] with the biggest contributor related to bowel continence.[109]

BOWEL MANAGEMENT

In both ARM and HD patients, the goal is to determine the consistency of stool for the patient to have bowel movements under voluntary control. Patients are first categorized as constipated or incontinent, with the understanding that incontinent patients may be suffering from overflow incontinence due to severe constipation, and in fact have normal pelvic floor and sphincter function. One must then determine which patients with incontinence are able to have a voluntary bowel movement, which defines true incontinence, and is managed differently depending on if they are dilated-constipated or nondilated-loose (see **Fig. 5**).

Patients with pseudoincontinence seem to be incontinent but are instead suffering from constipation and overflow incontinence. The first step is to determine if the patient has pseudoincontinence or true incontinence. Patients without the capacity for a voluntary bowel movement have true incontinence. X-ray in patients with pseudoincontinence will show constipation, and stimulant laxatives should show improvement. If soiling is worsened with laxatives, one needs to consider the alternative diagnosis of true incontinence-dilated/constipated.

Patients with true incontinence cannot have a voluntary bowel movement. They require medical therapy with a combination of dietary modifications, bulking agents, antimotility medications and enemas, which should be tailored so that they can be clean for 24 hours until the next enema. Contrast enema will reveal a dilated colon, typically rectosigmoid, with constipation, which suggests hypomotility and overflow as the cause, or a nondilated colon, which suggests normal motility and absent rectosigmoid reservoir with poor sphincter tone as the cause.

Patients with incontinence-dilated/constipation are incontinent, have abnormal sphincters and radiographic evidence of constipation with a dilated neorectum. They should be treated with daily enemas, with either saline or phosphate (typically 350–750 mL saline, with 10–40 mL of glycerin or 10–40 mL soap suds added if needed) to result in a bowel movement 30 to 45 minutes afterward. This should be supplemented with daily abdominal X-rays. Adjustments are made to the enema until the patient is clean and without accidents for 24 hours after the bowel movement and the rectosigmoid colon is clear on radiography.

Patients with incontinence-nondilated/loose are incontinent and have abnormal sphincters but with radiographically normal neorectum, without fecal burden or dilation. They initially require a constipating diet, avoidance of stimulating foods, bulking agents (eg, pectin), and possible oral antimotility agents (eg, loperamide, diphenoxylate/atropine) to slow stool passage throughout the colon. This should be supplemented by daily enema to empty the colon and radiographs to confirm a clear rectosigmoid, as above. Many patients have suffered despite various bowel management regimens for years. Although most can become clean with the above strategies, many still have significant effects on their quality of life and may require an appendicovesicostomy or cecostomy for antegrade enemas.

Patients with HD, in the absence of sphincter damage, should not have true fecal incontinence but rather constipation or pseudoincontinence with associated overflow. The exception to this rule is the rare patient with HD who undergoes total or near subtotal colectomy with ileoanal pull-through, who should be treated similar to any patient who has undergone a colectomy with an ileoanal anastomosis, with diet adjustments, oral antimotility agents, and bulking agents. Enemas should not be required because the pelvic floor musculature and anorectal sphincter complex of these patients are normal.

SUMMARY

ARM involves an abnormally located rectum, with a possible fistulous connection to skin or genitourinary tract. Repair requires separation of the rectum from the involved organ, where applicable, and placement of the rectum within the center of the anal sphincter complex. The intestine in HD is properly positioned, but inherently abnormal in function, and repair requires resection of abnormal intestine with anastomosis of normal intestine to the distal anal canal, within the anal sphincter complex. These diseases overlap in many aspects of long-term management.

Important complications associated with ARM include ROOF, fistula recurrence, ureteral reflux with associated CRI, cryptorchidism in men, and gynecologic anomalies in women, with associated sexual dysfunction and fertility challenges. However, women with ARM can become pregnant and have healthy babies, by either Cesarean section or vaginal delivery, although they may require ART.

Complications of HD include acquired or persistent aganglionosis, which may require repeat pull-through, and internal sphincter achalasia, which can be treated with topical therapies, injections, or sphincterotomy and myectomy, although these should be reserved for refractory cases because surgical interventions can worsen continence.

Mechanical obstruction, stricture, and prolapse are seen in both conditions. Bowel dysfunction and difficulties with continence can be severe in both diseases, particularly in ARM with "high"/severe anomalies and is the primary detractor in terms of quality of life in these patients. Bowel management is critical and consists of a varied combination of stool softeners, antimotility agents, bulking agents, diet changes, and antegrade or retrograde enemas. With a careful and specific approach to bowel management, almost all patients can achieve social continence.

CLINICS CARE POINTS

- Most patients with anorectal malformations (ARM) and Hirschsprung disease (HD) will require bowel management long-term

- Patients with "higher" ARM, abnormal sphincters or sphincter injury will require more intensive bowel management

- Contrary to historical belief, many patients with HD will require bowel management, and their concerns should not be ignored

- Patients who continue to suffer despite aggressive bowel management may benefit from cecostomy tube maturation, which allows them more control via antegrade enemas, and in a less invasive manner, which is important to many

- Neurologic, psychological, and behavioral comorbidities can contribute to difficulties with continence, particularly pertaining to stool-holding behaviors, social concerns, and participation in care

- Women with repaired ARM can have children, and can do so via vaginal delivery, but may need vaginal reconstruction to do so, and may need assistance from reproductive technologies

- A multidisciplinary approach is key in patients with urologic and gynecologic comorbidities

DISCLOSURE

The authors have nothing to disclose.

REFERENCES

1. Boemers TM, Beek FJ, van Gool JD, et al. Urologic problems in anorectal malformations. Part 1: Urodynamic findings and significance of sacral anomalies. J Pediatr Surg 1996;31(3):407–10.
2. Belman AB, King LR. Urinary tract abnormalities associated with imperforate anus. J Urol 1972;108(5):823–4.
3. Munn R, Schillinger JF. Urologic abnormalities found with imperforate anus. Urology 1983;21(3):260–4.
4. Hoekstra WJ, Scholtmeijer RJ, Molenaar JC, et al. Urogenital tract abnormalities associated with congenital anorectal anomalies. J Urol 1983;130(5):962–3.
5. McLorie GA, Sheldon CA, Fleisher M, et al. The genitourinary system in patients with imperforate anus. J Pediatr Surg 1987;22(12):1100–4.
6. Cortes D, Thorup JM, Nielsen OH, et al. Cryptorchidism in boys with imperforate anus. J Pediatr Surg 1995;30(4):631–5.
7. Fanjul M, Lancharro A, Molina E, et al. Gynecological anomalies in patients with anorectal malformations. Pediatr Surg Int 2019;35(9):967–70.
8. Vilanova-Sanchez A, McCracken K, Halleran DR, et al. Obstetrical Outcomes in Adult Patients Born with Complex Anorectal Malformations and Cloacal Anomalies: A Literature Review. J Pediatr Adolesc Gynecol 2019;32(1):7–14.
9. Bischoff A, Peña A, Levitt MA. Laparoscopic-assisted PSARP - the advantages of combining both techniques for the treatment of anorectal malformations with recto-bladderneck or high prostatic fistulas. J Pediatr Surg 2013;48(2):367–71.
10. Georgeson K. Laparoscopic-assisted anorectal pull-through. Semin Pediatr Surg 2007;16(4):266–9.
11. Coran AG, Adzick NS, Krummel TM, et al, editors. Pediatric surgery. 7th edition. Philadelphia: Mosby; 2012.
12. Hong AR, Acuña MF, Peña A, et al. Urologic injuries associated with repair of anorectal malformations in male patients. J Pediatr Surg 2002;37(3):339–44.
13. Rentea RM, Halleran DR, Vilanova-Sanchez A, et al. Diagnosis and management of a remnant of the original fistula (ROOF) in males following surgery for anorectal malformations. J Pediatr Surg 2019;54(10):1988–92.
14. Pathak M, Saxena AK. Postoperative "complications" following laparoscopic-assisted anorectoplasty: A systematic review. Pediatr Surg Int 2020;36(11):1299–307.
15. Grimsby GM, Fischer AC, Baker LA. Autologous buccal mucosa graft for repair of recurrent rectovaginal fistula. Pediatr Surg Int 2014;30(5):533–5.
16. Grimsby GM, Baker LA. The use of autologous buccal mucosa grafts in vaginal reconstruction. Curr Urol Rep 2014;15(8):428.
17. Nikolaev Vv. Recurrent rectourethral fistula repair: A novel technique of gracilis muscle interposition. J Pediatr Surg 2020;55(9):1974–8.
18. Bjoersum-Meyer T, Kaalby L, Lund L, et al. Long-term Functional Urinary and Sexual Outcomes in Patients with Anorectal Malformations-A Systematic Review. Eur Urol Open Sci 2021;25:29–38.
19. Skerritt C, DaJusta DG, Fuchs ME, et al. Long-term urologic and gynecologic follow-up and the importance of collaboration for patients with anorectal malformations. Semin Pediatr Surg 2020;29(6):150987.
20. Warne SA, Wilcox DT, Ledermann SE, et al. Renal outcome in patients with cloaca. J Urol 2002;167(6):2548–51 [discussion: 2551].
21. Caldwell BT, Wilcox DT. Long-term urological outcomes in cloacal anomalies. Semin Pediatr Surg 2016;25(2):108–11.

22. Trovalusci E, Rossato M, Gamba P, et al. Testicular function and sexuality in adult patients with anorectal malformation. J Pediatr Surg 2020;55(9):1839–45.
23. Borg H, Holmdahl G, Doroszkievicz M, et al. Longitudinal study of lower urinary tract function in children with anorectal malformation. Eur J Pediatr Surg 2014; 24(6):492–9.
24. Fuchs ME, Halleran DR, Bourgeois T, et al. Correlation of anorectal malformation complexity and associated urologic abnormalities. J Pediatr Surg 2021;56(11): 1988–92.
25. Levitt MA, Stein DM, Peña A. Gynecologic concerns in the treatment of teenagers with cloaca. J Pediatr Surg 1998;33(2):188–93.
26. Warne SA, Wilcox DT, Creighton S, et al. Long-term gynecological outcome of patients with persistent cloaca. J Urol 2003;170(4 Pt 2):1493–6.
27. Couchman A, Creighton SM, Wood D. Adolescent and adult outcomes in women following childhood vaginal reconstruction for cloacal anomaly. J Urol 2015;193(5 Suppl):1819–22.
28. Sharma S, Gupta DK. Early vaginal replacement in cloacal malformation. Pediatr Surg Int 2019;35(2):263–9.
29. Vilanova-Sanchez A, Halleran DR, Reck CA, et al. Factors predicting the need for vaginal replacement at the time of primary reconstruction of a cloacal malformation. J Pediatr Surg 2020;55(1):71–4.
30. Demehri FR, Halaweish IF, Coran AG, et al. Hirschsprung-associated enterocolitis: pathogenesis, treatment and prevention. Pediatr Surg Int 2013;29(9): 873–81.
31. Teitelbaum DH, Qualman SJ, Caniano DA. Hirschsprung's disease. Identification of risk factors for enterocolitis. Ann Surg 1988;207(3):240–4.
32. Hackam DJ, Filler RM, Pearl RH. Enterocolitis after the surgical treatment of Hirschsprung's disease: risk factors and financial impact. J Pediatr Surg 1998;33(6):830–3.
33. Seo S, Miyake H, Hock A, et al. Duhamel and Transanal Endorectal Pull-throughs for Hirschsprung' Disease: A Systematic Review and Meta-analysis. Eur J Pediatr Surg 2018;28(1):81–8.
34. West KW, Grosfeld JL, Rescorla FJ, et al. Acquired aganglionosis: a rare occurrence following pull-through procedures for Hirschsprung's disease. J Pediatr Surg 1990;25(1):104–8 [discussion: 108–9].
35. White F v, Langer JC. Circumferential distribution of ganglion cells in the transition zone of children with Hirschsprung disease. Pediatr Dev Pathol 2000;3(3): 216–22.
36. Ghose SI, Squire BR, Stringer MD, et al. Hirschsprung's disease: problems with transition-zone pull-through. J Pediatr Surg 2000;35(12):1805–9.
37. Southwell BR, Clarke MCC, Sutcliffe J, et al. Colonic transit studies: normal values for adults and children with comparison of radiological and scintigraphic methods. Pediatr Surg Int 2009;25(7):559–72.
38. di Lorenzo C, Solzi GF, Flores AF, et al. Colonic motility after surgery for Hirschsprung's disease. Am J Gastroenterol 2000;95(7):1759–64.
39. Mazziotti M v, Langer JC. Laparoscopic full-thickness intestinal biopsies in children. J Pediatr Gastroenterol Nutr 2001;33(1):54–7.
40. Feichter S, Meier-Ruge WA, Bruder E. The histopathology of gastrointestinal motility disorders in children. Semin Pediatr Surg 2009;18(4):206–11.
41. Davidson M, Bauer C. Studies of distal colonic motility in children. IV. Achalasia of the distal rectal segment despite presence of ganglia in the myenteric plexuses of this area. Pediatrics 1958;21(5):746–61.

42. Minkes RK, Langer JC. A prospective study of botulinum toxin for internal anal sphincter hypertonicity in children with Hirschsprung's disease. J Pediatr Surg 2000;35(12):1733–6.
43. de Caluwé D, Yoneda A, Akl U, et al. Internal anal sphincter achalasia: outcome after internal sphincter myectomy. J Pediatr Surg 2001;36(5):736–8.
44. Heikkinen M, Lindahl H, Rintala RJ. Long-term outcome after internal sphincter myectomy for internal sphincter achalasia. Pediatr Surg Int 2005;21(2):84–7.
45. Kaymakcioglu N, Yagci G, Can MF, et al. Role of anorectal myectomy in the treatment of short segment Hirschsprung's disease in young adults. Int Surg 2005;90(2):109–12.
46. Abbas Banani S, Forootan H. Role of anorectal myectomy after failed endorectal pull-through in Hirschsprung's disease. J Pediatr Surg 1994;29(10):1307–9.
47. Wildhaber BE, Pakarinen M, Rintala RJ, et al. Posterior myotomy/myectomy for persistent stooling problems in Hirschsprung's disease. J Pediatr Surg 2004; 39(6):920–6 [discussion: 920–6].
48. Lucha PA, Fticsar JE, Francis MJ. The strictured anastomosis: successful treatment by corticosteroid injections–report of three cases and review of the literature. Dis Colon Rectum 2005;48(4):862–5.
49. van Leeuwen K, Teitelbaum DH, Elhalaby EA, et al. Long-term follow-up of redo pull-through procedures for Hirschsprung's disease: efficacy of the endorectal pull-through. J Pediatr Surg 2000;35(6):829–33 [discussion: 833–4].
50. Mueller CM, Beaunoyer M, St-Vil D. Topical mitomycin-C for the treatment of anal stricture. J Pediatr Surg 2010;45(1):241–4.
51. Anderson KD, Newman KD, Bond SJ, et al. Diamond flap anoplasty in infants and children with an intractable anal stricture. J Pediatr Surg 1994;29(9): 1253–7.
52. Balci B, Yildiz A, Leventoglu S, et al. Diamond-shaped flap anoplasty for severe anal stenosis - a video vignette. Colorectal Dis 2021;23(7):1941.
53. Belizon A, Levitt M, Shoshany G, et al. Rectal prolapse following posterior sagittal anorectoplasty for anorectal malformations. J Pediatr Surg 2005;40(1): 192–6.
54. de La Torre L, Zornoza M, Peña A, et al. Transanal rectal mucosectomy and muscular plication: A new technique for rectal prolapse in patients with an anorectal malformation. J Pediatr Surg 2020;55(11):2531–5.
55. Brisighelli G, di Cesare A, Morandi A, et al. Classification and management of rectal prolapse after anorectoplasty for anorectal malformations. Pediatr Surg Int 2014;30(8):783–9.
56. Witvliet MJ, van Gasteren S, van den Hondel D, et al. Predicting sexual problems in young adults with an anorectal malformation or Hirschsprung disease. J Pediatr Surg 2018;53(8):1555–9.
57. Kyrklund K, Pakarinen MP, Rintala RJ. Long-term bowel function, quality of life and sexual function in patients with anorectal malformations treated during the PSARP era. Semin Pediatr Surg 2017;26(5):336–42.
58. van den Hondel D, Sloots CEJ, Bolt JM, et al. Psychosexual Well-Being after Childhood Surgery for Anorectal Malformation or Hirschsprung's Disease. J Sex Med 2015;12(7):1616–25.
59. Rintala R, Mildh L, Lindahl H. Fecal continence and quality of life for adult patients with an operated high or intermediate anorectal malformation. J Pediatr Surg 1994;29(6):777–80.
60. Grano C, Aminoff D, Lucidi F, et al. Long-term disease-specific quality of life in adult anorectal malformation patients. J Pediatr Surg 2011;46(4):691–8.

61. Kyrklund K, Taskinen S, Rintala RJ, et al. Sexual Function, Fertility and Quality of Life after Modern Treatment of Anorectal Malformations. J Urol 2016;196(6): 1741–6.

62. Bicelli N, Trovalusci E, Zannol M, et al. Gynecological and psycho-sexual aspects of women with history of anorectal malformations. Pediatr Surg Int 2021; 37(8):991–7.

63. Learner HI, Creighton SM, Wood D. Augmentation vaginoplasty with buccal mucosa for the surgical revision of postreconstructive vaginal stenosis: a case series. J Pediatr Urol 2019;15(4):402.e1-7.

64. Neuvonen MI, Kyrklund K, Rintala RJ, et al. Bowel Function and Quality of Life After Transanal Endorectal Pull-through for Hirschsprung Disease: Controlled Outcomes up to Adulthood. Ann Surg 2017;265(3):622–9.

65. Neuvonen M, Kyrklund K, Taskinen S, et al. Lower urinary tract symptoms and sexual functions after endorectal pull-through for Hirschsprung disease: controlled long-term outcomes. J Pediatr Surg 2017;52(8):1296–301.

66. Iacusso C, Iacobelli BD, Morini F, et al. Assisted Reproductive Technology and Anorectal Malformation: A Single-Center Experience. Front Pediatr 2021;9: 705385.

67. Breech L. Gynecologic concerns in patients with anorectal malformations. Semin Pediatr Surg 2010;19(2):139–45.

68. Cardamone S, Creighton S. A gynaecologic perspective on cloacal malformations. Curr Opin Obstet Gynecol 2015;27(5):345–52.

69. Huibregtse ECP, Draaisma JMT, Hofmeester MJ, et al. The influence of anorectal malformations on fertility: a systematic review. Pediatr Surg Int 2014;30(8): 773–81.

70. Kawaguchi H, Matsumoto F, Okamoto Y, et al. Pregnancy Outcomes in 2 Women Born with Complex Anorectal Malformations: Challenges and Considerations. J Pediatr Adolesc Gynecol 2021;34(3):424–6.

71. Greenberg JA, Hendren WH. Vaginal delivery after cloacal malformation repair. Obstet Gynecol 1997;90(4 Pt 2):666–7.

72. Salvi N, Arthur I. A case of successful pregnancy outcome in a patient born with cloacal malformation. J Obstet Gynaecol 2008;28(3):343–5.

73. Nethercliffe J, Trewick A, Samuell C, et al. False-positive pregnancy tests in patients with enterocystoplasties. BJU Int 2001;87(9):780–2.

74. Danielson J, Karlbom U, Graf W, et al. Outcome in adults with anorectal malformations in relation to modern classification - Which patients do we need to follow beyond childhood? J Pediatr Surg 2017;52(3):463–8.

75. Rintala RJ, Lindahl H. Is normal bowel function possible after repair of intermediate and high anorectal malformations? J Pediatr Surg 1995;30(3):491–4.

76. Fabbro MA, Chiarenza F, D'Agostino S, et al. Anorectal malformations (ARM): quality of life assessed in the functional, urologic and neurologic short and long term follow-up. Pediatr Med Chir 2011;33(4):182–92.

77. Kyrklund K, Pakarinen MP, Taskinen S, et al. Bowel function and lower urinary tract symptoms in males with low anorectal malformations: an update of controlled, long-term outcomes. Int J Colorectal Dis 2015;30(2):221–8.

78. Levitt MA, Peña A. Pediatric fecal incontinence: a surgeon's perspective. Pediatr Rev 2010;31(3):91–101.

79. Peña A, Levitt MA. Colonic inertia disorders in pediatrics. Curr Probl Surg 2002; 39(7):666–730.

80. Peña A. Anorectal malformations. Semin Pediatr Surg 1995;4(1):35–47.

81. Levitt MA, Kant A, Peña A. The morbidity of constipation in patients with anorectal malformations. J Pediatr Surg 2010;45(6):1228–33.
82. Holcomb GW III, Murphy JP, Ostlie DJ, et al, editors. Ashcraft's Pediatric surgery. 6th edition. London: Elsevier Saunders; 2014.
83. Kapuller V, Arbell D, Udassin R, et al. A new job for an old device: a novel use for nerve stimulators in anorectal malformations. J Pediatr Surg 2014;49(3):495–6.
84. Rintala RJ, Pakarinen MP. Long-term outcomes of Hirschsprung's disease. Semin Pediatr Surg 2012;21(4):336–43.
85. Catto-Smith AG, Trajanovska M, Taylor RG. Long-term continence after surgery for Hirschsprung's disease. J Gastroenterol Hepatol 2007;22(12):2273–82.
86. Jarvi K, Laitakari EM, Koivusalo A, et al. Bowel function and gastrointestinal quality of life among adults operated for Hirschsprung disease during childhood: a population-based study. Ann Surg 2010;252(6):977–81.
87. Tomuschat C, Zimmer J, Puri P. Laparoscopic-assisted pull-through operation for Hirschsprung's disease: a systematic review and meta-analysis. Pediatr Surg Int 2016;32(8):751–7.
88. Kyrklund K, Neuvonen MI, Pakarinen MP, et al. Social Morbidity in Relation to Bowel Functional Outcomes and Quality of Life in Anorectal Malformations and Hirschsprung's Disease. Eur J Pediatr Surg 2018;28(6):522–8.
89. Leitner J, Kirchler E, Mantovan F. Quality of life of children and adolescents with congenital anorectal malformations. Kinderkrankenschwester 2017;36(3):85–90.
90. Grano C, Fernandes M, Bucci S, et al. Self-efficacy beliefs, faecal incontinence and health-related quality of life in patients born with anorectal malformations. Colorectal Dis 2018;20(8):711–8.
91. Nah SA, Ong CCP, Saffari SE, et al. Anorectal malformation & Hirschsprung's disease: A cross-sectional comparison of quality of life and bowel function to healthy controls. J Pediatr Surg 2018;53(8):1550–4.
92. Stenström P, Kockum CC, Benér DK, et al. Adolescents with anorectal malformation: physical outcome, sexual health and quality of life. Int J Adolesc Med Health 2014;26(1):49–59.
93. Kyrklund K, Pakarinen MP, Koivusalo A, et al. Long-term bowel functional outcomes in rectourethral fistula treated with PSARP: controlled results after 4-29 years of follow-up: a single-institution, cross-sectional study. J Pediatr Surg 2014;49(11):1635–42.
94. Kyrklund K, Pakarinen MP, Rintala RJ. Manometric findings in relation to functional outcomes in different types of anorectal malformations. J Pediatr Surg 2017;52(4):563–8.
95. Grano C, Bucci S, Aminoff D, et al. Transition from childhood to adolescence: Quality of life changes 6 years later in patients born with anorectal malformations. Pediatr Surg Int 2015;31(8):735–40.
96. Judd-Glossy L, Ariefdjohan M, Curry S, et al. A survey of adults with anorectal malformations: perspectives on educational, vocational, and psychosocial experiences. Pediatr Surg Int 2019;35(9):953–61.
97. Grano C, Bucci S, Aminoff D, et al. Quality of life in children and adolescents with anorectal malformation. Pediatr Surg Int 2013;29(9):925–30.
98. Versteegh HP, van den Hondel D, IJsselstijn H, et al. Cloacal malformation patients report similar quality of life as female patients with less complex anorectal malformations. J Pediatr Surg 2016;51(3):435–9.

99. Niramis R, Watanatittan S, Anuntkosol M, et al. Quality of life of patients with Hirschsprung's disease at 5 - 20 years post pull-through operations. Eur J Pediatr Surg 2008;18(1):38–43.
100. Tran VQ, Mahler T, Dassonville M, et al. Long-Term Outcomes and Quality of Life in Patients after Soave Pull-Through Operation for Hirschsprung's Disease: An Observational Retrospective Study. Eur J Pediatr Surg 2018;28(5):445–54.
101. Drissi F, Meurette G, Baayen C, et al. Long-term Outcome of Hirschsprung Disease: Impact on Quality of Life and Social Condition at Adult Age. Dis Colon Rectum 2019;62(6):727–32.
102. Dai Y, Deng Y, Lin Y, et al. Long-term outcomes and quality of life of patients with Hirschsprung disease: a systematic review and meta-analysis. BMC Gastroenterol 2020;20(1):67.
103. Meinds RJ, van der Steeg AFW, Sloots CEJ, et al. Long-term functional outcomes and quality of life in patients with Hirschsprung's disease. Br J Surg 2019;106(4):499–507.
104. Collins L, Collis B, Trajanovska M, et al. Quality of life outcomes in children with Hirschsprung disease. J Pediatr Surg 2017;52(12):2006–10.
105. Townley OG, Lindley RM, Cohen MC, et al. Functional outcome, quality of life, and "failures" following pull-through surgery for hirschsprung's disease: A review of practice at a single-center. J Pediatr Surg 2020;55(2):273–7.
106. Gunnarsdóttir A, Sandblom G, Arnbjörnsson E, et al. Quality of life in adults operated on for Hirschsprung disease in childhood. J Pediatr Gastroenterol Nutr 2010;51(2):160–6.
107. Yanchar NL, Soucy P. Long-term outcome after Hirschsprung's disease: patients' perspectives. J Pediatr Surg 1999;34(7):1152–60.
108. Menezes M, Corbally M, Puri P. Long-term results of bowel function after treatment for Hirschsprung's disease: a 29-year review. Pediatr Surg Int 2006;22(12):987–90.
109. Bai Y, Chen H, Hao J, et al. Long-term outcome and quality of life after the Swenson procedure for Hirschsprung's disease. J Pediatr Surg 2002;37(4):639–42.

Abdominal Tumors
Wilms, Neuroblastoma, Rhabdomyosarcoma, and Hepatoblastoma

Jennifer T. Castle, MD[a], Brittany E. Levy, MD[a],
David A. Rodeberg, MD[b],*

KEYWORDS

- Childhood cancer survivors • Long-term sequelae • Complications
- Pediatric solid tumors • Follow-up care

KEY POINTS

- Owing to increased longevity, pediatric cancer survivors are now transitioning to adult practitioners who are faced with managing long-term consequences/morbidity of their childhood cancer and treatment protocols.
- Childhood cancer survivors are at increased risk of secondary malignancies, neuropathies, chronic pain, cardiomyopathies, and more long-term systemic effects from their cancer treatments that can persist or arise well into adulthood.
- Staying apprised of the long-term effects of childhood cancer treatments allows for adult providers to appropriately screen for conditions that predispose childhood cancer survivors to an increased operative risk.

INTRODUCTION

Outcomes for pediatric patients with cancer have greatly improved due, in part, to advancements in protocolized multimodal treatment plans. Today, the 5-year survival rate for all pediatric patients with cancer is greater than 80%, a significant increase compared with the decades past.[1] However, these improved outcomes are frequently at the cost of intensified therapy. Owing to these improved outcomes, pediatric cancer survivors are now transitioning to adult practitioners who are faced with managing long-term consequences/morbidity of their childhood cancer and treatment protocols. Adult providers caring for pediatric cancer survivors must account for physiologic and anatomic differences in this growing patient population. Two large studies have provided the foundation of knowledge concerning outcomes and treatment-

[a] Department of Surgery, University of Kentucky College of Medicine, 800 Rose Street, Lexington, KY 40536, USA; [b] Division of Pediatric Surgery, University of Kentucky College of Medicine, 800 Rose Street, Lexington, KY 40536, USA
* Corresponding author.
E-mail address: David.Rodeberg@uky.edu

Surg Clin N Am 102 (2022) 715–737
https://doi.org/10.1016/j.suc.2022.07.006
0039-6109/22/© 2022 Elsevier Inc. All rights reserved.

surgical.theclinics.com

related morbidity in these long-term survivors. The Childhood Cancer Survivor Study (CCSS) and the British Childhood Cancer Survivor Study (BCCSS) are both multi-institutional studies that analyzed long-term outcomes and general health in pediatric cancer patients in the North America and Britain, respectively.[2,3] The information gained from these studies has given insight into the long-term effects of childhood cancer treatments and the health risks survivors experience as adults.

This article discuss four common pediatric cancers including Wilms tumor, neuro-blastoma (NB), rhabdomyosarcoma (RMS), and hepatoblastoma. Particular attention is given to the long-term health consequences associated with the treatments commonly used in these pediatric diseases. The goal of this article is to educate adult surgical providers regarding these malignancies and best practices regarding screening as well as subsequent anatomic, and physiologic sequela that can impact the delivery of care to the adult survivors of childhood cancers.

WILMS TUMOR
Overview of Wilms Tumor

Wilms tumor, or nephroblastoma, is the most common renal cancer in children younger than 5 year old, typically presenting as an asymptomatic abdominal mass.[4] Although Wilms tumors can be an isolated phenomenon, nearly 5% of patients have bilateral tumors and roughly 10% are associated with other congenital abnormalities.[4] There are more than 20 different syndromic conditions associated with an increased risk of developing Wilms tumors (**Table 1**).[5] In addition, approximately 1% to 8% of Wilms tumor patients acquire von Willebrand disease, necessitating routine testing before surgical or procedural interventions.[6] This associated coagulopathy does not persist following the surgical excision of the tumor. [7]

Patients presenting with Wilms tumor should have appropriate workup for all associated anomalies and genetic syndromes. Many of these syndromic diseases are associated with complex comorbid conditions or chronic medical conditions that impact patients' health throughout adulthood. Any patient presenting with suspicion for Wilms tumor should not routinely undergo a biopsy to confirm the diagnosis and should instead be referred to a pediatric oncology center. Biopsy of the tumor mass may result in pathologic upstaging of the tumor.[8]

Clinical Emergencies

Tumor rupture and/or hemorrhage
The majority of patients with Wilms tumors will present with asymptomatic abdominal masses. Rarely, patients can present with tumor rupture and associated abdominal pain. Tumor rupture will upstage the disease, but it is not a medical or surgical emergency. For instance, ruptures can be asymptomatic, contained within the retroperito-neum, or associated with self-limited bleeding. In either instance, appropriate medical therapy is indicated before surgical intervention. Less than 1% of patients require immediate surgery or embolization for ongoing bleeding. Patients with hemodynamically stable tumor ruptures should be evaluated at a children's cancer center for the extent of disease before surgical intervention.[9]

Inferior vena cava (IVC) thrombus
Between 4% and 8% of Wilms tumor patients present with thrombus or intravascular tumor extension into the inferior vena cava and a subset of this population exhibits extension into the right atrium.[10] Fortunately, these patients also do not constitute a medical or surgical emergency but should be treated carefully and cautiously. Although exceedingly rare, patients can suffer from embolism to the pulmonary artery

Table 1
A subset of the syndromic diseases associated with Wilms tumors and a brief description of each

Syndrome	Description
WAGR syndrome	Wilms tumor, aniridia, genitourinary anomaly, and mental retardation
Denys–Drash syndrome	Renal disease and pseudohermaphroditism
Perlman syndrome	High neonatal mortality, fetal overgrowth, renal dysplasia, and mental retardation
Beckwith–Wiedemann syndrome	Asymmetric bodily growth, associated with Wilms tumor as well as rhabdomyosarcoma and hepatoblastoma
Li–Fraumeni syndrome	TP53 genetic mutation with increased risk of a multitude of malignancies including Wilms tumors

and even cardiac arrest. Thus, patients should be evaluated for intravascular extension of the tumor when diagnosed and managed accordingly. This tumor thrombus is usually treated with standard chemotherapy.[11] The use of anticoagulation in these patients is controversial and, therefore, decisions on anticoagulation should be made by a multidisciplinary pediatric oncology team who will evaluate each patient's individual risk profile.[12]

Treatment History

Wilms tumors are treated based on the tumor stage, histology, and molecular signature. The Children's Oncology Group (COG) treatment protocols are predominately used in North America, whereas European countries are guided in treatment by the International Society of Pediatric Oncology (SIOP) guidelines. Protocols from these groups are different but do agree on emphasizing care from a multidisciplinary team and the need for multimodality therapy. This section will focus on what treatments patients may undergo for Wilms tumor and will minimally discuss the differences in treatment guidelines between COG and SIOP.

Surgery and Transplant

Surgical resection can be curative in low-stage diseases or used in combination with adjuvant or neoadjuvant therapy. The sequence of surgery and medical therapy differs between COG and SIOP protocols. However, COG and SIOP are in agreement that patients with high surgical risk are better treated with neoadjuvant therapy. Typically, a nephrectomy is performed with lymph node harvesting using a transabdominal or thoracoabdominal open approach. Care is taken to resect the whole tumor and involved surrounding tissue en bloc to prevent tumor spillage, including avoiding any form of biopsy, which can upstage the cancer. There are infrequent cases where nephrectomy may not be appropriate (ie, single kidney, bilateral tumors, horseshoe kidney, impaired renal function), and these patients should be managed on an individual basis including the option for nephron-sparing resections.[13] However, kidney salvage is not always possible in bilateral tumors or solitary kidneys and cancer therapy may lead to kidney dysfunction resulting in the need for renal dialysis and transplant. Patients with Denys–Drash syndrome are recommended to undergo bilateral nephrectomy with subsequent transplant because of the high risk of developing Wilms tumors. This is extremely rare as combined Wilms tumor and Denys–Drash syndrome only accounts for 1% of the end-stage renal disease in the pediatric population.[14]

Chemotherapy

Depending on what treatment protocol is being used, patients may receive adjuvant or neoadjuvant chemotherapy. COG recognizes the need for neoadjuvant therapy in patients with bilateral tumors, solitary kidneys, extensive involvement of surrounding structures, Inferior vena cava (IVC) thrombus extending beyond the level of the hepatic veins, and in some cases of metastatic disease.[15] Contrarily, SIOP protocols use neoadjuvant with or without adjuvant therapy in most Wilms tumor patients.[15]

Whether before or after surgical resection, most patients are treated with a combination of vincristine, dactinomycin, and doxorubicin.[16] Cyclophosphamide, etoposide, and carboplatin may also be used in select cases.[5]

Radiation

As with the other aspects of treatment for Wilms tumor, the need for radiation therapy (RT) is dependent on tumor stage, histology, and molecular signature.[17] RT can be used to treat metastatic disease and the primary tumor to help provide local control.[14] Wilms tumors are very radiosensitive and therefore RT should be started within 14-days after surgery. Delay in initiation of RT is associated with increased mortality.[18]

AFTER TREATMENT
Recurrence

Recurrence most often occurs within 2 years of diagnosis; however, recurrences have been documented as late as 17 years. Only 0.5% of patients have a late recurrence, (>5 years). The most common sites of late recurrence are the abdomen, lungs, and contralateral kidney.[19]

Follow-up

After completion of treatment, the surveillance for recurrence is done with renal ultrasound with or without chest x-ray. Duration of surveillance does not typically extend past 5 years unless the patient is at higher risk for recurrence.[20] Patients with Beckwith–Wiedemann, familial Wilms, and some other syndromic diseases are at a higher risk for recurrence and therefore will continue surveillance for 7 to 8 years after treatment completion. Early surveillance is done by the primary cancer treatment team and then transitioned to survivorship care as patients age into adult care.[5] Transitions to adulthood require appropriate patient handoff to a designated program with the resources and experience to conduct appropriate follow-up care.

Long-Term Mortality

Wilms tumor patients have a 5-year 90% survival rate with an estimated 15-year survival rate of 99% in those who already survived 5 years.[4] Beyond the long-term effects of treatment, Wilms tumors patients are at increased risk of chronic medical comorbidities as adults, particularly if their tumors are part of a syndromic disease. Wilms tumor survivors experience a fivefold increased mortality than expected for their age group at 30 and 50 years follow-up with secondary malignancies and cardiac disease being the two main causes of premature mortality.[4]

Survivors of Wilms tumor are at an increased risk of end-stage renal disease particularly in those with Denys–Drash syndrome, WAGR, bilateral tumors, associated genitourinary anomalies, and those who received radiation to the contralateral kidney.[21] Wilms tumors with syndromic diseases are also associated with an increased risk of hypertension.[5]

Neuroblastoma

Overview of neuroblastoma

NB is the most common extracranial solid tumor in childhood and the most common cancer in children less than 1-year-old.[4] NBs can arise almost anywhere in the body but are most commonly found in the adrenal gland. As treatment modalities have improved, an increasing number of these children are surviving into adulthood.[4] From 1975 to 2009, the 5-year survival rate of NB increased from 54% to 79%.[4]

This disease is unique in that its prognosis varies tremendously from spontaneous regression without intervention in the lowest risk patients to overall survival of 5% in the highest risk patients.[22] Thus, treatment depends on the risk profile of the NB at diagnosis with factors such as older age at diagnosis, MYCN amplification, and location of primary tumor all determining the risk stratification and subsequent optimal treatment.[23]

Clinical Emergencies

In NB patients, there are only two rare medical emergencies related to tumor burden. The first is spinal cord compression caused by the tumor invading the spinal foramina which can lead to permanent neurologic deficits.[24] The second is respiratory distress from hepatomegaly caused by metastatic tumor burden in very young patients.[25] If patients present with symptoms of either of these complications with a mass near the spinal cord or in the liver, they should be transferred to an inpatient pediatric oncology unit for immediate intervention and cancer treatment. In either instance, the transfer should not be delayed for diagnostic confirmation of NB by biopsy.

Treatment History

Patient treatment for NB depends on a multitude of variables established at the time of diagnosis. As knowledge of this disease has advanced, the staging has been modified to standardize staging, risk stratification, and treatment. This section will not go into the details of the most current staging system but will instead give a brief description of the typical treatments used for low, intermediate, and high-risk patients.[26]

OBSERVATION AND/OR SURGERY

A select subset of NB tumors has a high likelihood of spontaneous regression without intervention. A prospective study of patients less than 6 month old with small adrenal masses demonstrated a 100% survival at 3 year with 81% of these patients having been spared any surgical or medical intervention.[27] Although observation with close surveillance is appropriate for a very select group of NB patients, this decision should be made in conjunction with a multidisciplinary pediatric oncology board.[28] Other low-risk, isolated tumors can be cured with surgical resection alone. Feasibility and safety of resection is based on location and size of the tumor; however, the majority of low-risk tumors use surgical resection as the primary therapeutic modality.[29]

If surgery is not anticipated to be curative or if the tumor demonstrates intermediate or high-risk characteristics, surgery can be coupled with adjunctive treatment modalities.

Chemotherapy

Chemotherapy is not typically used in low-risk tumors unless the patient is symptomatic and cannot undergo immediate resection (eg, spinal cord compression, respiratory distress) or has a relapse following resection. In intermediate and high-risk tumors, chemotherapy can be used as neoadjuvant therapy preceding surgical resection.[30] The chemotherapeutic agents most commonly used in the treatment of NB are doxorubicin, cyclophosphamide, carboplatin/platinum-based drug, and etoposide.[28] Treatment most frequently uses a variable combination of these agents for a variable duration depending on the risk stratification of the tumor.

Radiation

RT is used in low and intermediate-risk tumors only when the patient is symptomatic and not responding to chemotherapy or is unable to undergo resection. In contrast, the treatment of high-risk tumors includes RT in all patients both to the primary tumor location, and to metastatic lesions.[30] The radiation technique used has changed with the advancement in radiation delivering technologies.[31] Thus, someone with this disease treated in the 80s will have a different radiation exposure compared with someone treated now and in the future.

IMMUNOTHERAPY, ISOTRETINOIN, AND STEM-CELL TRANSPLANT

Immunotherapy, isotretinoin, and stem-cell transplant are reserved for the treatment of high-risk tumors and relapse. These agents are not used as single modality therapy.[28] Typically, all are used sequentially as a part of or following myeloablative therapy and radiation. These treatment modalities have improved the outcomes for patients with high-risk tumors.[32]

AFTER TREATMENT
Recurrence

Recurrence of NB usually occurs within 5 years after initial diagnosis with a median time to recurrence of only 18 months.[33] Given this short time frame, most recurrences are detected on routine surveillance. Treatment of recurrence is dependent on multiple patient and disease-specific factors and requires a multidisciplinary approach as recurrence is the most common cause of late mortality in NB patients.[34] If a patient with a history of NB presents with concerns for recurrence outside of their primary treatment center, they should be directed back to their primary treatment center for evaluation and treatment.

Follow-Up

Following completion of treatment for NB, patient surveillance is variable based on each patient's risk stratification. The primary treatment team manages early surveillance using imaging, as well as urine and serum tumor markers.[35] Imaging typically consists of computed tomography (CT), MRI, or ultrasound, whereas laboratory evaluation includes homovanillic acid (HVA) and vanillylmandelic acid (VMA), plus potentially others as required.[35] The need for surveillance imaging and marker assessment past 5 years is not routine but may be beneficial in select patients. Survivorship clinics and adult community providers who assume care of survivors should be aware of the individual risk of that patient for recurrence and the initial tests for surveillance. If concern for recurrence arises in a survivor, the initial treatment team should be contacted, or the patient referred to their care for further evaluation.

Long-Term Mortality

NB survivors who survive 5 years have an estimated 94% 15-year survival rate.[4] However, an analysis from the CCSS looking at long-term outcomes in NB survivors found that survivors had as high as a 23% increase in their 25-year cumulative mortality, with the most common causes being disease recurrence and secondary malignancies.[34]

Survivors also had a greater cumulative risk of musculoskeletal, neurologic, endocrine, and sensory complications compared with their siblings. Amongst survivors, those treated with multimodal therapy had twofold greater risk of developing chronic health conditions compared with survivors treated only with surgery.[34]

RHABDOMYOSARCOMA
Overview of Rhabdomyosarcoma

RMS, composed of both embryonal (FOXO fusion negative) and alveolar (FOXO fusion-positive) subtypes, continues to be the most common soft-tissue malignancy in the pediatric patient.[36] Long-term survival rates are varied, with greater than 70% survival in patients with localized disease and poor outcomes in children with metastatic or recurrent disease. RMS has multiple potential primary tumor sites as it is derived from mesenchymal tissue. The site of the primary tumor is critical to determining stage and risk stratification and thereby the treatment regimen.[37]

Clinical Emergencies

No clinical emergencies exist for patients with RMS. Therefore, if clinical concern for RMS arises, referral to a pediatric care center for workup and management is indicated.

Treatment History

Treatment strategies for RMS largely depend on risk stratification that is composed stage, resection status, and FOXO fusion status. Key components of staging include the primary tumor site, tumor size, presence of tumor invasion, regional lymph node involvement, and distant metastasis. The extent of surgical resection and pathologic evaluation for nodes and margin that occurs before the initiation of chemotherapy determine the clinical group for the patient. In addition, genetic factors such as the presence of a PAX/FOXO$_1$ fusion are a negative prognostic factor and denote aggressive disease.[37] Using the stage, group, and genetic analysis, a risk group is determined and used to identify therapeutic regimens.

CHEMOTHERAPY

Chemotherapy-based treatment regimens are largely composed of vincristine, dactinomycin, cyclophosphamide, irinotecan, and temsirolimus in differing combinations depending on the risk group.[38]

Surgical Resection

Surgical resection is encouraged at diagnosis before the initiation of chemotherapy, if complete resection is anticipated without loss of vital structures or significant deformity.[38,39] If unable to resect the tumor completely, without compromising form or function, an incisional biopsy should be performed for histologic and molecular genetic diagnosis.[38]

If there is tumor remaining after the initial resection (biopsy or incomplete resection) and yet the surgeon thinks they would be able to completely remove the tumor safely then a re-excision can be performed.[40] Alternatively, following induction of chemotherapy, a delayed excision of the primary tumor can be performed depending on tumor respectability after induction chemotherapy.[41] Debulking surgery is not advised.

Lymph node involvement is a poor prognostic indicator and may be identified either on physical examination or diagnostic imaging.[42] Surgical evaluation is needed in patients older than 10 year old with paratesticular primary tumors, extremity or trunk tumors, those with enlarged nodes to confirm pathologic disease, or those that are FOXO fusion positive to best stage the patient's disease and inform future therapy.[43]

RADIATION

The role of RT is limited to FOX_1 fusion negative patients with residual tumor, and all FOX_1 fusion-positive patients.[44] Therefore, although not indicated for all patients, if indicated it should be pursued to reduce the risk of local recurrence.[45]

AFTER TREATMENT
Recurrence

Survival rates for patients with recurrent, metastatic, or otherwise high-risk RMS range from 20% to 30%.[46] Molecular genetic analysis regarding PAX/FOX1 fusion is a crucial prognostic factor for patients with recurrence, or metastatic disease.[47] Additional molecular markers, such as HRAS mutations, may impact outcomes; however, its significance is unclear.[47] Recurrence can be detected either by clinical symptoms or routine imaging. Clinical symptoms detect 60% of recurrence, with a median time frame of 12 months.[48] Routine screening imaging detects recurrence about 20% of the time, half within 8 months and all within 2.5 years.[48]

FOLLOW-UP

Recurrence of RMS is most common within 3 years of diagnosis. Therefore, following 3 years further surveillance is not routinely performed. Cancer predisposition syndromes have genetic variants that are associated with RMS (**Table 2**).[49] Therefore, appropriate prolonged surveillance for cancer predisposition syndromes is necessary. In addition, for patients who undergo abdominal RT, the decreased age for colonoscopy surveillance should be considered at age 35 or10 years following completion of RT.[50]

LONG-TERM MORTALITY

Disease survival is largely based on the presence of metastatic disease, the FOXO fusion status of the tumor, and the patient's age at diagnosis. Younger children, less than 9 year old have an overall better prognosis.[46] Low-risk RMS has a 5-year survival rate of 70% to 90%, whereas high-risk RMS patients have a poor 5-year survival

Table 2	
Associated cancer syndromes with rhabdomyosarcoma	
Syndrome	**Genes**
Li- Fraumeni Syndrome	TP53 and CHEK2
Neurofibromatosis Type 1	NF1
Costello syndrome	HRAS
DICER1 syndrome	DICER1
Gorlin syndrome	PTCH1 and SUFU
Noonan syndrome	SOS1, PTPN11, RAF1, CBL, KRAS, NRAS, RITI, and SHOC2
Constitutional mismatch repair deficiency	MLH1, MSH2, MSH6, and PMS2
Beckwith–Wiedemann syndrome	CDKN1C
Rubinstein–Taybi syndrome	CREBBP

rate of 20% to 30%.[46] Therefore, those patients who are living into adulthood are those with low or intermediate risk disease. Outcomes having a bearing on their adulthood are largely related to the location of their original tumor. Males with a history of para-testicular RMS may have sexual dysfunction post puberty, whereas females with a history of pelvic radiation secondary to vulvovaginal RMS may experience bladder dysfunction, colonic strictures, or reproductive dysfunction.[51–53] Young children with head and neck RMS may experience craniofacial differences because of targeted therapy modalities, in addition to pituitary and thyroid dysfunction.[54–56]

Adults with a childhood history of RMS have higher all-cause mortality compared with the general population, largely because of a high secondary malignancy rate due to radiation exposure.[53] Therefore, when transitioning to adult care regular surveillance for adult malignancies should be a priority.

HEPATOBLASTOMA
Overview of Hepatoblastoma

Hepatoblastoma is the most common malignant liver tumor in the pediatric population, targeting children less than 5 years of age.[57] Often characterized by elevated alpha-fetoprotein (AFP), patients undergo axial imaging to best characterize the patient's anatomy for surgical planning.[58] Over the past 20 years, international collaborations have created the Pre-treatment Extent of Tumor (PRETEXT) staging system to better inform treatment strategies.[59] Using this staging system patients are recommended to undergo initial upfront resection, neoadjuvant chemotherapy followed by re-evaluation for potential resection, or liver transplantation. Standardization of treatment guidelines, based on the PRETEXT system risk classification, has improved outcomes and is being used in the ongoing Paediatric Hepatic International Tumour Trial (PHITT).[59]

CLINICAL EMERGENCIES

There are case reports detailing potential tumor thrombus or tumor extension through the inferior vena cava into the right atrium.[60,61] Fortunately, extensive tumor thrombus does not denote a surgical emergency and the patient should be transferred to a pediatric oncologic center for further workup and evaluation regarding the underlying pathology.

Treatment History

Chemotherapy treatments
Cisplatin-based chemotherapy regimens remain a key component of hepatoblastoma treatment algorithms.[62] COG recommends cisplatin, 5-fluorouracil, and vincristine as the standard regimen with some patients receiving doxorubicin for intermediate or high-risk disease.[58] European centers have been providing neoadjuvant chemotherapy to all children with hepatoblastoma since the 1990s.

Surgical Resection and Liver Transplantation

Owing to the advances in surgical techniques, postoperative care, and the improved ability to perform vascular reconstruction as well as pediatric liver transplantations, the rates of successful surgical treatment of disease have increased over time.[63] Depending on the location of the hepatoblastoma tumor, liver resection may include an extended hemi-hepatectomy, a hemi-hepatectomy, a segmentectomy, or sectionectomy.[63,64] In patients, who cannot achieve full resection because of vascular involvement or inadequate remnant liver after neoadjuvant chemotherapy, a liver transplant should be considered.[64] Patients require early consultation with a tertiary care center with liver transplantation capabilities and are considered for either a living or deceased donor liver transplant.[65]

AFTER TREATMENT
Recurrence

Recurrence of hepatoblastoma occurs in less than 12% of children, more than 50% of these patients will undergo a salvage transplantation or re-resection of their liver and achieve secondary remission. Patients who receive a delayed, salvage transplantation have worse outcomes than those who undergo primary transplantation; therefore, patients should be seen at tertiary care centers with transplant capabilities early in their disease diagnosis when it is clear they are not amenable to resection.[66]

Follow-up

Patients with a molecular diagnosis or family diagnosis of familial adenomatous polyposis (FAP) should be screened for hepatoblastoma. All patients diagnosed with hepatoblastoma should undergo molecular testing to determine if an APC germline mutation is present to aid decision-making regarding colonoscopy timing for the patient and prompt genetic work up and subsequent screening initiation for affected family members.[67] Patients with FAP require early and frequent colonoscopy starting at age 10 to 12 years, and this surveillance should continue throughout their life.[67]

LONG-TERM MORTALITY

The long-term survival of hepatoblastoma has increased over the past decade because of standardized PRETEXT staging and treatment algorithms, in addition to a more aggressive approach regarding surgical resection and transplantation within the management algorithms.[68] To date, hepatoblastoma 5-year survival approaches 80%, and is well more than 80% in surgically treated patients.[69]

LONG-TERM TREATMENT CONCERNS
Surgery Long-Term Considerations

Adhesive disease
Laparotomy for the resection of all these tumors remains a common surgical approach. Small bowel obstruction (SBO) from adhesive disease occurs in a mean of 6.2% of neonates and 4.7% in older children who have undergone laparotomy.[70] There are diseases that have an increased risk of adhesive SBO (ie, intestinal surgery/resection, malrotation, gastroschisis) with occurrences as high as 14.2%; however, in children who have a laparotomy for cancer adhesion related SBO is approximately 5.5% to 14%.[70,71] In patients with a history of an open abdominal operation in childhood, concerns regarding the adhesive disease, SBO, and the standard risks of a re-operative abdomen should be considered for future surgical procedures.

POST-TRANSPLANT

Similar to adults, pediatric transplant recipients will require lifelong immunosuppression and are subject to the typical risks associated with prolonged immunosuppression including infections and immunosuppression-related malignancy. Pediatric transplant recipients are at an increased risk of severe viral illness as their immune system is typically naïve to these pathogens at time of transplant.[72] Thus, it is important for these patients to receive age-appropriate vaccinations both before and after transplantation. In addition, unique to this population is an increased emphasis on education regarding family planning as unintended pregnancies can be devastating while taking teratogenic immunosuppressive medications.[73]

Pediatric patients who undergo renal transplant have a 38% or 52% 10-year graft survival for deceased or living donor grafts, respectively.[72] Pediatric renal transplant recipients have a 90% to 95% 10-year survival.[72] They, unfortunately, have an increased risk of cardiovascular disease as adults that account for over a third of deaths in pediatric transplant recipients.[72] These patients are also at an increased risk of hypertension, obesity, growth delay, and diabetes.[74]

Pediatric liver transplant survival is greater than 80% at 20 years with late graft loss being very uncommon.[75] These patients are at increased risk of renal dysfunction and approximately 30% of recipients will eventually develop chronic renal failure.[75] Two-thirds of late mortality following pediatric liver transplant are from complications of immunosuppression. This mortality has resulted in studies and protocols to address graft tolerance and the ability to decrease or withdraw immunosuppression in this population.[76,77] Currently, the standard of care remains life-long immunosuppression. Immunosuppression withdrawal may be appropriate in some individuals, which should only be determined by the individual's transplant team.

Chemotherapy Long-Term Considerations

Doxorubicin

Although the toxicities of doxorubicin are widely appreciated, it remains a frequently prescribed chemotherapy agent for pediatric cancer because of its broad efficacy in different malignancies. Cardiotoxicity is a well-established complication of doxorubicin in the adult cancer population, with differing, but severe, cardiotoxic effects in the pediatric population who have young, growing hearts.[78] In the 1970s, roughly 8% of pediatric patients receiving doxorubicin developed acute severe cardiotoxic side effects.[79] This dose-dependent toxicity led to the adoption of decreased doxorubicin dosages in treatment protocols, resulting in decreased cardiotoxicity to approximately 1.7%.[79,80] However, doxorubicin exposure in childhood remains an independent risk factor for heart failure later in life in 7% of patients within 30 years following cancer diagnosis and is associated with a 50% mortality.[80–82] Risk-prediction models and surveillance guidelines are available to help health care providers employ appropriate screening for cardiotoxic side effects in childhood cancer survivors.[2,80]

DACTINOMYCIN

During treatment, dactinomycin is associated with severe hepatotoxicity, myelosuppression, mucositis, and rarely sinusoidal obstruction syndrome.[83,84] However, there are very few instances of long-term toxicity from dactinomycin. Some reports suggest that concurrent dactinomycin administration may exacerbate radiation toxicity.[85] In addition, it may be associated with premature ovarian failure suggested by abnormal ovarian reserve markers, but the clinical impact of these findings is unknown; in addition, dactinomycin is typically associated with little to no risk of gonadotoxicity.[86,87] Therefore, despite the dose-limiting effects of dactinomycin during treatment, there are minimal long-term concerns.

VINCRISTINE

Vincristine is the most common chemotherapeutic agent used in the treatment of pediatric cancers (ie, Wilms, NB, RMS, leukemia, etc.).[88–90] Peripheral neuropathy is a well-described long-term sequelae of vincristine treatments in childhood.[89] In adult survivors greater than 10 years from diagnosis, 17.5% have a lasting motor impairment.[90] Clinical scoring tools to quantify the severity of neuropathy, such as the Total Neuropathy Score-Pediatric Vincristine (TNS-PV) are often used in pediatric patients during or immediately after treatment.[91] Utilization of the Total Neuropathy Score (TNS) in adults can be easily correlated with the pediatric scale, and thereby can identify progression of neuropathy throughout life.[92]

PLATINUM DRUGS (CARBOPLATIN, CISPLATIN)

The platinum drugs have multiple complications both acute and chronic impacting different bodily systems. Cisplatin is responsible for long-term neuropathy, at a greater incidence than vincristine, with a greater prevalence of sensory deficits.[90,92] High-dose cisplatin for the treatment of NB is associated with hearing loss.[34] Ototoxicity (eg, hearing loss, tinnitus, vertigo) has also been observed in survivors of other tumors particularly head and neck tumors because of the concurrent use of cranial RT.[85,93] These sensory deficits because of cisplatin have been associated with decreased endurance and impaired mobility in adulthood resulting in significant disability.[92] In addition, cisplatin causes acute kidney injury and subsequent chronic kidney disease in 60% to 80% of childhood cancer survivors.[94] The long-term effects of cisplatin on the cardiovascular system in childhood cancer survivors is unclear. Several studies demonstrate an increased risk of cardiovascular dysfunction, myocardial infarction, hypertension, and metabolic syndrome, whereas others demonstrate no cardiac dysfunction up to 30 years after cisplatin exposure.[95–97] Given the ambiguity, any provider caring for a childhood cancer survivor who was treated with cisplatin should have a high clinical suspicion for cardiac dysfunction.

ETOPOSIDE

Etoposide is not typically associated with neurologic or physiologic deficits in the long-term. The most concerning long-term effect of etoposide exposure is the increased risk of secondary malignancies. There is a unique form of secondary acute myeloid leukemia significantly associated with prior etoposide treatments.[85,98] In addition, the use of etoposide in combination with RT is associated with an increased risk of secondary central nervous system malignancies.[99]

IMMUNOTHERAPY AND SCT LONG-TERM CONSIDERATIONS

Long-term effects of immunotherapy are not currently well documented in childhood cancer survivors. The long-term outcomes studies from the CCSS cohorts do not typically include immunotherapy in their analysis as there were few patients in those cohorts that were treated with immunotherapy.[100] It is documented that immunotherapy, like many of the other agents discussed, is nephrotoxic and 20% of childhood cancer survivors treated with immunotherapy develop chronic kidney disease by 5 years follow-up.[101]

In comparison, stem cell transplants (SCT) are associated with a multitude of long-term effects that have been well documented. Direct causality is difficult to define as stem cell transplant is accompanied by toxic conditioning agents (ie, total body irradiation, highly alkylating agents, etc.), which contribute to the observed effects. As the process of conditioning and SCT are relatively inextricable, we will group these long-term outcomes together for simplicity. One of the most clinically significant long-term effects of SCT is pulmonary toxicity. Up to 40% of childhood SCTs develop some degree of pulmonary fibrosis which is associated with increased morbidity and mortality.[85] Other long-term effects include increased risk of secondary malignancy, infertility, diabetes, growth delays, osteoporosis, thyroid disorders, cardiac abnormalities, and chronic graft versus host disease, which has its own list of sequelae such as liver impairment.[85,102–104] The risk of these outcomes varies depending on different variables (ie, conditioning agent used, age of transplant, prior radiation and/or chemotherapeutics used, etc.). However, any provider caring for an adult childhood cancer survivor who underwent SCT should be aware of these possible effects and the survivor should be assessed appropriately.

Radiation Long-Term Considerations

Long-term complications of RT are largely site specific. Pediatric patients receiving head and neck radiation have an increased risk of thyroid dysfunction, or thyroid cancer.[105] In addition, growth hormone deficiency is associated with pediatric cranial RT because of the hypothalamic-pituitary axis.[106] This may lead to reduced bone growth, which may affect stature.[107] In addition, radiation exposure to long bones may lead to avascular necrosis.[108,109] Hearing loss and visual impairments, secondary to cranial radiation, can also occur.[110] Radiation exposure to the chest results in cardiac toxicity. Paravertebral radiation renders a risk of vertebral abnormalities causing scoliosis, kyphosis, and short stature.[111] Similarly, RT results in impaired growth of vascular tissues and abnormal arterial compliance.[112]

Long-term complications related to abdominal/pelvic RT have implications for future fertility and child rearing. Patients with a childhood history of radiation have over a threefold increased rate of spontaneous abortion.[113] In addition, future pregnancies are subject to lower birth weight and preterm birth.[114]

All radiation exposure confers an increased risk of secondary malignancy. The CCSS identified a 20.5% incidence of secondary neoplasm following the primary childhood cancer, with a 7.9% incidence of malignancy.[115] The BCCSS identified similar results, concluding there was a 4x higher incidence ratio for secondary malignancy in childhood cancer survivors.[116] In those with a history of abdominal radiation, the incidence of colon cancer reached 1.4% by 50 year old, which is 0.2% higher incidence than those with a strong family history.[116,117]

SOCIODEMOGRAPHIC AND COGNITIVE OUTCOMES

The difficulties associated with being treated for cancer as a child do not just affect survivors' health as adults but also their livelihoods. Childhood cancer survivors are less likely to graduate college, less likely to be employed full-time, and have lower income.[118,119] Younger adult survivors show psychosexual developmental delay and are less likely to be married.[118] Of great concern is that 8% to 20% of survivors develop posttraumatic stress syndrome as adults which is associated with an increased risk of suicidal ideation.[118,120] As childhood cancer survivors demonstrate increased risks of poorer social, psychological, neurocognitive, and economic outcomes, the need to support survivors on all fronts is important to the care they are provided as a whole.

LONG-TERM PAIN

Pediatric chemotherapy regimens include vincristine and platinum-based agents, which significantly affect the neurologic system. Therefore, patients treated with these agents in childhood are at higher risk for chronic and recurrent pain syndromes as adults.[121] Patients treated with cranial RT see a similar effect, with a proportional increase in chronic pain scores in relation to Gray (Gy) dosages used during initial therapy.[121] It is well established that individuals suffering from chronic pain are at an increased risk for opioid abuse.[122] In fact, childhood cancer survivors have a greater risk (4.5 times) of opioid use.[123] For the adult surgeon, this is important to recognize as chronic pain and opioid tolerance is associated with hyperalgesia and subsequent poor pain control, greater postoperative complications, greater postoperative length of stay, greater readmission rates, and higher costs.[124]

Secondary Malignancies

Pediatric patients treated for a malignancy in childhood are more likely to experience a second malignancy in their lifetime. Although only 3% to 10% of survivors develop a secondary malignancy, they have a mortality rate of 38.2%.[125] Some disease and treatment-specific factors confer differing risks in the development of a secondary malignancy. For instance, secondary gastrointestinal cancers are associated with abdominal, pelvic, lower spine, or total body radiation exposure, thereby conferring a need for early and frequent colonoscopy compared with the general risk public recommendations.[126] Patients with this history of radiation are recommended to undergo endoscopic surveillance starting at 30 year old, or 5 years following completion of therapy (whichever is younger), per COG recommendations.[126] RT to the abdomen is also associated with secondary renal cancer, whereas RT to the chest (or abdominal radiation where the breast tissue was in the treatment field) are at greater risk for breast cancer.[103,114] Besides RT, certain chemotherapeutics (ie, etoposide, doxorubicin) and stem cell transplant also confer greater risk for the development of secondary malignancies in survivors.[98,103,127] Other secondary malignancies include thyroid cancer, central nervous system tumors, soft-tissue sarcomas, bone cancer, and leukemia.[125,127] It is important to recognize that the median time to development of a secondary malignancy is greater than 20 years from treatment, meaning these cancers are developing in adulthood.[125,128] Thus, health care providers should remain vigilant for signs and symptoms of possible secondary malignancies when caring for survivors.

DISCUSSION

As more childhood cancer survivors live longer into adulthood, the long-term consequences of the disease and treatment become increasingly important to adult providers. Many of these long-term effects will alter the care needed for survivors compared with the general surgical population. Some will need earlier screening for cancers (eg, colonoscopies, mammograms). Patients may require a more detailed cardiac assessment before an operation if treated with a cardiotoxic agent (eg, doxorubicin, chest radiation). Straight-forward operations may be more complicated and time-consuming due to extensive adhesions. Some will need personalized postoperative pain management plans that optimize adjunct pain relievers to account for the chronic use of opioids. All the outcomes discussed are dependent both on the specific cancer and treatment, so it is important to inquire about both when assessing a survivor. If the survivor is unsure, it is best to reach out to their previous cancer care team who can provide detailed treatment information and can also guide adult providers in appropriate screening and general follow-up care. In addition, the COG provides long-term survivorship guidelines that outline recommendations with risk-specific care.[126] What is known now about risk and long-term effects may change as treatment regimens shift. Thus, whenever caring for a childhood cancer survivor, it is advised to review updated guidelines and risk profiles. Whenever uncertainty arises in the care of childhood care survivors, it is always appropriate to contact the original cancer care team for guidance. In certain situations, it may be most appropriate to refer the survivor back to their care team. For instance, concern for disease recurrence or the development of a secondary malignancy that is typically considered a pediatric disease would be more appropriately treated by a pediatric cancer care team.

SUMMARY

Childhood cancer survivors encompass a new challenging cohort of adult surgical patients. Although many will have minimal to no long-lasting effects from their treatments, some will require specialized care personalized to their risk profiles. As more survivors live longer into adulthood, the knowledge and understanding of the long-term effects from both standard and newer treatment modalities will become more important. Fortunately, there are multiple sources, such as the COG, who provide updated guidelines for providers to help determine optimal care for survivors. Staying appraised of the long-term effects of childhood cancer treatments allows adult providers to appropriately screen for conditions that predispose these individuals to an increased perioperative risk.

CLINICS CARE POINTS

- The 5-year survival rate for all pediatric cancer patients is greater than 80%, a rate that has increased greatly in the past three decades
- Childhood cancer treatments are associated with a variety of long-term sequelae that can develop well into adulthood
- Certain childhood cancer survivors may be appropriate for earlier colonoscopies, mammograms, and cardiac stress testing based on treatments they received as children
- Childhood cancer survivors have an increased risk of PTSD, suicidality, social impairment, and economic disadvantage that can complicate their care

DISCLOSURE

J.T. Castle is funded by the NIH Training Grant T32CA160003.

REFERENCES

1. Erdmann F, Frederiksen LE, Bonaventure A, et al. Childhood cancer: Survival, treatment modalities, late effects and improvements over time. Cancer Epidemiol 2021;71(Pt B). https://doi.org/10.1016/J.CANEP.2020.101733.
2. Landier W, Skinner R, Wallace WH, et al. Surveillance for Late Effects in Childhood Cancer Survivors. J Clin Oncol 2018;36(21):2216–22.
3. Hawkins MM, Lancashire ER, Winter DL, et al. The British Childhood Cancer Survivor Study: Objectives, methods, population structure, response rates and initial descriptive information. Pediatr Blood Cancer 2008;50(5):1018–25.
4. Ward E, DeSantis C, Robbins A, et al. Childhood and adolescent cancer statistics. CA Cancer J Clin 2014;64(2):83–103.
5. PDQ Pediatric Treatment Editorial Board. Wilms Tumor and Other Childhood Kidney Tumors Treatment (PDQ®): Health Professional Version. PDQ Cancer

Information Summaries. 2002. Available at: https://pubmed.ncbi.nlm.nih.gov/26389282/. Accessed April 10, 2022.

6. Callaghan MU, Wong TE, Federici AB. Treatment of acquired von Willebrand syndrome in childhood. Blood 2013;122(12):2019–22.

7. Scott JP, Montgomery RR, Tubergen DG, et al. Acquired von Willebrand's disease in association with Wilm's tumor: regression following treatment. Blood 1981;58(4):665–9.

8. Ehrlich PF, Chi YY, Chintagumpala MM, et al. Results of Treatment for Patients With Multicentric or Bilaterally Predisposed Unilateral Wilms Tumor (AREN0534): A report from the Children's Oncology Group. Cancer 2020; 126(15):3516–25.

9. Zhang Y, Song HC, Fang YY, et al. Preoperative Wilms tumor rupture in children. Int Urol Nephrol 2021;53(4):619–25.

10. Khanna G, Rosen N, Anderson JR, et al. Evaluation of diagnostic performance of CT for detection of tumor thrombus in children with Wilms tumor: a report from the Children's Oncology Group. Pediatr Blood Cancer 2012;58(4):551–5.

11. Qureshi SS, Bhagat M, Smriti V, et al. Intravascular extension of Wilms tumor: Characteristics of tumor thrombus and their impact on outcomes. J Pediatr Urol 2021;17(1):69.e1–8.

12. Agarwal S, Mullikin D, Scheurer ME, et al. Role of anticoagulation in the management of tumor thrombus: A 10-year single-center experience. Pediatr Blood Cancer 2021;68(9). https://doi.org/10.1002/PBC.29173.

13. Aldrink JH, Heaton TE, Dasgupta R, et al. Update on Wilms tumor. J Pediatr Surg 2019;54(3):390–7.

14. Kist-Van Holthe JE, Ho PL, Stablein D, et al. Outcome of renal transplantation for Wilms' tumor and Denys-Drash syndrome: a report of the North American Pediatric Renal Transplant Cooperative Study. Pediatr Transpl 2005;9(3):305–10.

15. Bhatnagar S. Management of Wilms' tumor: NWTS vs SIOP. J Indian Assoc Pediatr Surg 2009;14(1):6–14.

16. Treger TD, Chowdhury T, Pritchard-Jones K, et al. The genetic changes of Wilms tumour. Nat Rev Nephrol 2019;15(4):240–51.

17. Stokes CL, Stokes WA, Kalapurakal JA, et al. Timing of radiation therapy in pediatric wilms tumor: a report from the national cancer database. Int J Radiat Oncol Biol Phys 2018;101(2):453–61.

18. Pater L, Melchior P, Rübe C, et al. Wilms tumor. Pediatr Blood Cancer 2021; 68(S2):e28257.

19. Malogolowkin MH, Spreafico F, Dome JS, et al. Incidence and outcomes of patients with late recurrence of Wilms' tumor. Pediatr Blood Cancer 2013;60(10): 1612–5.

20. Scott RH, Walker L, Olsen E, et al. Surveillance for Wilms tumour in at-risk children: pragmatic recommendations for best practice. Arch Dis Child 2006; 91(12):995–9.

21. Breslow NE, Collins AJ, Ritchey ML, et al. End stage renal disease in patients with Wilms tumor: results from the National Wilms Tumor Study Group and the United States Renal Data System. J Urol 2005;174(5):1972–5.

22. Yan P, Qi F, Bian L, et al. Comparison of incidence and outcomes of neuroblastoma in children, adolescents, and adults in the United States: a surveillance, epidemiology, and end results (SEER) Program Population Study. Med Sci Monit 2020;26. https://doi.org/10.12659/MSM.927218.

23. Mossé YP, Deyell RJ, Berthold F, et al. Neuroblastoma in older children, adolescents and young adults: a report from the International Neuroblastoma Risk Group project. Pediatr Blood Cancer 2014;61(4):627–35.
24. Katzenstein HM, Kent PM, London WB, et al. Treatment and outcome of 83 children with intraspinal neuroblastoma: the Pediatric Oncology Group experience. J Clin Oncol 2001;19(4):1047–55.
25. Weintraub M, Waldman E, Koplewitz B, et al. A sequential treatment algorithm for infants with stage 4s neuroblastoma and massive hepatomegaly. Pediatr Blood Cancer 2012;59(1):182–4.
26. Irwin MS, Naranjo A, Zhang FF, et al. Revised Neuroblastoma Risk Classification System: A Report From the Children's Oncology Group. J Clin Oncol 2021; 39(29):3229–41.
27. Nuchtern JG, London WB, Barnewolt CE, et al. A prospective study of expectant observation as primary therapy for neuroblastoma in young infants: a Children's Oncology Group study. Ann Surg 2012;256(4):573–80.
28. PDQ Screening and Prevention Editorial Board. Neuroblastoma Screening (PDQ®): Health Professional Version. PDQ Cancer Information Summaries. 2002. Available at: http://www.ncbi.nlm.nih.gov/pubmed/26389460. Accessed April 10, 2022.
29. Perez CA, Matthay KK, Atkinson JB, et al. Biologic variables in the outcome of stages I and II neuroblastoma treated with surgery as primary therapy: a children's cancer group study. J Clin Oncol 2000;18(1):18–26.
30. Whittle SB, Smith V, Doherty E, et al. Overview and recent advances in the treatment of neuroblastoma. Expert Rev Anticancer Ther 2017;17(4):369–86.
31. Gains JE, Moroz V, Aldridge MD, et al. A phase IIa trial of molecular radiotherapy with 177-lutetium DOTATATE in children with primary refractory or relapsed high-risk neuroblastoma. Eur J Nucl Med Mol Imaging 2020;47(10): 2348–57.
32. Atherine K, Atthay KM, Udith J, et al. Treatment of high-risk neuroblastoma with intensive chemotherapy, radiotherapy, autologous bone marrow transplantation, and 13-cis-retinoic acid. Children's Cancer Group. N Engl J Med 1999;341(16): 1165–73.
33. London WB, Bagatell R, Weigel BJ, et al. Historical time to disease progression and progression-free survival in patients with recurrent/refractory neuroblastoma treated in the modern era on Children's Oncology Group early-phase trials. Cancer 2017;123(24):4914–23.
34. Laverdiére C, Liu Q, Yasui Y, et al. Long-term outcomes in survivors of neuroblastoma: a report from the Childhood Cancer Survivor Study. J Natl Cancer Inst 2009;101(16):1131–40.
35. Lee KL, Ma JF, Shortliffe LD. Neuroblastoma: management, recurrence, and follow-up. Urol Clin North Am 2003;30(4):881–90.
36. Beverly Raney R, Anderson JR, Barr FG, et al. Rhabdomyosarcoma and undifferentiated sarcoma in the first two decades of life: a selective review of intergroup rhabdomyosarcoma study group experience and rationale for Intergroup Rhabdomyosarcoma Study V. J Pediatr Hematol Oncol 2001;23(4): 215–20.
37. Rhee DS, Rodeberg DA, Baertschiger RM, et al. Update on pediatric rhabdomyosarcoma: A report from the APSA Cancer Committee. J Pediatr Surg 2020;55(10):1987–95.
38. PDQ Pediatric Treatment Editorial Board. Childhood Rhabdomyosarcoma Treatment (PDQ®): Health Professional Version. PDQ Cancer Information

Summaries. 2002. Available at: https://pubmed.ncbi.nlm.nih.gov/26389243/. Accessed April 10, 2022.

39. Lawrence W, Hays DM, Heyn R, et al. Surgical lessons from the Intergroup Rhabdomyosarcoma Study (IRS) pertaining to extremity tumors. World J Surg 1988;12(5):676–84.

40. Cecchetto G, Guglielmi M, Inserra A, et al. Primary re-excision: The Italian experience in patients with localized soft-tissue sarcomas. Pediatr Surg Int 2001; 17(7):532–4.

41. Lautz TB, Chi YY, Li M, et al. Benefit of delayed primary excision in rhabdomyosarcoma: A report from the Children's Oncology Group. Cancer 2021;127(2): 275–83.

42. Lobeck I, Dupree P, Karns R, et al. Quality assessment of lymph node sampling in rhabdomyosarcoma: A surveillance, epidemiology, and end results (SEER) program study. J Pediatr Surg 2017;52(4):614–7.

43. Routh JC, Dasgupta R, Chi YY, et al. Impact of local control and surgical lymph node evaluation in localized paratesticular rhabdomyosarcoma: A report from the Children's Oncology Group Soft-tissue Sarcoma Committee. Int J Cancer 2020;147(11):3168–76.

44. Bradley JA, Kayton ML, Chi YY, et al. Treatment Approach and Outcomes in Infants With Localized Rhabdomyosarcoma: A Report From the Soft-tissue Sarcoma Committee of the Children's Oncology Group. Int J Radiat Oncol Biol Phys 2019;103(1):19–27.

45. Million L, Anderson J, Breneman J, et al. Influence of noncompliance with radiation therapy protocol guidelines and operative bed recurrences for children with rhabdomyosarcoma and microscopic residual disease: a report from the Children's Oncology Group. Int J Radiat Oncol Biol Phys 2011;80(2):333–8.

46. Siegel RL, Miller KD, Fuchs HE, et al. Cancer Statistics, 2021. CA Cancer J Clin 2021;71(1):7–33.

47. Shern JF, Selfe J, Izquierdo E, et al. Genomic Classification and Clinical Outcome in Rhabdomyosarcoma: A Report From an International Consortium. J Clin Oncol 2021;39(26):2859–71.

48. Vaarwerk B, Mallebranche C, Affinita MC, et al. Is surveillance imaging in pediatric patients treated for localized rhabdomyosarcoma useful? The European experience. Cancer 2020;126(4):823–31.

49. Li H, Sisoudiya SD, Martin-Giacalone BA, et al. Germline Cancer Predisposition Variants in Pediatric Rhabdomyosarcoma: A Report From the Children's Oncology Group. J Natl Cancer Inst 2021;113(7):875–83.

50. Daniel CL, Kohler CL, Stratton KL, et al. Predictors of colorectal cancer surveillance among radiation-treated survivors of childhood cancer: a report from the childhood cancer survivor study. Cancer 2015;121(11):1856.

51. Heyn R, Beverly Roney R, Hays DM, et al. Late effects of therapy in patients with paratesticular rhabdomyosarcoma. Intergroup Rhabdomyosarcoma Study Committee. J Clin Oncol 1992;10(4):614–23.

52. Piver MS, Rose PG. Long-term follow-up and complications of infants with vulvovaginal embryonal rhabdomyosarcoma treated with surgery, radiation therapy, and chemotherapy. Obstet Gynecol 1988;71(3 Pt 2):435–7. Available at: https://europepmc.org/article/med/3347430. Accessed April 10, 2022.

53. Youn P, Milano MT, Constine LS, et al. Long-term cause-specific mortality in survivors of adolescent and young adult bone and soft-tissue sarcoma: A population-based study of 28,844 patients. Cancer 2014;120(15):2334–42.

54. Vaarwerk B, Hol MLF, Schoot RA, et al. AMORE treatment as salvage treatment in children and young adults with relapsed head-neck rhabdomyosarcoma. Radiother Oncol 2019;131:21–6.
55. Mattos VDA de, Ferman S, Magalhães DMA, et al. Dental and craniofacial alterations in long-term survivors of childhood head and neck rhabdomyosarcoma. Oral Surg Oral Med Oral Pathol Oral Radiol 2019;127(4):272–81.
56. Schoot RA, Hol MLF, Merks JHM, et al. Facial asymmetry in head and neck rhabdomyosarcoma survivors. Pediatr Blood Cancer 2017;64(10). https://doi.org/10.1002/PBC.26508.
57. Darbari A, Sabin KM, Shapiro CN, et al. Epidemiology of primary hepatic malignancies in U.S. children. Hepatology 2003;38(3):560–6.
58. Kremer N, Walther AE, Tiao GM. Management of hepatoblastoma: an update. Curr Opin Pediatr 2014;26(3):362–9.
59. Towbin AJ, Meyers RL, Woodley H, et al. 2017 PRETEXT: radiologic staging system for primary hepatic malignancies of childhood revised for the Paediatric Hepatic International Tumour Trial (PHITT). Pediatr Radiol 2018;48(4):536–54.
60. Huang YL, Shih SL, Liu HC, et al. Hepatoblastoma with tumor extension through the inferior vena cava into the right atrium. J Pediatr Gastroenterol Nutr 2010;50(6):577.
61. Shimizu S, Sakamoto S, Fukuda A, et al. The extracorporeal circulation with transdiaphragmatic approach in living-donor liver transplantation for HB with atrial extension of tumor thrombus: A case report. Pediatr Transpl 2021;25(7). https://doi.org/10.1111/PETR.13948.
62. Meyers R, Hiyama E, Czauderna P, et al. Liver tumors in pediatric patients. Surg Oncol Clin N Am 2021;30(2):253–74.
63. PDQ Pediatric Treatment Editorial Board. Childhood Adrenocortical Carcinoma Treatment (PDQ®): Health Professional Version. PDQ Cancer Information Summaries. 2002. Available at: http://www.ncbi.nlm.nih.gov/pubmed/31661213. Accessed April 10, 2022.
64. Caicedo LA, Sabogal A, Serrano O, et al. Hepatoblastoma: transplant versus resection experience in a latin american transplant center. Transpl Direct 2017;3(6):e165.
65. Kueht M, Thompson P, Rana A, et al. Effects of an early referral system on liver transplantation for hepatoblastoma at Texas Children's Hospital. Pediatr Transpl 2016;20(4):515–22.
66. Yang T, Whitlock RS, Vasudevan SA. Surgical management of hepatoblastoma and recent advances. Cancers (Basel) 2019;11(12). https://doi.org/10.3390/CANCERS11121944.
67. Trobaugh-Lotrario AD, López-Terrada D, Li P, et al. Hepatoblastoma in patients with molecularly proven familial adenomatous polyposis: Clinical characteristics and rationale for surveillance screening. Pediatr Blood Cancer 2018;65(8):e27103.
68. Triana Junco P, Cano EM, Dore M, et al. Prognostic Factors for Liver Transplantation in Unresectable Hepatoblastoma. Eur J Pediatr Surg 2019;29(1):28–32.
69. Cruz RJ, Ranganathan S, Mazariegos G, et al. Analysis of national and single-center incidence and survival after liver transplantation for hepatoblastoma: new trends and future opportunities. Surgery 2013;153(2):150–9.
70. Lakshminarayanan B, Hughes-Thomas AO, Grant HW. Epidemiology of adhesions in infants and children following open surgery. Semin Pediatr Surg 2014;23(6):344–8.

71. Fredriksson F, Christofferson RH, Lilja HE. Adhesive small bowel obstruction after laparotomy during infancy. Br J Surg 2016;103(3):284–9.

72. Winterberg PD, Garro R. Long-term outcomes of kidney transplantation in children. Pediatr Clin North America 2019;66(1):269–80.

73. Perez-Aytes A, Marin-Reina P, Boso V, et al. Mycophenolate mofetil embryopathy: A newly recognized teratogenic syndrome. Eur J Med Genet 2017;60(1):16–21.

74. McDonald SP, Craig JC. Long-term survival of children with end-stage renal disease. New Engl J Med 2004;350(26):2654–62.

75. Vimalesvaran S, Souza LN, Deheragoda M, et al. Outcomes of adults who received liver transplant as young children. EClinicalMedicine 2021;38:100987.

76. Miloh T, Barton A, Wheeler J, et al. Immunosuppression in pediatric liver transplant recipients: Unique aspects. Liver Transplant 2017;23(2):244–56.

77. Feng S, Bucuvalas JC, Mazariegos Gv, et al. Efficacy and safety of immunosuppression withdrawal in pediatric liver transplant recipients: moving toward personalized management. Hepatology 2021;73(5):1985–2004.

78. Lipshultz SE, Adams MJ, Colan SD, et al. Long-term cardiovascular toxicity in children, adolescents, and young adults who receive cancer therapy: pathophysiology, course, monitoring, management, prevention, and research directions: a scientific statement from the American Heart Association. Circulation 2013;128(17):1927–55.

79. Longhi A, Ferrari S, Bacci G, et al. Long-term follow-up of patients with doxorubicin-induced cardiac toxicity after chemotherapy for osteosarcoma. Anti-Cancer Drugs 2007;18(6):737–44.

80. Armenian SH, Hudson MM, Mulder RL, et al. Recommendations for cardiomyopathy surveillance for survivors of childhood cancer: A report from the International Late Effects of Childhood Cancer Guideline Harmonization Group. The Lancet Oncol 2015;16(3):e123–36.

81. Mancilla TR, Iskra B, Aune GJ. Doxorubicin-induced cardiomyopathy in children. Compr Physiol 2019;9(3):905–31.

82. Harake D, Franco VI, Henkel JM, et al. Cardiotoxicity in childhood cancer survivors: Strategies for prevention and management. Future Cardiol 2012;8(4):647–70.

83. Langholz B, Skolnik JM, Barrett JS, et al. Dactinomycin and vincristine toxicity in the treatment of childhood cancer: a retrospective study from the Children's Oncology Group. Pediatr Blood Cancer 2011;57(2):252–7.

84. DM G, P N, NE B, et al. Severe hepatic toxicity after treatment with vincristine and dactinomycin using single-dose or divided-dose schedules: a report from the National Wilms' Tumor Study. J Clin Oncol 1990;8(9):1525–30.

85. Oeffinger KC, Hudson MM. Long-term complications following childhood and adolescent cancer: foundations for providing risk-based health care for survivors. CA: A Cancer J Clinicians 2004;54(4):208–36.

86. van den Berg MH, Overbeek A, Lambalk CB, et al. Long-term effects of childhood cancer treatment on hormonal and ultrasound markers of ovarian reserve. Hum Reprod 2018;33(8):1474–88.

87. Salama M, Woodruff TK. Anticancer treatments and female fertility: clinical concerns and role of oncologists in oncofertility practice. Expert Rev Anticancer Ther 2017;17(8):687–92.

88. Al-Mahayri ZN, AlAhmad MM, Ali BR. Long-term effects of pediatric acute lymphoblastic leukemia chemotherapy: can recent findings inform old strategies? Front Oncol 2021;11. https://doi.org/10.3389/FONC.2021.710163/TEXT.

89. Mora E, Lavoie Smith EM, Donohoe C, et al. Vincristine-induced peripheral neuropathy in pediatric cancer patients. Am J Cancer Res 2016;6(11):2416–30. Available at: https://pubmed.ncbi.nlm.nih.gov/27904761/.

90. Ness KK, Jones KE, Smith WA, et al. Chemotherapy-related neuropathic symptoms and functional impairment in adult survivors of extracranial solid tumors of childhood: results from the St. Jude Lifetime Cohort Study. Arch Phys Med Rehabil 2013;94(8):1451–7.

91. Smith EML, Li L, Hutchinson RJ, et al. Measuring vincristine-induced peripheral neuropathy in children with acute lymphoblastic leukemia. Cancer Nurs 2013; 36(5). https://doi.org/10.1097/NCC.0B013E318299AD23.

92. Kandula T, Farrar MA, Cohn RJ, et al. Chemotherapy-induced peripheral neuropathy in long-term survivors of childhood cancer clinical, neurophysiological, functional, and patient-reported outcomes. JAMA Neurol 2018;75(8):980–8.

93. Shim HJ, Kim HJ, Hwang JE, et al. Long term complications and prognostic factors in locally advanced nasopharyngeal carcinoma treated with docetaxel, cisplatin, 5-fluorouracil induction chemotherapy followed by concurrent chemoradiotherapy: A retrospective cohort study. Medicine 2020;99(49):e23173.

94. Skinner R. Late renal toxicity of treatment for childhood malignancy: risk factors, long-term outcomes, and surveillance. Pediatr Nephrol 2018;33(2):215–25.

95. Altena R, de Haas EC, Nuver J, et al. Evaluation of sub-acute changes in cardiac function after cisplatin-based combination chemotherapy for testicular cancer. Br J Cancer 2009;100(12):1861–6.

96. Chovanec M, Abu Zaid M, Hanna N, et al. Long-term toxicity of cisplatin in germ-cell tumor survivors. Ann Oncol 2017;28(11):2670–9.

97. Bjerring AW, Fosså SD, Haugnes HS, et al. The cardiac impact of cisplatin-based chemotherapy in survivors of testicular cancer: a 30-year follow-up. Eur Heart J - Cardiovasc Imaging 2021;22(4):443–50.

98. Kobayashi K, Ratain MJ. Pharmacodynamics and long-term toxicity of etoposide. Cancer Chemother Pharmacol 1994;34(1 Suppl). https://doi.org/10.1007/BF00684866.

99. Weaver L, Samkari A. Neurological Complications of Childhood Cancer. Semin Pediatr Neurol 2017;24(1):60–9.

100. Gibson TM, Mostoufi-Moab S, Stratton KL, et al. Temporal patterns in the risk of chronic health conditions in survivors of childhood cancer diagnosed 1970–99: a report from the Childhood Cancer Survivor Study cohort. Lancet Oncol 2018; 19(12):1590–601.

101. Lee M, Wang Q, Wanchoo R, et al. Chronic Kidney Disease in Cancer Survivors. Adv Chronic Kidney Dis 2021;28(5):469–76.e1.

102. Hudson MM. Reproductive outcomes for survivors of childhood cancer. Obstet Gynecol 2010;116(5):1171–83.

103. Ishida Y, Maeda M, Adachi S, et al. Secondary cancer after a childhood cancer diagnosis: viewpoints considering primary cancer. Int J Clin Oncol 2018;23(6): 1178–88.

104. Wasilewski-Masker K, Kaste SC, Hudson MM, et al. Bone mineral density deficits in survivors of childhood cancer: Long-term follow-up guidelines and review of the literature. Pediatrics 2008;121(3). https://doi.org/10.1542/PEDS.2007-1396.

105. Inskip PD, Veiga LHS, Brenner Av, et al. Hypothyroidism following radiation therapy for childhood cancer: a report from the childhood cancer survivor study. Radiat Res 2018;190(2):117.

106. Sklar CA, Antal Z, Chemaitilly W, et al. Hypothalamic-pituitary and growth disorders in survivors of childhood cancer: An Endocrine Society Clinical Practice Guideline. J Clin Endocrinol Metab 2018;103(8):2761–84.

107. Lerner SE, Huang GJM, McMahon D, et al. Growth hormone therapy in children after cranial/craniospinal radiation therapy: sexually dimorphic outcomes. J Clin Endocrinol Metab 2004;89(12):6100–4.

108. Hanif I, Mahmoud H, Pui C-H. Avascular femoral head necrosis in pediatric cancer patients. Med Pediatr Oncol 1993;21(9):655–60.

109. Madadi F, Shamsian BS, Alavi S, et al. Avascular necrosis of the femoral head in children with acute lymphoblastic leukemia: A 4- to 9-year follow-up study. Orthopedics 2011;34(10). https://doi.org/10.3928/01477447-20110826-07.

110. Wong KL, Song TT, Wee J, et al. Sensorineural hearing loss after radiotherapy and chemoradiotherapy: A single, blinded, randomized study. J Clin Oncol 2006;24(12):1904–9.

111. Jussila MP, Remes T, Anttonen J, et al. Late vertebral side effects in long-term survivors of irradiated childhood brain tumor. PLoS ONE 2018;13(12). https://doi.org/10.1371/JOURNAL.PONE.0209193.

112. Arnold N, Merzenich H, Wingerter A, et al. Promotion of arterial stiffness by childhood cancer and its characteristics in adult long-term survivors. J Am Heart Assoc 2021;10(5):1–21.

113. Wright KD, Green DM, Daw NC. Late effects of treatment for wilms tumor. Pediatric hematology oncology journal 2009;26(6):407–13.

114. Wong KF, Reulen RC, Winter DL, et al. Risk of adverse health and social outcomes up to 50 years after wilms tumor: The British childhood cancer survivor study. J Clin Oncol 2016;34(15):1772–9.

115. Friedman DL, Whitton J, Leisenring W, et al. Subsequent neoplasms in 5-year survivors of childhood cancer: the childhood cancer survivor study. JNCI J Natl Cancer Inst 2010;102(14):1083.

116. Reulen RC, Frobisher C, Winter DL, et al. Long-term risks of subsequent primary neoplasms among survivors of childhood cancer. JAMA - J Am Med Assoc 2011;305(22):2311–9.

117. Daniel CL, Kohler CL, Stratton KL, et al. Predictors of colorectal cancer surveillance among survivors of childhood cancer treated with radiation: A report from the Childhood Cancer Survivor Study. Cancer 2015;121(11):1856–63.

118. Brinkman TM, Recklitis CJ, Michel G, et al. Psychological symptoms, social outcomes, socioeconomic attainment, and health behaviors among survivors of childhood cancer: Current state of the literature. J Clin Oncol 2018;36(21):2190–7.

119. Gunnes MW, Lie RT, Bjørge T, et al. Economic independence in survivors of cancer diagnosed at a young age: A Norwegian national cohort study. Cancer 2016;122(24):3873–82.

120. Crochet E, Tyc VL, Wang M, et al. Posttraumatic stress as a contributor to behavioral health outcomes and health care utilization in adult survivors of childhood cancer: a report from the Childhood Cancer Survivor Study. J Cancer Survivorship 2019;13(6):981–92.

121. Karlson CW, Alberts NM, Liu W, et al. Longitudinal pain and pain interference in long-term survivors of childhood cancer: A report from the Childhood Cancer Survivor Study. Cancer 2020;126(12):2915–23.

122. Kaye AD, Jones MR, Kaye AM, et al. Prescription opioid abuse in chronic pain: an updated review of opioid abuse predictors and strategies to curb opioid abuse (Part 2). Pain Physician 2017;20(2):S111–33.

123. Smitherman AB, Mohabir D, Wilkins TM, et al. Early Post-Therapy Prescription Drug Usage among Childhood and Adolescent Cancer Survivors. J Pediatr 2018;195:161–8.e7.

124. Charipova K, Gress KL, Urits I, et al. Management of patients with chronic pain in ambulatory surgery Centers. Cureus 2020;12(9). https://doi.org/10.7759/CUREUS.10408.

125. Zichová A, Eckschlager T, Ganevová M, et al. Subsequent neoplasms in childhood cancer survivors. Cancer Epidemiol 2020;68. https://doi.org/10.1016/j.canep.2020.101779.

126. Children's Oncology Group. Available at: http://www.survivorshipguidelines.org/. Accessed May 10, 2022.

127. Erdmann F, Frederiksen LE, Bonaventure A, et al. Childhood cancer: Survival, treatment modalities, late effects and improvements over time. Cancer Epidemiol 2021;71. https://doi.org/10.1016/j.canep.2020.101733.

128. Taylor AJ, Winter DL, Pritchard-Jones K, et al. Second primary neoplasms in survivors of Wilms' tumour - A population-based cohort study from the British Childhood Cancer Survivor Study. Int J Cancer 2008;122(9):2085–93.

Congenital Diaphragmatic Hernia
Considerations for the Adult General Surgeon

Xiao-Yue Han, BS, MD[a], Leigh Taryn Selesner, BA, MD[a],
Marilyn W. Butler, MD, MPH, MPhil[b],*

KEYWORDS

- Congenital diaphragmatic hernia • CDH • Bochdalek hernia • Morgagni hernia

KEY POINTS

- CDH is a surgical disease primarily of the newborn infant, often diagnosed prenatally on screening ultrasound and presenting at birth with acute respiratory distress with abdominal viscera in the chest on plain x-rays.
- Management involves immediate endotracheal intubation with gentle ventilation, placement of an OGT or NGT, judicious fluid resuscitation, and timely echocardiographic evaluation to assess the degree of pulmonary hypertension and diagnose any associated congenital heart anomalies.
- Pulmonary hypertension is medically optimized prior to definitive operative repair, some infants needing extracorporeal life support.
- Infants with repaired CDH often have ongoing morbidities, including chronic lung disease, neurocognitive deficits, hearing loss, gastroesophageal reflux, bowel obstruction, chest wall deformities, and vascular anomalies in the neck if they have undergone ECMO.
- Cases of previously occult CDH may present acutely in the older child or adult with nonspecific gastrointestinal or pulmonary symptoms.

The problem of congenital diaphragmatic hernia in infancy is quite different from that of diaphragmatic hernia in later life.
— *William E. Ladd, MD and Robert E. Gross, MD in 1940 case series published in The New England Journal of Medicine.*[1]

---

[a] Department of Surgery, Oregon Health and Science University, 3181 Southwest Sam Jackson Park Road, Mail Code L223, Portland, OR 97239, USA; [b] Department of Surgery, Division of Pediatric Surgery, Oregon Health and Science University, 501 North Graham Street, Suite 300, Portland, OR 97227-2008, USA
* Corresponding author.
E-mail address: butlerm@ohsu.edu

Surg Clin N Am 102 (2022) 739–757
https://doi.org/10.1016/j.suc.2022.07.007
0039-6109/22/© 2022 Elsevier Inc. All rights reserved.

surgical.theclinics.com

LEARNING OBJECTIVES
Newborns with Congenital Diaphragmatic Hernia

- Identify the signs and symptoms of an infant with congenital diaphragmatic hernia (CDH).
- Understand the initial resuscitation, evaluation, and management of an infant with CDH.
- Recognize the importance of early transfer for definitive treatment of CDH in infants.
- Be familiar with the definitive repair options for CDH.

Adults with Congenital Hiaphragmatic Hernia

- Understand the medical and surgical morbidity after CDH repair and the lifelong implications of surgical repair in infancy.
- Be familiar with the consequences of extracorporeal life support in the newborn infant.
- Recognize common surgical presentations secondary to previously occult CDH.

INTRODUCTION

Congenital diaphragmatic hernia (CDH) is a surgical disease primarily diagnosed in newborn infants, with an incidence of approximately 1/5000 births in the United States.[2] CDH is thought to arise from errors in embryologic development during the first trimester where a fault in pleuroperitoneal fold maturation leads to failed separation of the developing chest and abdomen, leading to pathologic herniation of abdominal viscera into the chest.[3] Although the anatomic findings of abdominal viscera herniated into the chest can be dramatic, resultant bilateral lung hypoplasia and pulmonary hypertension represent the greatest immediate threats to life after birth.[4] Survival in CDH infants has significantly improved with contemporary management prioritizing medical stabilization before urgent or elective operative repair, and current survival rates approach 74.2% of live births.[5,6] The presence of other structural abnormalities involving the heart, kidneys, and neural tube add significant additional physiologic burdens to the newborn infant and may complicate management.[7,8]

Most CDH defects affect the posterolateral diaphragm (Bochdalek hernias): approximately 80% are left-sided, 20% are right sided, and 2% are bilateral. Hernias range in size from small defects involving less than 10% of the diaphragm to agenesis, involving complete or near complete absence of the hemidiaphragm. Larger defects are typically associated with worse mortality and morbidity and allow for greater herniation of abdominal organs, particularly the liver.[9] Left-sided hernias commonly contain small bowel, descending colon, stomach, and spleen. Right-sided hernias almost always involve the liver and may involve small bowel and colon. In contrast, anterior parasternal diaphragm defects (Morgagni hernias) and central diaphragm defects are rare and are not commonly diagnosed in infancy.[10]

The contemporary pillars of CDH management include prenatal diagnosis for multidisciplinary care coordination and counseling, medical optimization after birth, and elective (not emergent) operative repair after stabilization, allowing for improvement in pulmonary hypertension and maturation of lungs. Lung hypoplasia and pulmonary hypertension in infants with CDH represent a *medical* emergency, not one that necessitates immediate surgery (**Box 1**).

Box 1
Principles of newborn management of patients with congenital diaphragmatic hernia

Chest X-ray to confirm diagnosis

Immediate intubation if hypoxic; avoid bag value mask ventilation

Orogastric or nasogastric tube decompression

Umbilical artery and umbilical vein placement, judicious fluid resuscitation

Gentle ventilation: Peak inspiratory pressure <24 mm Hg, PEEP <5 cm H_2O, tidal volume <5 mL/kg

Target parameters: Mean arterial pressure >50 mm Hg, $Paco_2$ <65 mm Hg, preductal SaO_2 >85%

Echocardiogram to assess pulmonary hypertension and exclude congenital heart disease diagnoses

---

NEWBORNS WITH CONGENITAL DIAPHRAGMATIC HERNIA
Newborn Presentation: Characterized by Pulmonary Hypoplasia and Pulmonary Hypertension

Newborn case presentation
You are a general surgeon in a rural community hospital called by the pediatric hospitalist to assist with the care of a term newborn infant. On arrival to the Labor and Delivery resuscitation suite, you encounter an infant in acute respiratory distress, with a physical examination notable for cyanosis, absent left-sided breath sounds, and a scaphoid abdomen. You are concerned for CDH. The hospitalist is careful not to use bag valve mask ventilation, and the anesthesiologist intubates the patient. You ask the team to place an orogastric tube (OGT) to minimize bowel dilation and further cardiopulmonary embarrassment by air-filled abdominal viscera. The patient is started on gentle ventilation with a peak inspiratory pressure less than 24 mm Hg and less than 5 mL/kg tidal volume. Umbilical vein and artery catheters are placed, and the hospitalist begins resuscitating the patient with intravenous fluids. An X-ray confirms the diagnosis of a left-sided CDH with small bowel evident in the left chest, mediastinal shift to the right, and an abnormal course of the nasogastric tube (NGT) deflected away from its typical course and instead pointing toward the left shoulder. An echocardiogram is completed, which shows severe pulmonary hypertension but no congenital heart disease, and the patient is transferred to a tertiary level center for definitive management (**Fig. 1**).

Newborn case learning points

- CDH often presents as acute respiratory distress in the newborn infant.
- Physical examination may reveal a cyanotic infant with a scaphoid abdomen and absent ipsilateral lung sounds; diagnosis is confirmed with plain films demonstrating herniation of abdominal viscera into the chest, oftentimes associated with contralateral mediastinal shift.
- Treatment is immediate endotracheal intubation in the hypoxic infant, orogastric decompression, gentle ventilation, and judicious fluid resuscitation. *Avoiding unsecured positive pressure ventilation via bag valve mask is key to minimizing bowel dilation and further cardiopulmonary embarrassment.*
- Patients should undergo expedited transfer to a tertiary care center for definitive management. Echocardiography helps assess the severity of pulmonary hypertension and evaluate for associated cardiac anomalies.

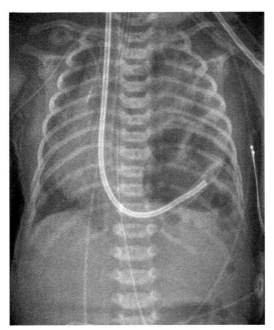

Fig. 1. Chest X-ray of a patient with left congenital diaphragmatic hernia (CDH). Chest X-ray shows air-filled loops of bowel in the left chest, mediastinal shift to the right, and OGT traversing above the left diaphragm.

Prenatal Diagnosis and Prognostication

Most cases of CDH are detected prenatally due to abnormal findings on first trimester screening ultrasound. These abnormal findings might include polyhydramnios, mediastinal shift, and inability to demonstrate the normal stomach bubble. Such abnormal findings prompt further workup with a more thorough diagnostic ultrasound, which might reveal absent bowel in the abdomen, intrathoracic herniation of the liver, spleen, stomach, or intestines, and peristalsis in the chest.

Typical measurements obtained on ultrasound include lung head ratio (LHR) or observed to expected (O/E) LHR. LHR is the ratio of the contralateral lung area to head circumference. Normal fetal LHR for the right lung ranges from 0.25 to 6.0, whereas normal fetal LHR for the left lung ranges from 0.25 to 3.5. For patients with CDH, fetal LHR less than 1.0 carries a poor prognosis, whereas LHR greater than 1.5 suggests a favorable outcome.[11]

Because the rate of lung growth exceeds that of head growth in utero, O/E LHR corrects for gestational age. Low O/E LHR ratios (ie, <15%) represent severe lung hypoplasia, whereas higher ratios (ie, >45%) represent mild lung hypoplasia. O/E LHR is an important prenatal parameter, because severity of lung hypoplasia correlates with increased mortality risk, with survival ranging from 15% to 30% for O/E LHR less than 25% to 85% to 100% for O/E LHR greater than 46%.[12,13] Findings of "liver up" is also a negative prognostic indicator, with survival dropping from 93% to 43% when liver is in the left chest.[14]

With the diagnosis of CDH made, prenatal MRI is frequently used to understand the anatomic defect, the presence and extent of abdominal visceral herniation, and a measurement of O/E total fetal lung volume, a more accurate measure of lung hypoplasia predictive of survival.[15] Considered together, these prenatal parameters assist with prognostication during family counseling and can help the multidisciplinary care team anticipate postdelivery needs, including extracorporeal membrane oxygenation (ECMO), clinical trajectory, and strategies for repair.[12] Fetuses with known CDH should be delivered at a tertiary level center because this independently improves the odds of survival.[16]

Fetal Interventions

With poor survivability for infants with CDH found to have poor prognostic indicators on prenatal testing, fetal interventions have garnered ongoing attention to alter disease natural history in utero. Animal models of CDH demonstrated that open CDH repair of a fetus through a hysterotomy improved lung hypoplasia and vascular abnormalities, which drive pulmonary hypertension.[17] Unfortunately, despite careful patient selection, early attempts at human CDH repair in utero did not improve survival, and fetal CDH repair has since been abandoned.[18]

With the lack of improved survival in fetal CDH repair, focus shifted toward minimally invasive approaches to mitigate lung hypoplasia. In animal models with CDH, tracheal occlusion via fetal endoscopic tracheal occlusion (FETO) reduced lung hypoplasia and improved survival; this was thought to be due to the retention of luminal pulmonary fluid driving pneumocyte maturation and changes of pulmonary vasculature toward normal.[19,20] An initial prospective randomized controlled trial in infants with severe left-sided CDH as defined by LHR less than 1.4 revealed no mortality or morbidity benefit with FETO; however, a subsequent randomized controlled trial from the Tracheal Occlusion to Accelerate Lung Growth (TOTAL) trial investigators evaluated the efficacy of the procedure in experienced FETO centers and found improved survival to discharge for infants with severe left-sided CDH as defined by O/E LHR less than 25%.[21,22] The efficacy seen with the more recent trial is thought to be due to improved patient selection by using more robust measures of CDH severity; in contrast, a similar trial evaluating FETO in moderate CDH as defined by an O/E LHR greater than 25% showed no benefit.[23] At present, FETO should only be performed at centers experienced with the technique, using TOTAL criteria.

Resuscitation at Birth and Stabilization

If hypoxic at birth, the newborn infant is intubated immediately *without* the use of bag valve mask ventilation. Bag valve mask ventilation may increase the dilation of the bowel resulting in cardiopulmonary embarrassment during resuscitation, difficulty with lung-protective ventilation after intubation, and problematic closure of the abdomen at repair.[24,25] An NGT or OGT tube is also inserted and placed to low wall suction to further prevent bowel distention. Umbilical vein and artery catheters are placed to enable arterial blood gas sampling, fluid resuscitation, and blood pressure support medications to maintain a mean arterial pressure greater than 50 mm Hg. The patient is placed on gentle ventilation, as described in later discussion. A chest X-ray confirms the diagnosis of CDH and assesses mediastinal shift, as well as confirms proper position of the endotracheal tube, the NGT or OGT, and lines. A transthoracic echocardiogram is obtained to assess for associated congenital heart defects and to evaluate the severity of pulmonary hypertension. A standardized approach to resuscitation and medical management with the principles of gentle ventilation and stepwise approach to management of pulmonary hypertension is thought to drive improvements in outcomes of infants with CDH.[26,27]

Gentle Ventilation

Conventional pressure-controlled ventilation with a peak inspiratory pressure less than 24 mm Hg, Positive end-expiratory pressure (PEEP) less than 5 cm H_2O, and tidal volume less than 5 mL/kg minimizes barotrauma and improves survival in infants with CDH by allowing permissive hypercapnia.[28] Preductal SaO_2 should ideally be greater than 85%, although up to 2 hours of 70% can be tolerated, as long as it is improving, urine output is adequate, and lactate is less than 3 mmol/L. $Paco_2$ of 45 to 70 mm Hg and pH 7.2 to 7.4 can be expected with gentle ventilation.[11]

For infants who require escalating ventilatory support, high-frequency oscillating ventilators (HFOV) can be used as a rescue therapy to improve oxygenation and ventilation while minimizing barotrauma. Of note, an international multicenter randomized controlled trial demonstrated that there was no survival benefit of HFOV when compared with conventional ventilation for infants with prenatally diagnosed CDH and that conventional ventilation was associated with shorter ventilator duration and less risk for needing ECMO.[29] Nonetheless, HFOV is often used for patients with persistent hypercapnia with $Paco_2$ greater than 70 mm Hg or hypoxemia with preductal O_2 saturations less than 85% despite maximizing conventional ventilation settings.[11]

Nitric Oxide

Inhaled nitric oxide (iNO), which causes pulmonary smooth muscle relaxation and dilation, has been effective in the treatment of persistent pulmonary hypertension of the newborn, and its use is widespread in patients with CDH. There is, however, no randomized trial that demonstrates decreased mortality or need for ECMO when iNO is used to treat hypoxemia in CDH, and many are now questioning its cost effectiveness.[30]

Extracorporeal Membrane Oxygenation

ECMO is a form of extracorporeal life support used in infants with CDH for which maximal medical therapy and ventilatory strategies are unable to maintain physiologic parameters compatible with ongoing survival (ie, worsening metabolic acidosis with pH < 7.2, poor oxygenation with preductal SaO_2 persistently less than 85%, hypercarbia with $Paco_2$ persistently greater than 70 mm Hg, heart failure with persistent hypotension, and inadequate tissue perfusion with lactate greater than 5 mmol/L). ECMO enables additional time for the treatment and improvement of pulmonary hypertension, while avoiding barotrauma. Although there is a paucity of large prospective randomized controlled trials for the use of ECMO in CDH, large retrospective cohort analysis of the CDH Study Group (CDHSG) consortium revealed improved survival in high-risk infants with CDH when ECMO is initiated at high-volume centers.[31]

Veno-arterial (VA) ECMO is the most common form of ECMO in infants with CDH with venous access using the right internal jugular vein and arterial access using the right carotid artery, often resulting in ligation of these vessels unless a percutaneous approach is used. Although there are many benefits to VA-ECMO—including hemodynamic support for the patient by improving forward flow of oxygenated blood—there has been increasing awareness of the neurologic complications including seizures and cerebral infarction from arterial emboli on VA-ECMO. Veno-venous (VV) ECMO using the right internal jugular vein preserves the right carotid artery and has a lower neurologic complication profile when compared with VA-ECMO. VV-ECMO, however, can be technically challenging to initiate due to size mismatch between the VV-ECMO cannula and the internal jugular vein and due to difficulties with reliably maintaining cannula position. There is no difference in survival between VA-ECMO and VV-ECMO.[32]

Timing of Congenital Diaphragmatic Hernia Repair

Much has changed since Drs Ladd and Gross published their CDH case series in 1940 advocating for early emergent surgery:

> *The policy of waiting until the child gets older and stronger is apparently responsible for the loss of a great many lives that might have been saved by a timely operation...infants in the first forty-eight hours of life stand major surgical procedures extremely well – in fact, far better than at the end of a week or ten days.*

Luckily, much more is understood about the physiology of pulmonary hypertension, and infants with CDH today benefit from the many advances in medical therapy and ventilation that have developed since the era of Drs Ladd and Gross. Priorities now are on resuscitation and stabilization at birth followed by a period of medical optimization to allow for the resolution or improvement of pulmonary hypertension and lung hypoplasia before elective repair of the diaphragmatic defect, sometimes days or weeks after birth.[1,5] Most surgeons will wait until an infant is able to be weaned off ECMO and decannulated before repairing the CDH, although some centers perform CDH repair while the patient remains on ECMO. Ethical dilemmas arise when babies cannot be weaned off ventilatory or ECMO support and are deemed to have hypoplastic lungs incompatible with life.

Techniques of Surgical Repair

Many options are available for CDH repair, depending on the stability of the patient, skillset of the surgeon, and comfort level of the anesthesiologist. Regardless of approach—chest versus abdomen, open versus minimally invasive—the key operative steps include positioning, access to the body cavity, reduction of the hernia, dissection of the diaphragmatic rim, hernia repair, and closure of the body cavity.

According to a CDHSG study of a 2014-2019 cohort of patients, an open abdominal repair is performed 81.6% of the time.[33] With this approach, the patient is placed in a supine position, and a small ipsilateral bump may be used. A subcostal or transverse incision is made approximately 1 cm below the ipsilateral costal margin, followed by careful manual reduction of bowel and any solid organs that may be involved in the hernia. Care with manual reduction of the liver and spleen is necessary to avoid injury and hemorrhage. The rim of the defect is then carefully dissected to maximize mobilization of the diaphragmatic remnant with particular attention to the posterior and medial aspects to unfurl any remnant muscular diaphragm; this increases the probability of primary repair and minimizes the size of flap or patch necessary for coverage of large defects. The hernia is then repaired with nonabsorbable sutures (often pledgeted), and the access incision closed.[34] Sutures sometimes need to be placed around the ribs when there is no posterior rim for closure. Loss of abdominal domain and dilated bowel may prevent primary closure of the abdominal fascia; skin closure alone or silo placement with secondary repair may be necessary.

For large CDH defects, a prosthetic patch, typically polytetrafluoroethylene (Gore-Tex Soft Tissue Patch, Flagstaff, AZ), may be needed for the diaphragm repair or to supplement or reinforce a repair that can only be partially approximated primarily without tension. Mesh repairs have historically been associated with higher rates of postoperative adhesive bowel obstructions and recurrences; however, some recent studies have not found a significant increase in the risk of recurrence with patch repair.[35–38] Many have abandoned using biologic mesh alone due to high rates of recurrence.[37,39]

Some surgeons use split abdominal muscle flaps to cover large defects, with such an approach associated with decreased rates of hernia recurrence when compared with the patch repair.[40] In order to use this autologous tissue flap, an ipsilateral transverse incision is performed at the level of the umbilicus or lower. After reduction of the hernia contents, the internal oblique and transversus abdominal muscles are separated from the external oblique muscle using gentle manual dissection along an avascular plane; the flap is then reflected to the diaphragmatic defect and secured.[41] Retrospective evaluations of large CDH repairs using muscle flaps have shown long-term outcomes with acceptable degrees of musculoskeletal deformities (eg, scoliosis), low rates of recurrence, and rare instances of abdominal wall hernias requiring repair.[42,43]

Interest in minimally invasive surgical (MIS) repair has been driven by findings that such an approach minimizes hospital length of stay, ventilator duration, and the risk of postoperative adhesive bowel obstruction.[44] Patient selection and surgeon experience remain key considerations for this operative approach. Infants who have been medically optimized with smaller defects seem to be preferential candidates for minimally invasive approaches; studies have found that patients undergoing MIS repair also had higher birth weights, had lower rates of ECMO utilization, used patches less frequently, and had higher rates of survival.[11] The thoracoscopic approach is more frequently used than the laparoscopic approach to CDH repair in infants due to improved visualization of the operative field through the chest and assistance of CO_2 insufflation for the reduction of the hernia contents. With the thoracoscopic approach, however, the posterior edge of the diaphragmatic defect can be difficult to fully dissect and unfurl. A Gore-Tex patch may be used for thoracoscopic repairs but some centers use a monofilament polypropylene mesh inguinal hernia repair plug (Bard PerFix Plug, C. R. Bard Inc., Franklin Lakes, NJ).[45,46] Others have found that reinforcing primary repairs with biologic mesh reduces the rate of recurrence and adhesions.[47] Minimally invasive CDH repair is associated with an increased rate of recurrence, and there is a higher rate of conversion from thoracoscopic to open repair for right-sided hernias.[44,48]

Survival

Overall survival of liveborn CDH patients is currently 74.2%, in the latest cohort of patients in a study that included 5203 patients from 23 centers during 24 years in the CDHSG registry.[33] An earlier study from the CDHSG found that mortality is highest among patients with the largest diaphragmatic defects, with a survival rate of only 58%, whereas those with the smallest defects have a survival rate of 99%. Presence of a major cardiac anomaly raises the mortality regardless of the size of defect.[49] Mortality is also significantly higher when the abdomen cannot be closed primarily, necessitating a silo or abdominal wall patch.[39]

ADULTS WITH CONGENITAL DIAPHRAGMATIC HERNIA
Long-Term Considerations for Patients with Repaired Congenital Diaphragmatic Hernia

Many infants surviving CDH repair have significant morbidities that may persist into adulthood.

Lung Hypoplasia and Obstructive Lung Disease

The pulmonary hypoplasia that is a result of CDH contributes to significantly reduced pulmonary function in survivors of CDH. Ratios of forced expiratory volume in 1 second to forced vital capacity (FEV1/FVC) reveal obstructive lung disease with more significant obstructive pathologic conditions in those with ongoing gastroesophageal reflux disease (GERD).[50] Infants with repaired CDH have life-long reductions in exercise capacity; patients with longer hospitalizations and reduced diffusion capacity at the index repair are found to have greater reductions in exercise capacity.[51] Up to 10% of CDH patients have supplemental oxygen needs for greater than 6 months, and this number increases to 25% to 75% in patients needing ECMO.[52] CDH patients are more susceptible to respiratory infections, such as respiratory syncytial viral (RSV) bronchiolitis and pneumonia, occurring in approximately 7% of patients in the first year of life.[53] Asthma or reactive airway disease is seen in school-aged children in 10% to 50% of CDH patients, with higher rates of 25% to 75% in those needing ECMO.[52]

Gastroesophageal Reflux Disease

GERD is a highly prevalent consequence of repaired CDH and thought to be due to distortion of the lower esophageal sphincter (LES), impacting 45% to 90% of infants.[53] The LES involves a physiologic interplay of the muscular fibers of the esophagus, stomach, and diaphragm crura; the relationship of the structures of the LES is distorted with diaphragmatic repair in CDH.[54] Larger CDH defects, use of patch repair, and liver herniation into the chest are predictive of GERD.[55,56] Approximately 20% of infants with repaired CDH subsequently undergo antireflux surgery, most commonly during infancy due to feeding intolerance.[56] Despite medical and surgical therapy for GERD in CDH survivors, the presence of subclinical GERD—silent reflux—may be higher than previously understood and contribute to esophageal injury and dysplasia, prompting many to recommend attentive regular screening in these patients.[53,57]

Neurocognitive Deficiencies

The prevalence of developmental delay may be higher than 30% in survivors of CDH, with a higher prevalence among infants requiring ECMO.[58] This increased prevalence may be driven by increased risk of intraventricular hemorrhage in anticoagulated ECMO patients, ligation of the carotid artery in VA-ECMO, and thromboembolic phenomena.[59] Notably, neurocognitive injuries are also prevalent in adults who undergo ECMO, with 75% of VA-ECMO adult patients demonstrating cerebral infarction, microemboli, or hemorrhage compared with 17% of VV-ECMO adult patients.[60] Further studies are needed to understand whether neonatal ECMO cannulation mode affects long-term cognition through similar mechanisms.[61]

Hearing Loss

Approximately 1% of patients with CDH experience sensorineural hearing loss but rates of hearing loss can be as high as 50% in patients undergoing ECMO.[52] Hearing aids are needed in 5% to 10% of CDH patients needing ECMO, with hearing loss often affecting speech development in these patients.[52] Patch or flap repair, prolonged ventilation, and high neonatal furosemide exposure have the highest association with hearing loss.[62]

Recurrence

CDH recurrence occurs in 10% to 12% of repairs, most commonly occurring in infancy; prolonged length of stay, liver herniation, large defect size, diaphragmatic patch repair, and use of abdominal wall prostheses followed by staged abdominal wall closure seem to be associated with a greater risk of recurrence.[63,64] CDH recurrence in adulthood is rare, with only limited case reports.[65,66] Most surgeons approach recurrences through the abdomen, either open or laparoscopically; recurrences diagnosed late might result in significant adhesions of abdominal viscera in the chest.

Bowel Obstruction

The true incidence of bowel obstruction after CDH repair is unclear, with varying rates cited in the literature confounded by nonstandardized follow-up. Despite its apparent rarity, this remains an important factor in postoperative morbidity for CDH survivors.[67] Recent meta-analysis reveals that patch repair is associated with an increased risk of small bowel obstruction when compared with primary repair (relative risk 1.9).[68] Patients presenting with bowel obstruction with a history of CDH repair should be managed similarly to other patients with bowel obstruction. Consideration should be given to possible CDH recurrence, and if a patch repair was used, the adult general surgeon should expect dense adhesions to the patch and to the diaphragm.

Failure to Thrive and Gastrostomy Tube Dependence

Newborns with CDH who have prolonged preoperative or postoperative courses often have significantly delayed initiation of oral feeds, leading to poor oromotor coordination or oral aversion. In addition, increased respiratory efforts may lead to inadequate oral intake and failure to thrive, requiring supplemental feeds via an NGT or gastrostomy tube in up to 50% of CDH patients who needed ECMO.[52] Most gastrostomy tubes will have been removed by the time a patient is seen by an adult surgeon, but if a tube has been in place for many years, a persistent gastrocutaneous fistula might necessitate surgical closure, which can be accomplished via either an open or laparoscopic approach.

Chest Wall Deformities

Approximately 5% to 20% of patients who have undergone CDH repair in the newborn period have associated chest wall deformities, most commonly pectus excavatum.[37,52] The adult surgeon should understand that these chest wall deformities rarely, if ever, carry physiologic consequences in terms of pulmonary or cardiac function. Evaluation for repair should be considered for serious cosmetic concerns. In addition, up to 20% of patients will develop scoliosis following CDH repair.[37,52]

Vascular Considerations in Patients Who Have Undergone Extracorporeal Membrane Oxygenation

The adult surgeon should understand that patients who have undergone ECMO during the newborn resuscitation for CDH have abnormal right neck vasculature. The right internal jugular vein and, frequently, the right carotid artery may have been ligated. This might pose challenges for future central venous access and should prompt vascular diagnostic investigations before any planned interventions.

Congenital Diaphragmatic Hernia Presenting in Older Children and Adults: Delayed Diagnosis

Delayed presentation case

A 33-year-old man presents to a rural community hospital emergency room with 24 hours of worsening left-sided chest pain and dyspnea. He has no known medical problems and no history of trauma. He does, however, report a 20-year history of chronic epigastric pain, typically postprandial. He reports the pain he currently has is much worse than his chronic pain and is sharp, intermittent, and radiating to his left shoulder. His pain is associated with nausea, nonbilious emesis, and obstipation. His last bowel movement was 2 days before presentation. His vital signs show a heart rate of 104, blood pressure of 115/65, respiratory rate of 22, and no fever. On examination, bowel sounds are heard over the left hemithorax, and he is mildly tender to palpation in the left upper quadrant and epigastrium; there are no signs of peritonitis. Laboratory study reveals a mild leukocytosis and normal lactate and undetectable cardiac enzymes. Electrocardiogram (ECG) reveals sinus tachycardia without any ST changes or Q waves suggestive of myocardial infarct. Chest X-ray shows an elevation of the left hemidiaphragm and what seems to be a gastric bubble in the left hemithorax. A computerized tomography (CT) scan demonstrates a 5 cm defect in the left posterior hemidiaphragm with herniated stomach. You are the on-call general surgeon consulted for this patient and take him for a diagnostic laparoscopy. During the procedure, he is found to have stomach herniating into the chest. The adhesions are carefully released, and the herniated stomach is reduced. There are no ischemic changes to the stomach. The defect is measured to be approximately 5 × 6 cm in the posterolateral position. The defect area is covered with a 10 × 8 cm Gore-Tex patch and fixed with a laparoscopic fixation device. The patient recovers uneventfully on the floor and is discharged on postoperative day 5.

Delayed presentation learning points

- Adults with CDH may be asymptomatic or present with vague abdominal and pulmonary complains. Occasionally, a patient will present with a surgical emergency, such as a gastric volvulus or obstruction.
- The workup includes plain X-rays and a CT scan if the diagnosis is still uncertain.
- Minimally invasive approaches to repair can be attempted with minimal morbidity in the setting of hemodynamic stability. In general, most cases should be repaired before serious complications occur.

Presentation

Delayed presentation of CDH in adulthood is rare because the defect often has significant morbidity and mortality in infancy and is therefore detected shortly after birth, if not detected prenatally.[69] The reported prevalence of Bochdalek hernias in adults ranges from 0.17% to 12.5%, most of these involving the left hemidiaphragm.[70,71] Only a small number of case reports, case series, and systemic review articles of adult CDH are available in the literature. No cohort or randomized control studies regarding diagnosis or repair exist.

CDH in adults may either be diagnosed incidentally or with a range of symptoms. Due to the rarity of this condition in adults, misdiagnosis can easily occur, resulting in serious consequences for the patient. Concern for a hernia should be raised in a patient with vague abdominal complaints, such as pain, discomfort, and emesis, as well as pulmonary symptoms, such as dyspnea and cough. Symptoms may be sporadic, as herniated viscera may intermittently reduce. CDH can also present as a surgical emergency in the setting of bowel incarceration or strangulation.[72]

In a systemic review of 180 articles from 1955 to 2015, a total of 368 adults with Bochdalek hernias were identified. The most common symptoms were abdominal pain and discomfort (63%). This was followed by pulmonary symptoms of cough, chest pain, wheezing, and pneumonia (40%). Other symptoms observed were signs of bowel obstruction (36%) and strangulation (26%). Finally, 14.5% of cases were asymptomatic.[73] A review of 13,000 abdominal CT scans at one institution over a single year detected Bochdalek hernia in 0.17% of patients, none of which were symptomatic.[74]

Morgagni hernias are uncommon for any age group, comprising only 2% to 5% of all congenital diaphragmatic hernias; most defects involve the right hemidiaphragm.[69] Despite the congenital cause, Morgagni hernias commonly present beyond the neonatal years because these patients may be asymptomatic or have only nonspecific symptoms.

In terms of Morgagni hernias, a 2021 systemic review incorporating 189 studies and 310 patients found that patients predominantly presented with pulmonary symptoms (44.8%) followed by abdominal pain (39.7%), nausea and/or vomiting (30%), cardiac symptoms (6.8%), dysphagia (6.1%), and obstructive symptoms (7.4%). About 10.3% were found to be asymptomatic.[75]

Diagnostic Imaging

The diagnosis of CDH in the adult is made using various imaging modalities. Plain X-rays of the chest may show partial or complete opacification of a hemithorax, as well as deviation of the mediastinum; however, neither finding is specific. The finding of air-filled bowel in the chest is highly suggestive of a diaphragmatic defect, although eventration must also be considered, particularly following procedures where the phrenic nerve may have been injured. One shortcoming of chest X-rays is the potential for a false-negative result in the setting of intermittent reduction of hernia contents.[73]

Further imaging studies beyond plain films are sometimes obtained to confirm the diagnosis of a diaphragmatic hernia, as well as to clarify the location and extent of the defect. Computed tomography of the chest may be used to distinguish from other pathologic conditions, define the anatomic location of the defect, and help surgeons determine the most appropriate approach for repair. Other diagnostic tests, including esophagogastroduodenoscopy, ultrasound, and manometry, are less frequently used.[76] Because of the known association of malrotation with CDH, some recommend upper gastrointestinal contrast evaluation before surgical intervention. The presence of malrotation would warrant an abdominal approach, in order to perform a Ladd procedure at the time of hernia repair.[74]

Surgical Repair

Although well-studied in the pediatric population, less is found in the literature about indications and timing of surgery for CDH in adults. Consensus based on several different case series is that repair of CDH should be performed in both symptomatic and asymptomatic patients who are fit for surgery.[77–81] Patients with unrepaired CDH risk incarceration, which would require emergent operation, carrying significant morbidity and mortality.

In brief, surgical repair includes the reduction of intrathoracic contents, resection of the hernia sac (if present), and repair of the diaphragmatic defect. Unlike the pediatric population, some degree of adhesiolysis may need to be performed, and bowel resection may be needed in extreme cases. In almost all Morgagni hernias, the abdominal contents are encased within a peritoneal sac;however, hernia sacs are only occasionally present in Bochdalek hernias, with an incidence of 10% to 15% in one study.[82] When a sac is present, minimal adhesions exist between pleural and abdominal contents. If not resected, the sac may persist in the thorax and lead to seroma formation or recurrent hernia. Removal of the sac, however, is not always possible, particularly when it is fused to the pleura or the pericardium, and some surgeons prefer to leave all sacs in place, to avoid the risk of injury.[83]

The next step in the operation is to repair the diaphragmatic defect. The principle of a tension-free repair applies. Small defects can be repaired primarily with heavy braided nonabsorbable sutures. There are no data to suggest the superiority of running versus interrupted sutures.[84] A larger hernia may require a prosthetic patch to achieve a tension-free repair. There is controversy on what sizes of diaphragmatic hernia require patch repair. Many types of patches are available, including polypropylene, Gore-Tex, and biological grafts, and evidence is lacking regarding which patch material is best.[85] Polypropylene allows for indefinite support and tissue in-growth; however, there is a risk for erosion into bowel and enteric fistulae. Gore-Tex has a decreased risk for adhesions to viscera and is, therefore, generally the preferred synthetic patch.[73] Biologic patch overlays are helpful in reinforcing a primary repair and in protecting polypropylene from adhesions to bowel but using it alone to repair a defect carries a higher risk of recurrence.[47] Patches can be secured using sutures or with mechanical fixation devices. No studies exist reviewing the use of muscle flaps for repair of adult congenital diaphragmatic hernias.

The approach chosen for repair depends on the clinical presentation, as well as the size and laterality of the defect. In the setting of emergent presentation, laparotomy or posterolateral thoracotomy is the technique of choice. Midline, subcostal, or thoracoabdominal laparotomy incisions may be used.[74,86] Laparotomy has the advantage of being able to inspect herniated contents after reduction and perform a Ladd procedure if malrotation is present. Alternatively, thoracotomy is better for lysing adhesions between the pleura and herniated contents, as might be expected in longstanding CDH.

With the advent and improvements in minimally invasive techniques, the laparoscopic and thoracoscopic approaches to repairing CDH have become more prevalent. This is especially seen with elective repairs but may also be considered in more urgent cases. One benefit of laparoscopic repair is improved visualization of the diaphragmatic defect with an angled laparoscope. Studies have found that laparoscopic repair also results in improved clinical outcomes, including shorter lengths of stay.[83–87] The advantages of thoracoscopy mirror that of a thoracotomy, allowing lysis of adhesions between the pleura and the sac or abdominal contents. In addition, repair of right-sided defects is facilitated by thoracoscopy because the liver is not obscuring the view.[87] Given the lack of high-powered studies and randomized controlled trials, the decision to perform a minimally invasive versus open approach, or even an abdominal versus thoracic approach is at the individual surgeon's discretion, often based on the stability of the patient and the specific surgeon's skills and experience.

SUMMARY

CDH is a surgical disease primarily of the newborn infant. Most cases are diagnosed prenatally using screening ultrasound, enabling timely multidisciplinary consultation and planning at a tertiary care center. A minority of cases are diagnosed in the newborn period when infants with acute respiratory distress are found to have abdominal viscera in the chest on plain X-rays. For newborn infants, management involves immediate endotracheal intubation with gentle ventilation, placement of an OGT or NGT, judicious fluid resuscitation, and timely echocardiographic evaluation to assess the degree of pulmonary hypertension and to diagnose any associated congenital heart anomalies. Pulmonary hypertension is medically optimized before definitive operative repair. Some infants may need extracorporeal life support in cases of severe pulmonary hypertension or lung hypoplasia. Infants with large defects or hemidiaphragm agenesis may require prosthetic patches or abdominal wall muscle flap repair. Infants with repaired CDH often have ongoing morbidities, including chronic lung disease, neurocognitive deficits, hearing loss, gastroesophageal reflux, bowel obstruction, chest wall deformities, and vascular anomalies in the neck if they have undergone ECMO. Cases of previously occult CDH may present acutely in the older child or adult with gastrointestinal or pulmonary symptoms. The adult general surgeon must be able to recognize infants with CDH, help direct initial resuscitation and transfer to a higher level of care, be familiar with repair principles of CDH diagnosed in older children and adults, and understand the comorbidities and surgical implications of CDH patients who survive into adulthood.

CLINICS CARE POINTS

- In the cyanotic newborn with acute respiratory distress suspected to have CDH, secure the airway with an endotracheal tube before ventilation; noninvasive positive pressure ventilation may further distend bowel and worsen cardiopulmonary physiology. Confirm the diagnosis of CDH with a chest X-ray.

- Lung hypoplasia and pulmonary hypertension are the immediate threats to life in a newborn with CDH. Order a transthoracic echocardiogram to evaluate for the severity of pulmonary hypertension and to assess for the presence of congenital cardiac anomalies that may affect care. Support the patient with gentle ventilation, with ECMO if needed, and allow time for physiologic improvement before elective CDH repair.

- In adult survivors of CDH presenting with surgical pathologic conditions (ie, bowel obstruction, chest wall deformities, abdominal wall hernias, and recurrent CDH), a history that targets the patient's CDH course (ie, ECMO utilization, autologous muscle flaps, synthetic patches, need for fundoplication and/or gastrostomy tube, and associated cardiac abnormalities) and focused physical examination evaluating for the location and orientation of scars in the neck, chest, and abdomen are critical to understanding how CDH affects the current presentation and management. ECMO patients may have a ligated right internal jugular vein and/or right carotid artery, autologous muscle flaps may contribute to disrupted abdominal wall tissue planes, and synthetic patches increase the likelihood of dense adhesions.

DISCLOSURE

None of the authors has commercial or financial conflicts of interest; none has external funding.

REFERENCES

1. Ladd WE, Gross RE. Congenital diaphragmatic hernia. N Engl J Med 1940; 223(23):917–25.
2. Balayla J, Abenhaim HA. Incidence, predictors and outcomes of congenital diaphragmatic hernia: a population-based study of 32 million births in the United States. J Matern Fetal Neonatal Med 2014;27(14):1438–44.
3. Edel GG, Schaaf G, Wijnen RMH, et al. Cellular origin(s) of congenital diaphragmatic hernia. Front Pediatr 2021;9:804496.
4. Pierro M, Thebaud B. Understanding and treating pulmonary hypertension in congenital diaphragmatic hernia. Semin Fetal Neonatal Med 2014;19(6):357–63.
5. Boloker J, Bateman DA, Wung JT, et al. Congenital diaphragmatic hernia in 120 infants treated consecutively with permissive hypercapnea/spontaneous respiration/elective repair. J Pediatr Surg 2002;37(3):357–66. https://doi.org/10.1053/jpsu.2002.30834.
6. Gupta VS, Harting MT, Lally PA, et al. Mortality in Congenital Diaphragmatic Hernia: A Multicenter Registry Study of Over 5000 Patients Over 25 Years. Ann Surg 2021. https://doi.org/10.1097/SLA.0000000000005113.
7. Graziano JN, Congenital Diaphragmatic Hernia Study G. Cardiac anomalies in patients with congenital diaphragmatic hernia and their prognosis: a report from the Congenital Diaphragmatic Hernia Study Group. J Pediatr Surg 2005;40(6): 1045–9. https://doi.org/10.1016/j.jpedsurg.2005.03.025 ; discussion 1049-50.

8. Bojanic K, Pritisanac E, Luetic T, et al. Malformations associated with congenital diaphragmatic hernia: Impact on survival. J Pediatr Surg 2015;50(11):1817–22. https://doi.org/10.1016/j.jpedsurg.2015.07.004.
9. Congenital Diaphragmatic Hernia Study G, Lally KP, Lally PA, et al. Defect size determines survival in infants with congenital diaphragmatic hernia. Pediatrics 2007;120(3):e651–7. https://doi.org/10.1542/peds.2006-3040.
10. Cunniff C, Jones KL, Jones MC. Patterns of malformation in children with congenital diaphragmatic defects. J Pediatr 1990;116(2):258–61. https://doi.org/10.1016/s0022-3476(05)82884-7.
11. Gupta V, Lally K, Berman L, et al. Congenital diaphragmatic hernia. In: Pediatric Surgery NaT. American Pediatric Surgical Association; 2020. https://www.pedsurglibrary.com/apsa/view/Pediatric-Surgery-NaT/829001/all/About_the_Pediatric_Surgery_NaT.
12. Cordier AG, Russo FM, Deprest J, et al. Prenatal diagnosis, imaging, and prognosis in Congenital Diaphragmatic Hernia. Semin Perinatol Feb 2020;44(1):51163.
13. Jani J, Nicolaides K, Keller R, et al. Observed to expected lung area to head circumference ratio in the prediction of survival in fetuses with isolated diaphragmatic hernia. Ultrasound Obstet Gynecol 2007;30(1):67–71.
14. Albanese CT, Lopoo J, Goldstein RB, et al. Fetal liver position and perinatal outcome for congenital diaphragmatic hernia. Prenat Diagn 1998;18(11):1138–42 (199811)18:11<1138::aid-pd416>3.0.co;2-a.
15. Cannie M, Jani J, Meersschaert J, et al. Prenatal prediction of survival in isolated diaphragmatic hernia using observed to expected total fetal lung volume determined by magnetic resonance imaging based on either gestational age or fetal body volume. Ultrasound Obstet Gynecol 2008;32(5):633–9. https://doi.org/10.1002/uog.6139.
16. Nasr A, Langer JC, Canadian Pediatric Surgery N. Influence of location of delivery on outcome in neonates with congenital diaphragmatic hernia. J Pediatr Surg 2011;46(5):814–6. https://doi.org/10.1016/j.jpedsurg.2011.02.007.
17. Adzick NS, Outwater KM, Harrison MR, et al. Correction of congenital diaphragmatic hernia in utero. IV. An early gestational fetal lamb model for pulmonary vascular morphometric analysis. J Pediatr Surg 1985;20(6):673–80.
18. Harrison MR, Langer JC, Adzick NS, et al. Correction of congenital diaphragmatic hernia in utero, V. Initial clinical experience. J Pediatr Surg 1990;25(1):47–55 ; discussion 56-7.
19. Luks FI, Wild YK, Piasecki GJ, et al. Short-term tracheal occlusion corrects pulmonary vascular anomalies in the fetal lamb with diaphragmatic hernia. Surgery 2000;128(2):266–72.
20. Flageole H, Evrard VA, Piedboeuf B, et al. The plug-unplug sequence: an important step to achieve type II pneumocyte maturation in the fetal lamb model. J Pediatr Surg 1998;33(2):299–303.
21. Harrison MR, Keller RL, Hawgood SB, et al. A randomized trial of fetal endoscopic tracheal occlusion for severe fetal congenital diaphragmatic hernia. N Engl J Med 2003;349(20):1916–24.
22. Deprest JA, Nicolaides KH, Benachi A, et al. Randomized trial of fetal surgery for severe left diaphragmatic hernia. N Engl J Med 2021;385(2):107–18.
23. Deprest JA, Benachi A, Gratacos E, et al. Randomized trial of fetal surgery for moderate left diaphragmatic hernia. N Engl J Med 2021;385(2):119–29.
24. Maxwell D, Baird R, Puligandla P. Abdominal wall closure in neonates after congenital diaphragmatic hernia repair. J Pediatr Surg 2013;48(5):930–4.

25. Canadian Congenital Diaphragmatic Hernia C, Puligandla PS, Skarsgard ED, et al. Diagnosis and management of congenital diaphragmatic hernia: a clinical practice guideline. CMAJ. Jan 29 2018;190(4):E103-E112. doi:10.1503/cmaj.170206

26. Reiss I, Schaible T, van den Hout L, et al. Standardized postnatal management of infants with congenital diaphragmatic hernia in Europe: the CDH EURO Consortium consensus. Neonatology 2010;98(4):354–64. https://doi.org/10.1159/000320622.

27. Tracy ET, Mears SE, Smith PB, et al. Protocolized approach to the management of congenital diaphragmatic hernia: benefits of reducing variability in care. J Pediatr Surg Jun 2010;45(6):1343–8. https://doi.org/10.1016/j.jpedsurg.2010.02.104.

28. Garcia A, Stolar CJ. Congenital diaphragmatic hernia and protective ventilation strategies in pediatric surgery. Surg Clin North Am 2012;92(3):659–668, ix. https://doi.org/10.1016/j.suc.2012.03.003.

29. Snoek KG, Capolupo I, van Rosmalen J, et al. Conventional Mechanical Ventilation Versus High-frequency Oscillatory Ventilation for Congenital Diaphragmatic Hernia: A Randomized Clinical Trial (The VICI-trial). Ann Surg 2016;263(5):867–74. https://doi.org/10.1097/SLA.0000000000001533.

30. Campbell BT, Herbst KW, Briden KE, et al. Inhaled nitric oxide use in neonates with congenital diaphragmatic hernia. Pediatrics 2014;134(2):e420–6. https://doi.org/10.1542/peds.2013-2644.

31. Jancelewicz T, Langham MR, Brindle ME, et al. Survival benefit associated with the use of extracorporeal life support for neonates with congenital diaphragmatic hernia. Ann Surg 2022;275(1):e256–63.

32. Guner YS, Harting MT, Fairbairn K, et al. Outcomes of infants with congenital diaphragmatic hernia treated with venovenous versus venoarterial extracorporeal membrane oxygenation: A propensity score approach. J Pediatr Surg 2018;53(11):2092–9. https://doi.org/10.1016/j.jpedsurg.2018.06.003.

33. Gupta VS, Harting MT, Lally PA, et al. Mortality in congenital diaphragmatic hernia: a multicenter registry study of over 5000 patients over 25 years. Ann Surg 2021. https://doi.org/10.1097/sla.0000000000005113.

34. Zani A, Zani-Ruttenstock E, Pierro A. Advances in the surgical approach to congenital diaphragmatic hernia. Semin Fetal Neonatal Med 2014;19(6):364–9.

35. Fisher J, Haley M, Ruiz-Elizalde A, et al. Multivariate model for predicting recurrence in congenital diaphragmatic hernia. J Pediatr Surg 2009;44:1173–80.

36. Tsai J, Sulkowski J, Adzick NS, et al. Patch repair for congenital diaphragmatic hernia: is it really a problem? J Pediatr Surg 2012;47(4):637–41.

37. Jancelewicz T, Vu L, Keller R, et al. Long-term surgical outcomes in congenital diaphragmatic hernia: observations from a single institution. J Pediatr Surg 2010;45:155–60.

38. Moss RL, Chen CM, Harrison MR. Prosthetic patch durability in congenital diaphragmatic hernia: A long-term follow-up study. J Pediatr Surg 2001;36(1):152–4.

39. Jawaid W, Qasem E, Jones M, et al. Outcomes following prosthetic patch repair in newborns with congenital diaphragmatic hernia. The Br J Surg 2013;100:1833–7.

40. Barnhart DC, Jacques E, Scaife ER, et al. Split abdominal wall muscle flap repair vs patch repair of large congenital diaphragmatic hernias. J Pediatr Surg 2012;47(1):81–6.

41. Scaife ER, Johnson DG, Meyers RL, et al. The split abdominal wall muscle flap–a simple, mesh-free approach to repair large diaphragmatic hernia. J Pediatr Surg 2003;38(12):1748–51.

42. Molino JA, Garcia Martinez L, Guillen Burrieza G, et al. Outcomes after split abdominal wall muscle flap repair for large congenital diaphragmatic hernias. Eur J Pediatr Surg 2020;30(2):210–4.

43. Nasr A, Struijs M-C, Ein S, et al. Outcomes after muscle flap vs prosthetic patch repair for large congenital diaphragmatic hernias. J Pediatr Surg 2010;45:151–4.

44. Putnam LR, Tsao K, Lally KP, et al. Minimally invasive vs open congenital diaphragmatic hernia repair: is there a superior approach? J Am Coll Surg 2017; 224(4):416–22.

45. Saltzman DA, Ennis JS, Mehall JR, et al. Recurrent congenital diaphragmatic hernia: A novel repair. J Pediatr Surg 2001;36(12):1768–9.

46. Cho S, Krishnaswami S, McKee J, et al. Analysis of 29 consecutive thoracoscopic repairs of congenital diaphragmatic hernia in neonates compared to historical controls. J Pediatr Surg 2009;44(1):80–6.

47. Vandewalle R, Yalcin S, Clifton M, et al. Biologic mesh underlay in thoracoscopic primary repair of congenital diaphragmatic hernia confers reduced recurrence in neonates: a preliminary report. J Laparoendosc Adv Surg Tech 2019;29(10): 1212–5.

48. Putnam LR, Gupta V, Tsao K, et al. Factors associated with early recurrence after congenital diaphragmatic hernia repair. J Pediatr Surg 2017;52(6):928–32.

49. Harting M, Lally K. The Congenital Diaphragmatic Hernia Study Group registry update. Semin Fetal Neonatal Med 2014;19(6):370–5.

50. Peetsold MG, Heij HA, Nagelkerke AF, et al. Pulmonary function and exercise capacity in survivors of congenital diaphragmatic hernia. Eur Respir J 2009;34(5): 1140–7.

51. Toussaint-Duyster LCC, van der Cammen-van Zijp MHM, de Jongste JC, et al. Congenital diaphragmatic hernia and exercise capacity, a longitudinal evaluation. Pediatr Pulmonol 2019;54(5):628–36.

52. Berman L, Jackson J, Miller K, et al. Expert surgical consensus for prenatal counseling using the Delphi method. J Pediatr Surg 2017;53(8):1592–9.

53. American Academy of Pediatrics Section on S, American Academy of Pediatrics Committee on F, Newborn Lally KP, Engle W. Postdischarge follow-up of infants with congenital diaphragmatic hernia. Pediatrics 2008;121(3):627–32.

54. Peetsold MG, Kneepkens CM, Heij HA, et al. Congenital diaphragmatic hernia: long-term risk of gastroesophageal reflux disease. J Pediatr Gastroenterol Nutr 2010;51(4):448–53.

55. Sigalet DL, Nguyen LT, Adolph V, et al. Gastroesophageal reflux associated with large diaphragmatic hernias. J Pediatr Surg 1994;29(9):1262–5.

56. Verbelen T, Lerut T, Coosemans W, et al. Antireflux surgery after congenital diaphragmatic hernia repair: a plea for a tailored approach. Eur J Cardiothorac Surg 2013;44(2):263–7 ; discussion 268.

57. Morandi A, Macchini F, Zanini A, et al. Endoscopic Surveillance for Congenital Diaphragmatic Hernia: Unexpected Prevalence of Silent Esophagitis. Eur J Pediatr Surg 2016;26(3):291–5. https://doi.org/10.1055/s-0035-1552568.

58. Nobuhara KK, Lund DP, Mitchell J, et al. Long-term outlook for survivors of congenital diaphragmatic hernia. Clin Perinatol 1996;23(4):873–87.

59. D'Agostino JA, Bernbaum JC, Gerdes M, et al. Outcome for infants with congenital diaphragmatic hernia requiring extracorporeal membrane oxygenation: the first year. J Pediatr Surg 1995;30(1):10–5. https://doi.org/10.1016/0022-3468(95)90598-7.

60. Risnes I, Wagner K, Nome T, et al. Cerebral outcome in adult patients treated with extracorporeal membrane oxygenation. Ann Thorac Surg 2006;81(4):1401–6. https://doi.org/10.1016/j.athoracsur.2005.10.008.

61. Guner YS, Khemani RG, Qureshi FG, et al. Outcome analysis of neonates with congenital diaphragmatic hernia treated with venovenous vs venoarterial extracorporeal membrane oxygenation. J Pediatr Surg 2009;44(9):1691–701. https://doi.org/10.1016/j.jpedsurg.2009.01.017.

62. Amoils M, Crisham Janik M, Lustig LR. Patterns and predictors of sensorineural hearing loss in children with congenital diaphragmatic hernia. JAMA Otolaryngol Head Neck Surg 2015;141(10):923–6. https://doi.org/10.1001/jamaoto.2015.1670.

63. Fisher JC, Haley MJ, Ruiz-Elizalde A, et al. Multivariate model for predicting recurrence in congenital diaphragmatic hernia. J Pediatr Surg 2009;44(6):1173–9. https://doi.org/10.1016/j.jpedsurg.2009.02.043 ; discussion 1179-80.

64. Nagata K, Usui N, Terui K, et al. Risk factors for the recurrence of the congenital diaphragmatic hernia-report from the long-term follow-up study of Japanese CDH study group. Eur J Pediatr Surg 2015;25(1):9–14. https://doi.org/10.1055/s-0034-1395486.

65. Horiguchi K, Lee SW, Shimizu T, et al. Recurrence of a congenital diaphragmatic hernia 57 years postoperatively: a case report and review of the literature. Medicine (Baltimore) 2022;101(3):e28650. https://doi.org/10.1097/MD.0000000000028650.

66. Spoel M, Vlot J, van de Ven KP, et al. Recurrent diaphragmatic hernia in two young adults: Lung function before and after repair. The Air that we Breathe: Respiratory Morbidity in Children with Congenital Pulmonary Malformations 2012;119. https://pure.eur.nl/en/publications/4225d1a8-4c4b-457d-8e1d-800368e23855.

67. Sivarajah V, Bhatnagar P, Tom KN, et al. Late complication of congenital diaphragmatic hernia repair: recurrent small bowel obstruction. Pediatr Emerg Care 2022;38(2):e1028–9.

68. Heiwegen K, de Blaauw I, Botden S. A systematic review and meta-analysis of surgical morbidity of primary versus patch repaired congenital diaphragmatic hernia patients. Sci Rep 2021;11(1):12661.

69. Nasr A, Fecteau A. Foramen of Morgagni hernia: presentation and treatment. Thorac Surg Clin 2009;19(4):463–8. https://doi.org/10.1016/j.thorsurg.2009.08.010.

70. Brown SR, Horton JD, Trivette E, et al. Bochdalek hernia in the adult: demographics, presentation, and surgical management. Hernia 2011;15(1):23–30. https://doi.org/10.1007/s10029-010-0699-3.

71. Kinoshita F, Ishiyama M, Honda S, et al. Late-presenting posterior transdiaphragmatic (Bochdalek) hernia in adults: prevalence and MDCT characteristics. J Thorac Imaging 2009;24(1):17–22. https://doi.org/10.1097/RTI.0b013e31818c6bc8.

72. Millington TM. Congenital diaphragmatic hernias in adults: management of bochdalek and morgagni hernias. In: Sugarbaker DJ, Bueno R, Burt BM, et al, editors. Sugarbaker's adult chest surgery, 3e. New York: McGraw-Hill Education; 2020. p. 1357–60.

73. Machado NO. Laparoscopic repair of bochdalek diaphragmatic hernia in adults. N Am J Med Sci 2016;8(2):65–74.

74. Thomas S, Kapur B. Adult Bochdalek hernia–clinical features, management and results of treatment. Jpn J Surg 1991;21(1):114–9.

75. Katsaros I, Katelani S, Giannopoulos S, et al. Management of morgagni's hernia in the adult population: a systematic review of the literature. World J Surg 2021; 45(10):3065–72.
76. Perrone G, Giuffrida M, Annicchiarico A, et al. Complicated diaphragmatic hernia in emergency surgery: systematic review of the literature. World J Surg 2020; 44(12):4012–31.
77. Kocakusak A, Arikan S, Senturk O, et al. Bochdalek's hernia in an adult with colon necrosis. Hernia 2005;9(3):284–7.
78. Palanivelu C, Rangarajan M, Senthilkumaran S, et al. Safety and efficacy of laparoscopic surgery in pregnancy: experience of a single institution. J Laparoendosc Adv Surg Tech A 2007;17(2):186–90.
79. Gedik E, Tuncer MC, Onat S, et al. A review of Morgagni and Bochdalek hernias in adults. Folia Morphol (Warsz) 2011;70(1):5–12.
80. Slesser AA, Ribbans H, Blunt D, et al. A spontaneous adult right-sided Bochdalek hernia containing perforated colon. JRSM Short Rep 2011;2(7):54.
81. Islah MA, Jiffre D. A rare case of incarcerated bochdalek diaphragmatic hernia in a pregnant lady. Med J Malaysia 2010;65(1):75–6.
82. Liem NT. Thoracoscopic surgery for congenital diaphragmatic hernia: a report of nine cases. Asian J Surg 2003;26(4):210–2.
83. Hamid KS, Rai SS, Rodriguez JA. Symptomatic Bochdalek hernia in an adult. JSLS 2010;14(2):279–81.
84. Thoman DS, Hui T, Phillips EH. Laparoscopic diaphragmatic hernia repair. Surg Endosc 2002;16(9):1345–9.
85. Palanivelu C, Rangarajan M, Rajapandian S, et al. Laparoscopic repair of adult diaphragmatic hernias and eventration with primary sutured closure and prosthetic reinforcement: a retrospective study. Surg Endosc 2009;23(5):978–85.
86. Wadhwa A, Surendra JB, Sharma A, et al. Laparoscopic repair of diaphragmatic hernias: experience of six cases. Asian J Surg 2005;28(2):145–50.
87. Nakashima S, Watanabe A, Hashimoto M, et al. Advantages of video-assisted thoracoscopic surgery for adult congenital hernia with severe adhesion: report of two cases. Ann Thorac Cardiovasc Surg 2011;17(2):185–9.

Esophageal Atresia and Tracheoesophageal Fistula
Overview and Considerations for the General Surgeon

Ryan M. Walk, MD

KEYWORDS

- Esophageal atresia • Tracheoesophageal fistula • Complications
- Respiratory compromise • Gastroesophageal reflux • Long-term outcomes

KEY POINTS

- This condition is rarely definitively diagnosed in the prenatal period, but may be suspected based on a small stomach bubble with polyhydramnios on ultrasound.
- Infants with distal fistulas are at risk for the development of respiratory insufficiency or failure.
- If a respiratory emergency develops, ligation or occlusion of the tracheoesophageal fistula (TEF) will be required.
- Gastroesophageal reflux and dysphagia are exceptionally common in postoperative survivors, and these conditions may worsen with time rather than improve.
- The evaluation of postoperative issues should proceed in a stepwise fashion, and special consideration must be given to ruling out associated congenital anomalies.

INTRODUCTION

The evaluation and management of an infant with esophageal atresia (EA) and tracheoesophageal fistula (TEF) are one of the most challenging but rewarding scenarios in Pediatric Surgery. The condition is relatively common and only rarely conclusively identified during prenatal care. Therefore, General Surgeons may encounter afflicted neonates, particularly those practicing in rural or austere environments. Moreover, these patients are surviving into adulthood, even late adulthood, with increasing frequency. Therefore, the General Surgeon can expect to encounter patients with late sequelae of the disorder. Here, an overview of the condition and its treatment are provided, with special consideration given to scenarios that the nonsubspecialty surgeon may be expected to temporize or manage.

Uniformed Services University of the Health Sciences, Walter Reed National Military Medical Center, 4901 Jones Bridge Road, Bethesda, MD 20814, USA
E-mail address: ryan.walk@usuhs.edu

Surg Clin N Am 102 (2022) 759–778
https://doi.org/10.1016/j.suc.2022.07.008
0039-6109/22/Published by Elsevier Inc.

surgical.theclinics.com

HISTORY

Esophageal atresia (EA) was first recorded in 1670 by Durston, who documented the presence of an upper esophageal pouch in a female thoracopagus conjoined twin.[1] In 1697, Thomas Gibson provided the first detailed account of the classic blind-ending upper pouch in combination with a distal TEF. He described an infant who experienced choking fits with attempts at feeding and died at 3 days old. He provided a detailed description of the anomaly on postmortem examination.[1,2]

Owing largely to the surgical inaccessibility of a neonate's chest, the condition remained universally fatal until well into the twentieth century. In 1939, Ladd in Boston and Levin in St. Paul simultaneously and independently described the first long-term survivors of the condition.[2] Both surgeons described staged repairs, with initial extrapleural ligation of the TEF followed by the creation of a gastrostomy. The upper pouch was exteriorized through a proximal esophagostomy. Continuity was eventually restored through the creation of an extra-thoracic skin-lined tube on the anterior chest, connecting the esophagostomy with the gastrostomy.[2]

This staged approach to the anomaly proved short-lived. In March 1941, Cameron Haight of Ann Arbor, Michigan performed the first successful primary repair of an EA-TEF in an unusually robust 12-day-old infant female. He approached the anomaly through a left para-vertebral incision and completed an extra-pleural primary anastomosis. While the consequent postoperative course was less than straightforward, the child survived and is reported to have been the last patient he saw before his death in 1970.[2] By the end of the twentieth century, infants with this once-fatal condition born both larger than 2.5 kg and without additional congenital defects had a nearly 100% survival.[2]

EPIDEMIOLOGY

The spectrum of EA-TEF disorders is relatively common, occurring in roughly one in 2500 to 3500 infants.[1,3] There does not seem to be any geographic variation in frequency.[3] The anatomic variants are typically grouped as illustrated in **Fig. 1.**[4] Of these, proximal EA with a distal TEF is by far the most common, comprising more than 80% of cases.[3] More unusual variants. or variants in combination with other congenital esophageal defects, have been described.[5]

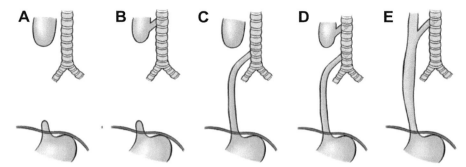

Fig. 1. Gross classification of EA-TEF anomalies: (A) Pure esophageal atresia. (B) Proximal pouch fistula with distal atresia (C) Proximal pouch atresia with distal fistula (D) Fistula to both upper and lower pouches (E) Tracheoesophageal fistula without atresia. (*Adapted from*: Rothenberg, S. S. Esophageal Atresia and Tracheoesophageal Fistula Malformations. In: Holcomb G, Murphy JP, St. Peter SD, eds. Holcomb and Ashcraft's Pediatric Surgery, 7th Ed. Philadelphia, PA, Elsevier Inc: 2019:437-458. Used with permission.)

In most series, roughly half of infants with EA-TEF will have another congenital defect.[6] Of these, perhaps the best known is the VACTERL association (**Table 1**), first described as the VATER association by Quan and Smith in 1973.[7] A recent review of the Pediatric Health Information System (PHIS) database demonstrated cardiac defects to be the most common VACTERL-associated anomaly, affecting approximately 60% of neonates.[8] Multiple genetic syndromes leading to EA-TEF have been identified, including Feingold syndrome, Rogers/AEG syndrome, Opitz G syndrome, and Fryns syndrome.[6]

Family studies of patients with EA-TEF have demonstrated a low incidence of recurrence in subsequent generations. Twin concordance is roughly 3%. Siblings of patients with EA-TEF have less than a 1% chance of being similarly afflicted.[3] Likewise, in a single study of 28 offspring of patients with EA-TEF, one child (3.6%) was found to have the anomaly.[9] Interestingly, one study has demonstrated that first-degree relatives of patients with EA-TEF have other VACTERL-associated anomalies at a higher than expected rate, at 5.8% versus 3.1% in healthy controls.[10]

PRENATAL ASSESSMENT

EA-TEF is rarely definitively identified on prenatal ultrasound. Rather, the diagnosis is more commonly suspected based on a combination of associated findings. These include polyhydramnios and a small or absent stomach bubble, particularly when anomalies of other VACTERL-associated organ systems have been identified. The so-called "pouch-sign" of a dilated cervical esophagus in combination with a small or absent stomach was felt to be pathognomonic for EA in the 1990s and early 2000s;[11] however, later prospective studies questioned the accuracy of this finding.[12] More recently, fetal MRI has been demonstrated to be more accurate than US, with both an improved specificity and positive predictive value.[13] Finally, the amniotic fluid biochemical analysis may be more accurate than either imaging modality.[14] This diagnostic technique has not been adopted widely, presumably due to the invasiveness of sampling.

In any case, the suspicion of EA-TEF in isolation does not have a significant impact on prenatal management. The diagnosis does not dictate either mode or timing of delivery. Moreover, given the combination of the nonspecific nature of the prenatal findings and the generally nonemergent nature of the postnatal diagnosis, there is no absolute requirement for delivery at a tertiary center. However, prenatal discussion regarding the possibility of the diagnosis and its potential management is meaningful. Expecting parents should be referred to a pediatric surgeon for counseling when able.

Table 1 Percentage of associated VACTERL defects in infants diagnosed with EA-TEF anomalies in the Pediatric Health Information System (PHIS) database between 2004 and 2012[8]	
Anomaly	Percentage of EA-TEF Patients
Vertebral	25.5%
Anorectal	11.6%
Cardiac	59.1%
Tracheoesophageal	—
Renal	21.8%
Limb	7.1%

POSTNATAL ASSESSMENT

Classically, infants with EA-TEF present with coughing and choking after their initial feeding.[1] The evaluating physician should demonstrate the presence or absence of esophageal patency by attempting to pass a Replogle tube (6–10 French) via the mouth into the stomach. The same step should be performed when evaluating the newborn with prenatal suspicion for the condition. The tube should be advanced only until resistance is met, at which point a plan film of the chest is obtained. Curling or arrest of the tube in the mediastinum is diagnostic (**Fig. 2**). Importantly, the tube should not progress into either hemithorax or beyond the carina. These findings decrease the probability of EA-TEF and should raise suspicion for an iatrogenic esophageal perforation, a well-known pitfall in the diagnosis and a particular risk in extremely low birthweight infants.[15] Other diagnostic considerations include tracheal rings, congenital esophageal stenoses, or even esophageal compression from congenital paraesophageal hernias. If the diagnosis is in question, a small amount of air or contrast injected via the oral-esophageal tube demonstrates the blind-ending esophageal pouch. If esophageal perforation is demonstrated in an otherwise stable infant, this can typically be managed conservatively with the removal of the tube, antibiotics, and a delay in oral feeding.

Once the diagnosis of EA has been made, the oral-esophageal tube should be left in place to prevent salivary aspiration. Importantly, the existence of a distal TEF (Gross-types C or D) can be inferred based on the presence or absence of bowel gas on the initial plain film. This finding has important implications, not only for the consequent operative approach but also for potential respiratory instability due to the aspiration of gastric acid into the tracheobronchial tree. Both of these will be discussed later in greater detail.

Special note is made of the evaluation for an isolated TEF, or a Gross Type-E anomaly. These infants will generally suffer from the aspiration of esophageal and gastric content, with exacerbation during feeds. If not identified in the neonatal period, these

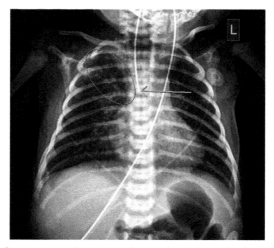

Fig. 2. Plan x-ray after attempted passage of an oral-esophageal tube in an infant with respiratory distress after the initial attempt at feeding. The tip of the tube arrests just above the level of the carina (arrow). An abberrant right upper lobe bronchus was identified on this x-ray (circle). Note the presence of intraluminal gas below the diaphragm, indicating the presence of a distal tracheoesophageal fistula.

can present with recurrent pulmonary infections. Unfortunately, diagnosis in these cases can be challenging. Oral-gastric tube passage will rule-out associated EA. Persistence of symptoms generally leads to the performance of a contrast esophagram as the initial diagnostic maneuver. Depending on both the diameter of the fistula and its level of entry into the trachea, this may or may not prove conclusive, as difficulty can arise in distinguishing contrast flow through the fistula from gastroesophageal reflux and spillage over the epiglottis. The classic radiographic study, the prone "pull-back" esophagram, can improve diagnostic yield. Even with this adjunct, false negatives are reported. Endoscopy, particularly rigid tracheo-bronchoscopy, will typically follow, both to establish the diagnosis and rule out a laryngotracheoesophageal cleft, which can present in an identical fashion. In cases whereby the diagnosis remains uncertain, cross-sectional imaging with computed tomography, or magnetic resonance imaging, has been described.[16]

Once the diagnosis of an EA-TEF anomaly has been established, the infant should subsequently be evaluated for VACTERL-associated diagnoses. Physical examination will demonstrate radial-limb anomalies as well as anorectal malformations. Plain films can identify vertebral anomalies. Renal and spinal ultrasounds are typically performed on the first day of life, although these are not urgent studies.

Echocardiography has typically been considered a compulsory step in the preoperative evaluation of an infant with EA-TEF. Recently, authors have questioned the necessity of this study in patients with otherwise normal clinical and x-ray findings.[17,18] Importantly, these selective imaging strategies overlook the potential for failing to identify a right-sided aortic arch, a variant present in roughly 6% of infants with EA-TEF,[18] as well as the presence of a vascular ring. If a vascular ring is identified, cross-sectional imaging can be pursued, as the ring may need to be addressed before esophageal reconstruction. The right-sided arch has important implications for the operative approach, as authors have typically advocated for repair via a left posterolateral thoracotomy when this variant is identified. Indeed, small studies have demonstrated improved outcomes when these patients are repaired from the left versus the standard right-sided approach.[19,20] On the other hand, advocates of a selective imaging strategy point out that echocardiography does not always identify the aberrant arch.[18] As such, when a right-sided arch is discovered only at the time of operation, conversion to a left thoracotomy should be considered only when the repair is prohibitivly difficult.[1]

RESPIRATORY CONSIDERATIONS

The potential for respiratory failure represents the most likely scenario requiring the involvement of a General Surgeon to treat a neonate in a rural or austere environment. As mentioned previously, of primary importance in the initial evaluation is the presence or absence of distal bowel gas on the plan x-ray. This indicates the presence of a distal fistula when present; most-likely the classic a type-C defect. Alternatively, the absence of bowel gas implies the presence of a type-A anomaly, pure EA, with a lower likelihood of a type-B configuration.

Due to the lack of associated reflux into the respiratory tree, infants with types A and B anomalies are typically stable from a respiratory standpoint. Oral-esophageal tubes are still necessary to prevent or limit salivary aspiration. Gasless abdomens in the presence of an occluded distal fistula have been reported.[5,21] Fortunately, these are rare; regardless, these patients should also demonstrate stable respiratory physiology. When isolated, infants with these defects do not require urgent intervention or transfer. Instability in this scenario should prompt investigation for an associated complex cardiac anomaly.

On the other hand, the presence of a distal fistula has important implications for the infant's respiratory function. In this circumstance, negative intra-thoracic pressure pulls the gastric contents directly into the trachea, typically leading to a progressive decline in respiratory status. For this reason, most pediatric surgeons will advocate repair within the first 2 or 3 days of life.[22] Unfortunately, the provision of positive-pressure ventilation, delivered either via an endotracheal tube or noninvasive means, can flow out of the fistula and into the gastrointestinal tract. This has the deleterious effect of inflating the neonatal abdomen and preventing lung inflation via diaphragmatic splinting. The combination perpetuates a vicious cycle of respiratory failure. Worse, gastric perforation has been described.[23] For that reason, should positive pressure support prove necessary, gentle low-pressure ventilation is of the utmost importance.[1,24]

Even with gentle ventilation, progressive respiratory failure is well-described. It is this specific scenario that can mandate emergent intervention. A number of adjuncts have been documented. High-frequency jet ventilation represents a simple escalation in ventilatory strategy, but is obviously not widely available.[25] Bronchoscopy and occlusion of the distal fistula with a Fogarty balloon catheter have been described.[26] This will typically require specialized neonatal equipment and expertise in rigid bronchoscopy; the size of a neonatal endotracheal tube will generally preclude passage of both a flexible fiberoptic scope and the balloon catheter. Attempts at blindly cannulating the fistula should be discouraged.

Needle decompression of the stomach to relieve abdominal distension may be attempted. This maneuver has typically been combined with so-called "water-seal gastrostomy[27]:" connection of the needle to tubing and a chest drain, which attempts to prevent loss of tidal volume through the gastric opening. Obviously, gastric decompression additionally necessitates eventual laparotomy with the repair of the gastrotomy.

Others have described laparotomy with occlusion of the distal esophagus at the diaphragmatic hiatus.[28] This represents a reasonable option for intervention when the surgeon lacks thoracic surgical experience. A generous left subcostal or upper midline incision should be performed. On entering the abdomen, marked gastric and intestinal distension can be anticipated; this may well require simultaneous performance of gastrostomy for decompression; again, the surgeon must balance the decompression with a loss of tidal volume through the enterotomy. If a gastrostomy is performed, the simplest maneuver for esophageal occlusion is a passage of a balloon catheter retrograde into the distal esophagus. If the surgeon is able to isolate the esophagus at the diaphragmatic hiatus, outflow through the fistula can be controlled with either an umbilical tape and Rummel tourniquet or a vessel loop. Neither the esophagus nor the stomach should be divided, as was historically described.[29]

In truth, however, these should all be considered temporizing maneuvers. In most cases, the definitive intervention is the ligation of the fistula via right posterolateral thoracotomy (**Fig. 3**). The infant is positioned in the left lateral decubitus position. A third or fourth-interspace posterolateral thoracotomy is performed. A muscle-sparing approach is optimal, but not compulsory. The lung is retracted anteriorly, and the azygos vein is identified. This landmark reliably approximates the location of the distal fistula. The vein is ligated. The vagus nerve is then identified on the surface of the fistula, which will generally be seen to inflate with the respiratory cycle. The fistula should be controlled with a vessel loop and dissected to its point of entry into the posterior trachea. This can generally be accomplished with blunt dissection and judicious use of electrocautery. The vagus nerve should be isolated and preserved. A test clamping of the fistula is performed, to ensure that neither a bronchus nor the aorta has been

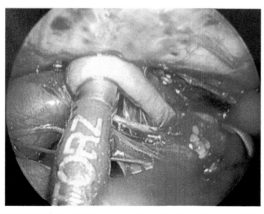

Fig. 3. Thoracoscopic view of an isolated distal tracheoesophageal fistula entering the posterior trachea. Note the vagus nerve isolated immediately inferior to the fistula. The distal esophagus remains inflated underneath its pleural investments. The divided azygos vein is not visible. (Photo courtesy of Frankie Fike, MD.)

mistakenly isolated. The fistula is then ligated. This is commonly performed 1–2 mm from the posterior wall of the trachea with the serial placement of interrupted permanent sutures. However, titanium or self-locking clips can be placed more efficiently, and concerns regarding their potential for migration seem to be largely overstated.[30] If the condition of the infant improves dramatically after ligation, and the surgeon is experienced, primary repair can be considered. Otherwise, the operation should be concluded, and the esophagus reconstructed in a staged fashion. Importantly, if the fistula is ligated without division, traditional teaching suggests that recanalization may occur within weeks.[1] Therefore, if the surgeon anticipates a longer period between operations, the fistula should be divided with the closure of the distal end. Sutured pexy of the distal fistula to the prevertebral fascia in the right chest prevents the retraction of the fistula into the abdominal cavity and facilitates its identification at re-exploration.

Simultaneous anorectal malformations can accelerate respiratory compromise. In this specific situation, the distal obstruction precludes any outflow of air from the gastrointestinal tract, which may precipitate the previously described vicious cycle of respiratory failure more rapidly. As such, this combination of defects should be managed on a more urgent timeline, typically within the first day of life.[31] In all cases, the initial step should be control of the TEF.[1,2]

Interestingly, the combination of EA-TEF and duodenal atresia is not necessarily associated with the same degree of respiratory instability, presumably because the proximal obstruction precludes marked abdominal distension and diaphragmatic excursion. Nevertheless, division of the TEF remains the priority.[1,2,31] Controversy surrounds the subsequent timing and sequence of gastrointestinal tract reconstruction. Some have advocated for repairing the duodenal atresia first.[32] This is based on the principle of avoiding an obstruction distal to an esophageal anastomosis, with the well-described postoperative delay in duodenal function an additional consideration. Others favor simultaneous repair.[1,31] Either decision must be tailored to the individual neonate's physiology. Regardless, the EA should not be repaired without a near-term plan for establishing gastric outflow, either via a duodenal anastomosis or gastrostomy.

SURGICAL CONSIDERATIONS

Once the appropriate preoperative evaluation has been completed, both type-specific and physiologic considerations will dictate consequent operative planning. These will be outlined in the following sections.

Infants with distal fistulas are generally taken to the operating room within the first 3-days of life.[22] For the most part, these are nonemergent operations, apart from the special circumstances outlined above. Typically, the initial operative step is the performance of a rigid tracheo-bronchoscopy (**Fig. 4**). This demonstrates the presence of the TEF, provides information regarding the level of the fistulous connection to the trachea, assesses for associated laryngotracheoesophageal clefts, and likely rules out concurrent proximal fistulas. However, this step is not compulsory. Surgeons who chose to forego endoscopy argue that concurrent proximal fistulas are rare, present in less than 5%, and may still be missed if small and proximal. Moreover, bronchoscopy may exacerbate an already delicate respiratory physiology and delay the division of the fistula.[33]

As alluded to previously, the operative approach is typically through the right chest. In the current era, most infants are repaired with thoracotomy, either trans- or extra-pleural.[34] Thoracoscopic repair was first described in 2000 and has gained widespread acceptance (**Fig. 5**). Studies comparing the 2 approaches have demonstrated roughly equivalent outcomes.[35,36] Not surprisingly, the thoracoscopic approach is technically demanding, and a learning curve has been demonstrated.[37] Therefore, experts have recommended limiting this approach to stable infants with isolated defects weighing greater than 2 kg.[30]

Following the division of the distal fistula, the decision to proceed with esophageal reconstruction will be broadly dependent on four factors. The primary consideration is the infant's physiologic status. If the ligation has been performed emergently to control respiratory compromise, additional operation should be performed only if there is a rapid and sustained improvement. Next, the presence of a more acute associated defect, such as a complex cardiac anomaly requiring neonatal palliation, may preclude immediate esophageal reconstruction. Third, the birthweight of the infant must be considered. Due to the associated polyhydramnios, preterm delivery of

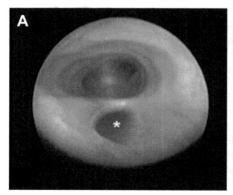 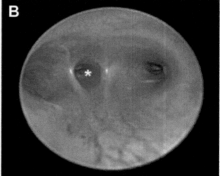

Fig. 4. Rigid bronchoscopy demonstrating distal tracheoesophageal fistulas (delineated by the stars) entering the mid-trachea (*A*) and at the level of the carina (*B*). (*Reproduced from*: Rothenberg, S. S. Esophageal Atresia and Tracheoesophageal Fistula Malformations. In: Holcomb G, Murphy JP, St. Peter SD, eds. Holcomb and Ashcraft's Pediatric Surgery, 7th Ed. Philadelphia, PA, Elsevier Inc: 2019:437-458. Used with permission.)

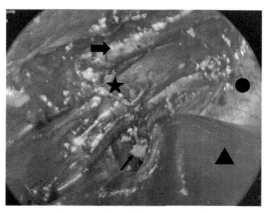

Fig. 5. Thoracoscopic repair of a type-C EA-TEF anomaly. Note the anastomosis (*star*), the divided azygos vein (*thin arrow*), the superior vena cava (*circle*) and the right upper lobe of the lung (*triangle*). The infant was noted to have an aberrant right subclavian artery on preoperative echocardiography, which was demonstrable on thoracoscopy (*thick arrow*).

infants with EA is common. Pediatric surgeons have long recognized the association between birthweight and outcomes.[38] A recent British study demonstrated that patients weighing less than 1500 g are less likely to achieve a primary anastomosis and have higher mortality. As such, the authors recommend delayed repair in these patients.[39] Their evidence-based recommendation is consistent with common practice.

The fourth, and perhaps most challenging, consideration for primary esophageal reconstruction is the gap between the upper and lower pouches. In infants with distal fistulas, this distance will not be conclusively apparent before the exploration of the chest. Two findings may provide clues but are nondefinitive. First, if the oral-esophageal tube arrests at the thoracic inlet or high mediastinum on preoperative chest x-ray, a longer-gap may be anticipated. Second, if bronchoscopy demonstrates a fistula at the carina, the so-called trifurcation fistula (see **Fig. 4**B), a longer-gap may be encountered.[30]

Infants with gasless abdomens can be confidently assessed to have either a type A or B defect. As has been discussed extensively, the initial management will be dependent on a number of factors, including the birthweight and presence of associated defects. However, these infants will typically be found to have long gaps; as such, they are usually managed in a delayed fashion.[40] In isolated cases, gastrostomies are performed initially to secure enteral feeding access, typically within the first week of life. Similar to the discussion regarding bronchoscopy for infants with distal fistulas, bronchoscopy can be performed at the initial operation to evaluate for a proximal fistula and rule out associated anomalies. Importantly, due to the lack of in utero amniotic fluid distension, these infant's stomachs are notoriously underdeveloped. Therefore, the placement of a standard gastrostomy balloon device can either prove impossible or lead to gastric outlet obstruction. As such, an 8 to 12 French Malecot tube provides an ideal solution. Alternatively, smaller Foley catheters can be used if necessary.

As was alluded to previously, the management of long-gap EA presents a notorious challenge. Notably, the length of defect required for a "long-gap" has not been precisely defined.[40] As applies to intra-operative decision making, this applies to any defect that cannot be bridged without excessive tension. For infants managed in a delayed fashion, combinations of preoperative fluoroscopy, endoscopy, and bougienage have been used to estimate gap length. Most authors accept a defect of more than 2 vertebral bodies as definitive.[40]

A number of adjuncts have been described to bridge these gaps. Intra-operative strategies include the creation of esophageal myotomies, either spiral[41] or circular.[42] If the gap is recognized before the creation of the proximal esophagostomy, additional upper pouch length can be gained through the use of an anterior flap in a manner analogous to a V to Y advancement.[43] Realistically, however, all three of these methods injure the native esophagus, and their long-term implications on esophageal function are unknown. Staged lengthening of the upper pouch through serial advancement of an esophagostomy from the neck down the anterior chest has been described. This strategy is rarely used in the modern era.[44]

Currently, the most commonly reported intra-operative strategy involves the stimulation of esophageal growth by placing traction on the ends of the pouches with sutures, either internal or external.[45,46] A thoracoscopic method has been likewise described.[47] Advocates of the technique point to a shorter duration to anastomosis and a lower complication rate.[46] However, these techniques, particularly those using serial external traction, are complex and resource intensive, and whether these results can be extrapolated to other centers remains to be established. Intriguingly, humanitarian approval of a novel magnetic device has recently been granted by the FDA.[48] Criteria for its use include a documented gap length of 4 cm or less and patient age of less than 1 year. Using this device, pressure necrosis of the pouch ends creates the esophagoesophagostomy.

In most circumstances, the gap-length decreases spontaneously as the infant grows. Bolus feeding of the stomach can stimulate the growth of the lower pouch into the chest. As such, most authors will advocate a period of observation and serial imaging before intervention.[40] The requirement for proximal esophageal tube decompression typically mandates in-patient care throughout. Periodic endoscopic or fluoroscopic dilations to hasten this nonoperative process have been described.[49] Once the defect is within 2 vertebral bodies on imaging, a primary anastomosis is likely feasible. If this is not achievable within 2 to 3 months, traction techniques can then be applied. Esophageal replacement using stomach, jejunum, or colon are also well-described adjuncts.[40,50] No conduit demonstrates conclusive superiority, nor is there any definitive algorithm for determining when to abandon the native esophagus. Currently, most experts agree that the native esophagus should be salvaged whenever possible.[40,50]

Finally, most Gross type E defects are repaired through the right neck. Typically, these lesions enter high on the trachea, at the level of either the low cervical or high thoracic vertebrae. The typical approach for this anomaly involves rigid bronchoscopy with the passage of a heavy guide wire across the fistula from the tracheal to the esophageal side. Endoscopy of the esophagus is then performed, and the guidewire is grasped and brought out of the mouth. Tension applied to the wire brings the fistula out of the thoracic inlet and facilitates its identification. If the preoperative imaging demonstrates a lower fistula, the lesion can be approached through the chest.[16] A thoracoscopic approach to ligation is well described.[51] Endoscopic management of this anomaly is also reported in small single-center series.[16]

EARLY COMPLICATIONS

Complications from EA-TEF can be categorized into early and late, and additionally classified as to whether morbidities are consequent to the nature of the anomaly or the technical outcome of the procedure. A recent multi-center retrospective review of 292 patients with EA-TEF demonstrated an eye-opening 62% rate of morbidity.[34] These complications included an 18% rate of anastomotic leak, a 43% rate of anastomotic stricture, a 5% rate of vocal cord injury, a 5% rate of recurrent fistula, and anastomotic dehiscence in an additional 2%. These rates are broadly consistent with outcomes reported in earlier single-center studies. The management of common early complications will be briefly discussed.

Given the nature of the disease process and the frequent need for the creation of an anastomosis under tension, the rates of anastomotic leak and stricture are perhaps unsurprising. Reported rates of anastomotic leak can vary, owing largely to different practice patterns regarding their detection and classification. Most surgeons leave a drain in the chest following esophageal reconstruction.[22] Provided that the leak is controlled, nearly all will resolve with time and antibiotics. Percutaneous placement of one or more additional drains is occasionally required, but reoperation is rarely indicated.

Early anastomotic strictures are even more common. Curiously, 3 papers have demonstrated that placement of transanastomotic feeding tubes is an independent risk factor for stricture formation.[34,52,53] Again, however, stricture rate will vary depending on whether the researchers include clinically apparent strictures versus those that are or only radiographically suspected. When clinically significant, most strictures will respond to endoscopic dilation, with series documenting a median of three dilations required for a sustained improvement.[34,54] If refractory, intralesional steroid or mitomycin-c injection can be considered. Strictures that develop outside of infancy are more commonly associated with reflux and esophageal acid exposure. These will be discussed in a later section.

The recurrent TEF is perhaps the most feared complication of EA repair. The complication is comparatively and fortunately rare, but can be immensely challenging and frustrating to manage, as chronic inflammation combines with the adjacent low-pressure respiratory system, predisposing to fistulization. Rerecurrences are well described, despite anastomotic revision and even muscle flap interposition. Several authors have described endoscopic attempts at the management of these lesions, with response rates varying in small single-center series.[55] Recently, the group at Boston Children's Hospital reported their results with repeat thoracotomy, rotational esophagoplasty, and posterior tracheopexy, with excellent results.[56]

Vocal cord injuries are increasingly recognized.[57–59] Mobilization of the upper esophageal pouch requires its separation from the posterior wall of the trachea and subsequent dissection in the tracheoesophageal grove. Recurrent laryngeal nerve injury can result from overaggressive dissection or overuse of electrocautery. For that reason, sharp dissection, directly on the wall of the esophagus, should be used at this stage of the operation.

Tracheomalacia is common comorbidity, independent of the conduct of the operation. Reported rates vary, ranging between 24% and 79%, and are increasingly common with decreasing gestational age.[59] The EA-TEF anomaly results in an increased width of the membranous portion of the trachea, with consequent loss of support from the C-shaped cartilaginous rings. This weakness allows tracheal collapse with expiration. The pathognomonic presentation is the so-called "barking" cough. The diagnosis must be considered in the evaluation and management of infants with otherwise unexplained respiratory distress or apneic events.[60] Aortopexy, either through an open or thoracoscopic approach, is the accepted surgical intervention for severely symptomatic infants,[60] but there is no widely accepted treatment algorithm, and institutional practices vary.

LATE COMPLICATIONS

The late complications of EA-TEF anomalies are, unfortunately, under-reported. Nevertheless, they represent the next most likely situation for a General Surgeon to encounter a patient with this disease process. As outcomes for EA-TEF have improved markedly over the past decades, these patients are likely to present with increasing frequency in the future. A number of considerations will be described in the following sections.

Gastroesophageal reflux disease (GERD) is a well-recognized comorbidity, affecting up to 60% of patients.[61] EA-TEF anomalies predispose to reflux due to intrinsically impaired esophageal motility.[62] Moreover, esophageal reconstruction, particularly conducted under tension, adversely impacts the lower esophageal sphincter complex. This combination is particularly apparent in infants with isolated EA (Gross type A), in whom reflux symptoms are nearly universal.[63] Importantly, in contrast to normal children, GERD in patients with EA-TEF should not be expected to improve over time; instead, studies have demonstrated an increasing incidence of symptomatic reflux with increasing age, with obvious lifelong implications.[64]

The evaluation of a postoperative patient with troublesome reflux should follow a similar, if not identical, algorithm to the non-EA/TEF patient,[63] using a combination of contrast studies, pH-probe, or multichannel intraluminal impedance, and endoscopy. However, important diagnostic considerations deserve mention.

In most cases, the initial study will be esophageal and upper gastrointestinal fluoroscopy. This allows for the identification of anastomotic stricture, associated distal congenital esophageal stenosis, hiatal hernia, and distal intestinal malformations.[8] As is well documented elsewhere, the presence or absence of reflux in the contrast study is of lesser importance.

Importantly, manometry will be abnormal in essentially all patients,[62,65–67] and may worsen over time.[67] Disordered motility is typically most notable in the lower esophagus,[62] and can even manifest as an achalasia-like absence of distal esophageal peristalsis.[68] Therefore, this study's overall contribution to the evaluation of reflux is debatable. Its use in the evaluation of dysphagia will be discussed in a later section.

Recent guidelines have advocated for either pH-probe or multi-channel intraluminal impedance evaluation of all patients with EA-TEF.[63] As applies to the evaluation of pathologic reflux, a lack of standardized pH-probe or impedance scores should not limit the application of these tests to younger patients, as reflux is just as likely to be non-acid, and simple symptom correlation to documented reflux events is felt to be the most important diagnostic indicator.[63] Finally, esophagogastroduodenoscopy (EGD) is compulsory in the evaluation of patients with EA-TEF with GERD, to demonstrate the presence of esophagitis, to rule out eosinophilic esophagitis, and to rule out Barrett's metaplasia, as will be discussed later.

Similar to patients with non-EA/TEF, medical management is the mainstay of treatment of GERD.[69] While regimens have historically varied, recent expert guidelines advocate for proton-pump inhibitors (PPIs) as first-line therapy.[63] Notably, these experts have additionally recommended that medication be continued for a minimum of 1-year in all postoperative patients, with pH- or impedance-probe testing used to determine whether asymptomatic individuals can discontinue therapy.

Rates of refractory GERD requiring fundoplication have varied in the literature,[30] perhaps reflecting well-recognized regional practice variations. Historically, up to 45% of all postoperative patients,[63] and more than 50% of patients with severe reflux, have undergone fundoplication.[64] Despite fears that complete fundoplication could exacerbate dysphagia due to the aforementioned impaired distal esophageal motility, meta-analysis does not demonstrate the superiority of partial fundoplication.[70] The currently accepted indications for fundoplication in patients with postoperative EA-TEF are failure of high-dose PPIs, recurrent or refractory strictures, dependence on postpyloric feeds, and brief resolved unexplained events in the absence of other causes.[63]

Consequent to reflux, Barrett's esophagus has been increasingly recognized in patients with postoperative EA-TEF.[61,65–67,71–73] Rates have varied, but a recent systematic review of the literature demonstrated a pooled 5% overall incidence, with a 12.6% rate in cohorts followed with prospective surveillance. Surprisingly, the earliest documented case is an 8-month-old infant. Conversely, a 56 year old has been identified as the oldest patient to receive an initial diagnosis of Barrett's esophagus, illustrating the need for life-long surveillance.[72]

As such, the aforementioned expert panel has offered screening guidelines. The initial endoscopy should be performed at the time of PPI discontinuation, typically at age 1 in asymptomatic patients with normal pH or impedance probe results. They recommend a second scope before age 10, and a third at the time of transition to adulthood. Thereafter, endoscopy should be performed at 5 to 10-year intervals.[63] In symptomatic patients or those with demonstrated pathology, the schedule should be accelerated as appropriate.

Curiously, and despite this recognized association with Barrett's esophagus, there are only thirteen reported cases of esophageal cancer in patients with EA-TEF.[72] Moreover, squamous cell cancer has been reported more than twice as often as adenocarcinoma, nine versus four cases, respectively.[72] Even more surprisingly, a large, prospectively monitored, population-based cohort in Finland has thus-far reported zero cases.[65] Nonetheless, as these anomalies have only been survivable for 80 years, there are concerns that esophageal cancer will be identified with increasing frequency as more patients with EA-TEF enter late adulthood. Furthermore, the median age at cancer diagnosis in reported patients is 40 years; the youngest was 20.[72] Taken together, these realities demonstrate the need for close surveillance.

Dysphagia is similarly well-recognized sequelae of the anomaly and its repair.[61,66,67,73–75] More than half of the respondents to 2 independently conducted surveys have reported swallowing difficulty.[74,75] When troublesome, evaluation delineates between anastomotic stricture,[66,73,74] associated congenital anomalies, and the aforementioned motility issues.[74] As mentioned previously, strictures generally respond well to either balloon or bougie dilation.[63] When strictures develop outside of infancy, they are most commonly consequent to GERD; this should be simultaneously evaluated and addressed. Importantly, dysphagia may be due to associated anomalies, including congenital esophageal stenosis and thoracic vascular anomalies. These are typically identified via fluoroscopy, endoscopy, or cross-sectional imaging, with intervention as appropriate. Fortunately, conservative management of intrinsic esophageal dysmotility is generally successful. Most patients are able to compensate by adjusting eating behaviors, such as taking sips of liquids with each swallow or avoiding troublesome foods.[74] One case of achalasia responding to myotomy has been reported,[68] but no long-term outcomes or comparison studies are available; this should be interpreted with caution. Esophageal replacement is required in only the most recalcitrant cases[63]

Chronic respiratory issues are likewise common.[59] These include issues with aspiration, pneumonia, choking, wheezing, cough, asthma, and reactive airways disease.[59,61,65,66,76] Endoscopy of the aerodigestive tract is the compulsory step in the evaluation of symptomatic patients.[63] This allows not only for the assessment of known sequelae of the operation and the anomaly, such as the previously mentioned vocal cord paralysis, recurrent TEF, anastomotic stricture, and tracheomalacia, but also for known associated congenital anomalies, such as laryngoesophageal clefts, vascular rings, and distal esophageal stenoses. Additionally, the presence of a tracheal diverticulum at the site of fistula ligation is a known potential nidus for infection.[76] Pharyngeal coordination should be assessed with a modified barium swallow when aspiration is suspected or demonstrated.[63] Importantly, while respiratory symptoms may represent extra-esophageal manifestations of GERD, their response to antireflux therapy, either medicinal or surgical, is not well accepted. For all of the above-listed reasons, empiric reflux treatment of respiratory symptoms should be avoided.[63]

Musculoskeletal issues described after thoracotomy for the repair of EA-TEF include scoliosis,[65,77] chest wall deformities,[78] breast deformities,[79] fused ribs,[65] winged scapulae,[80] and shoulder asymmetry.[80] These issues seem to have been more common in the past; it is unclear whether risks for musculoskeletal complications remain as high with the contemporary "muscle-sparing" thoracotomy technique.[81] Moreover, when present, these findings tend to be subtle; a systematic review of scoliosis after EA-TEF repair documents only rare cases whereby surgery is required.[77] Nonetheless, avoidance of these issues has been frequently touted as a major advantage of repair via a thoracoscopic approach.[30] Single-center reports on the efficacy of the thoracoscopic technique have routinely commented on the lack of musculoskeletal sequelae,[82,83] although these results are limited by the relative lack of long-term follow-up. Similarly, a 2009 paper reported musculoskeletal results in a single-center German cohort, with thoracoscopy demonstrating clear advantages over thoracotomy with a median follow-up of roughly 4 years.[80]

OUTCOMES

Outcomes for infants with EA-TEF have steadily improved over the past 80 years. Birthweight and cardiac anomalies, the prognostic indicators identified by Waterston in the 1960s[38] and modified by Spitz in the 1990s[84] remain relevant today.[85,86] For the most part, infants without complex cardiac malformations and birthweights over 2 kg should be expected to survive in the modern era. Conversely, outcomes remain dismal for infants with cardiac lesions and birthweights under 1 kg.

Longer-term outcomes are less well defined, as described in the late complications section. A 2015 review and meta-analysis focused on reported health-related quality of life in children and adults with the condition.[87] The authors found that the current literature indicates that survivors of EA-TEF spectrum anomalies, indeed, have a reduction in health-related quality of life. Importantly, however, their meta-analysis did not show any decrease in patients' mental health or social functioning, demonstrating that survivors go on to live meaningful lives.

SUMMARY

EA-TEF is among the most common congenital anomalies requiring surgical intervention in infancy. General surgeons practicing in rural or austere environments may encounter emergency situations requiring their involvement. Therefore, a practical understanding of the anomaly and its associated surgical pearls and pitfalls is necessary. As applies to a respiratory emergency in the neonatal period, the recommended approaches are the ligation of the fistula through the right chest or occlusion of the distal esophagus through the abdomen, depending on the comfort of the surgeon. Additionally, as more survivors of the condition reach late adulthood, General Surgeons can anticipate encountering these patients with greater frequency. An understanding of risk factors, common symptoms, associated anomalies, and the diagnostic evaluation will facilitate the care of these potentially complicated individuals.

CLINICS CARE POINTS

- Roughly 1 in 3000 infants is born with an EA-TEF anomaly
- The condition is rarely definitively diagnosed in the prenatal period, but may be suspected based on a small stomach bubble on ultrasound with polyhydramnios
- The initial step in newborn evaluation is an attempted passage of an oral-gastric tube into the stomach
- Approximately 50% of infants have an additional congenital anomaly; cardiac conditions are most common
- Plain x-rays of the abdomen will demonstrate the presence of a distal fistula if air has progressed into the abdominal cavity
- Infants with distal fistulas are at risk for the development of respiratory insufficiency or failure
- If a respiratory emergency develops, ligation or occlusion of the TEF will be required
- Infants with gasless abdomens do not have fistulas between the respiratory and distal gastrointestinal tracts, and should, therefore, remain stable
- Gastroesophageal reflux and dysphagia are exceptionally common in postoperative survivors, and these conditions may worsen with time rather than improve
- The evaluation should proceed in a stepwise fashion, and special consideration must be given to ruling out associated congenital anomalies
- Barrett's esophagus is recognized with increasing frequency, and life-long endoscopic surveillance is required

DISCLOSURE

The author has nothing to disclose.

REFERENCES

1. Spitz L. Esophageal atresia. Lessons I have learned in a 40-year experience. J Pediatr Surg 2006;41(10):1635–40.
2. Nakayama DK. The history of surgery for esophageal atresia. J Pediatr Surg 2020;55(7):1414–9.
3. Shaw-Smith C. Oesophageal atresia, tracheo-oesophageal fistula, and the VACTERL association: review of genetics and epidemiology. J Med Genet 2006;43(7): 545–54.
4. Rothenberg SS. Esophageal Atresia and Tracheoesophageal Fistula Malformations. In: George W, Holcomb JPM, Shawn D, et al, editors. Holcomb and Ashcraft's pediatric surgery. 7th edition. Philadelphia, PA: Elsevier Inc; 2019. p. 437–58.
5. Kluth D. Atlas of esophageal atresia. J Pediatr Surg 1976;11(6):901–19.
6. Genevieve D, de Pontual L, Amiel J, et al. An overview of isolated and syndromic oesophageal atresia. Clin Genet 2007;71(5):392–9.
7. Quan L, Smith DW. The VATER association. Vertebral defects, Anal atresia, T-E fistula with esophageal atresia, Radial and Renal dysplasia: a spectrum of associated defects. J Pediatr 1973;82(1):104–7.

8. Lautz TB, Mandelia A, Radhakrishnan J. VACTERL associations in children undergoing surgery for esophageal atresia and anorectal malformations: Implications for pediatric surgeons. J Pediatr Surg 2015;50(8):1245–50.
9. Warren J, Evans K, Carter CO. Offspring of patients with tracheo-oesophageal fistula. J Med Genet 1979;16(5):338–40.
10. Brown AK, Roddam AW, Spitz L, et al. Oesophageal atresia, related malformations, and medical problems: a family study. Am J Med Genet 1999;85(1):31–7.
11. Centini G, Rosignoli L, Kenanidis A, et al. Prenatal diagnosis of esophageal atresia with the pouch sign. Ultrasound Obstet Gynecol 2003;21(5):494–7.
12. Solt I, Rotmensch S, Bronshtein M. The esophageal 'pouch sign': a benign transient finding. Prenat Diagn 2010;30(9):845–8.
13. Ethun CG, Fallon SC, Cassady CI, et al. Fetal MRI improves diagnostic accuracy in patients referred to a fetal center for suspected esophageal atresia. J Pediatr Surg 2014;49(5):712–5.
14. Czerkiewicz I, Dreux S, Beckmezian A, et al. Biochemical amniotic fluid pattern for prenatal diagnosis of esophageal atresia. Pediatr Res 2011;70(2):199–202.
15. Sapin E, Gumpert L, Bonnard A, et al. Iatrogenic pharyngoesophageal perforation in premature infants. Eur J Pediatr Surg 2000;10(2):83–7.
16. Sampat K, Losty PD. Diagnostic and management strategies for congenital H-type tracheoesophageal fistula: a systematic review. Pediatr Surg Int 2021;37(5):539–47.
17. Nasr A, McNamara PJ, Mertens L, et al. Is routine preoperative 2-dimensional echocardiography necessary for infants with esophageal atresia, omphalocele, or anorectal malformations? J Pediatr Surg 2010;45(5):876–9.
18. Tanny SPT, King SK, Comella A, et al. Selective approach to preoperative echocardiography in esophageal atresia. Pediatr Surg Int 2021;37(4):503–9.
19. Lal DR, Gadepalli SK, Downard CD, et al. Infants with esophageal atresia and right aortic arch: Characteristics and outcomes from the Midwest Pediatric Surgery Consortium. J Pediatr Surg 2019;54(4):688–92.
20. Babu R, Pierro A, Spitz L, et al. The management of oesophageal atresia in neonates with right-sided aortic arch. J Pediatr Surg 2000;35(1):56–8.
21. Goh DW, Brereton RJ, Spitz L. Esophageal atresia with obstructed tracheoesophageal fistula and gasless abdomen. J Pediatr Surg 1991;26(2):160–2.
22. Lal DR, Gadepalli SK, Downard CD, et al. Perioperative management and outcomes of esophageal atresia and tracheoesophageal fistula. J Pediatr Surg 2017;52(8):1245–51.
23. Maoate K, Myers NA, Beasley SW. Gastric perforation in infants with oesophageal atresia and distal tracheo-oesophageal fistula. Pediatr Surg Int 1999;15(1):24–7.
24. Malone PS, Kiely EM, Brain AJ, et al. Tracheo-oesophageal fistula and preoperative mechanical ventilation. Aust N Z J Surg 1990;60(7):525–7.
25. Donn SM, Zak LK, Bozynski ME, et al. Use of high-frequency jet ventilation in the management of congenital tracheoesophageal fistula associated with respiratory distress syndrome. J Pediatr Surg 1990;25(12):1219–21.
26. Filston HC, Chitwood WR Jr, Schkolne B, et al. The Fogarty balloon catheter as an aid to management of the infant with esophageal atresia and tracheoesophageal fistula complicated by severe RDS or pneumonia. J Pediatr Surg 1982;17(2):149–51.
27. Fann JI, Hartman GE, Shochat SJ. Waterseal" gastrostomy in the management of premature infants with tracheoesophageal fistula and pulmonary insufficiency. J Pediatr Surg 1988;23(1 Pt 2):29–31.

28. Templeton JM Jr, Templeton JJ, Schnaufer L, et al. Management of esophageal atresia and tracheoesophageal fistula in the neonate with severe respiratory distress syndrome. J Pediatr Surg 1985;20(4):394–7.
29. Gamble HA. Tracheo-Esophageal Fistula: Description of a New Operative Procedure and Case Report. Ann Surg 1938;107(5):701–7.
30. Holcomb GW 3rd. Thoracoscopic surgery for esophageal atresia. Pediatr Surg Int 2017;33(4):475–81.
31. Ceccanti S, Midrio P, Messina M, et al. The DATE Association: A Separate Entity or a Further Extension of the VACTERL Association? J Surg Res 2019;241: 128–34.
32. Ein SH, Palder SB, Filler RM. Babies with esophageal and duodenal atresia: a 30-year review of a multifaceted problem. J Pediatr Surg 2006;41(3):530–2.
33. Taghavi K, Stringer MD. Preoperative laryngotracheobronchoscopy in infants with esophageal atresia: why is it not routine? Pediatr Surg Int 2018;34(1):3–7.
34. Lal DR, Gadepalli SK, Downard CD, et al. Challenging surgical dogma in the management of proximal esophageal atresia with distal tracheoesophageal fistula: Outcomes from the Midwest Pediatric Surgery Consortium. J Pediatr Surg 2018;53(7):1267–72.
35. Yang YF, Dong R, Zheng C, et al. Outcomes of thoracoscopy versus thoracotomy for esophageal atresia with tracheoesophageal fistula repair: A PRISMA-compliant systematic review and meta-analysis. Medicine (Baltimore) 2016; 95(30):e4428.
36. Way C, Wayne C, Grandpierre V, et al. Thoracoscopy vs. thoracotomy for the repair of esophageal atresia and tracheoesophageal fistula: a systematic review and meta-analysis. Pediatr Surg Int 2019;35(11):1167–84.
37. Lee S, Lee SK, Seo JM. Thoracoscopic repair of esophageal atresia with tracheoesophageal fistula: overcoming the learning curve. J Pediatr Surg 2014;49(11): 1570–2.
38. Waterston DJ, Bonham-Carter RE, Aberdeen E. Congenital tracheo-oesophageal fistula in association with oesophageal atresia. Lancet 1963;2(7298):55–7.
39. Folaranmi SE, Jawaid WB, Gavin L, et al. Influence of birth weight on primary surgical management of newborns with esophageal atresia. J Pediatr Surg 2021; 56(5):929–32.
40. Baird R, Lal DR, Ricca RL, et al. Management of long gap esophageal atresia: A systematic review and evidence-based guidelines from the APSA Outcomes and Evidence Based Practice Committee. J Pediatr Surg 2019;54(4):675–87.
41. Shoshany G, Kimura K, Jaume J, et al. A staged approach to long gap esophageal atresia employing a spiral myotomy and delayed reconstruction of the esophagus: an experimental study. J Pediatr Surg 1988;23(12):1218–21.
42. Livaditis A, Radberg L, Odensjo G. Esophageal end-to-end anastomosis. Reduction of anastomotic tension by circular myotomy. Scand J Thorac Cardiovasc Surg 1972;6(2):206–14.
43. Gough MH. Esophageal atresia–use of an anterior flap in the difficult anastomosis. J Pediatr Surg 1980;15(3):310–1.
44. Kimura K, Soper RT. Multistaged extrathoracic esophageal elongation for long gap esophageal atresia. J Pediatr Surg 1994;29(4):566–8.
45. Foker JE, Linden BC, Boyle EM Jr, et al. Development of a true primary repair for the full spectrum of esophageal atresia. Ann Surg 1997;226(4):533–41 [discussion: 541–3].
46. Nasr A, Langer JC. Mechanical traction techniques for long-gap esophageal atresia: a critical appraisal. Eur J Pediatr Surg 2013;23(3):191–7.

47. van der Zee DC, Gallo G, Tytgat SH. Thoracoscopic traction technique in long gap esophageal atresia: entering a new era. Surg Endosc 2015;29(11):3324–30.
48. Slater BJ, Borobia P, Lovvorn HN, et al. Use of Magnets as a Minimally Invasive Approach for Anastomosis in Esophageal Atresia: Long-Term Outcomes. J Laparoendosc Adv Surg Tech A 2019;29(10):1202–6.
49. Mahour GH, Woolley MM, Gwinn JL. Elongation of the upper pouch and delayed anatomic reconstruction in esophageal atresia. J Pediatr Surg 1974;9(3):373–83.
50. Shieh HF, Jennings RW. Long-gap esophageal atresia. Semin Pediatr Surg 2017; 26(2):72–7.
51. Rothenberg SS. Thoracoscopic management of non-type C esophageal atresia and tracheoesophageal atresia. J Pediatr Surg 2017. https://doi.org/10.1016/j.jpedsurg.2017.10.025.
52. Wang C, Feng L, Li Y, et al. What is the impact of the use of transanastomotic feeding tube on patients with esophageal atresia: a systematic review and meta-analysis. BMC Pediatr 2018;18(1):385.
53. LaRusso K, Joharifard S, Lakabi R, et al. Effect of transanastomotic feeding tubes on anastomotic strictures in patients with esophageal atresia and tracheoesophageal fistula: The Quebec experience. J Pediatr Surg 2022;57(1):41–4.
54. Sun LY, Laberge JM, Yousef Y, et al. The Esophageal Anastomotic Stricture Index (EASI) for the management of esophageal atresia. J Pediatr Surg 2015;50(1): 107–10.
55. Nazir Z, Khan MAM, Qamar J. Recurrent and acquired tracheoesophageal fistulae (TEF)-Minimally invasive management. J Pediatr Surg 2017;52(10): 1688–90.
56. Kamran A, Zendejas B, Meisner J, et al. Effect of Posterior Tracheopexy on Risk of Recurrence in Children after Recurrent Tracheo-Esophageal Fistula Repair. J Am Coll Surg 2021;232(5):690–8.
57. Mortellaro VE, Pettiford JN, St Peter SD, et al. Incidence, diagnosis, and outcomes of vocal fold immobility after esophageal atresia (EA) and/or tracheoesophageal fistula (TEF) repair. Eur J Pediatr Surg 2011;21(6):386–8.
58. Morini F, Iacobelli BD, Crocoli A, et al. Symptomatic vocal cord paresis/paralysis in infants operated on for esophageal atresia and/or tracheo-esophageal fistula. J Pediatr 2011;158(6):973–6.
59. Porcaro F, Valfre L, Aufiero LR, et al. Respiratory problems in children with esophageal atresia and tracheoesophageal fistula. Ital J Pediatr 2017;43(1):77.
60. Bergeron M, Cohen AP, Cotton RT. The Management of Cyanotic Spells in Children with Oesophageal Atresia. Front Pediatr 2017;5:106.
61. Connor MJ, Springford LR, Kapetanakis VV, et al. Esophageal atresia and transitional care–step 1: a systematic review and meta-analysis of the literature to define the prevalence of chronic long-term problems. Am J Surg 2015;209(4): 747–59.
62. Kawahara H, Kubota A, Hasegawa T, et al. Lack of distal esophageal contractions is a key determinant of gastroesophageal reflux disease after repair of esophageal atresia. J Pediatr Surg 2007;42(12):2017–21.
63. Krishnan U, Mousa H, Dall'Oglio L, et al. ESPGHAN-NASPGHAN Guidelines for the Evaluation and Treatment of Gastrointestinal and Nutritional Complications in Children With Esophageal Atresia-Tracheoesophageal Fistula. J Pediatr Gastroenterol Nutr 2016;63(5):550–70.
64. Koivusalo A, Pakarinen MP, Rintala RJ. The cumulative incidence of significant gastrooesophageal reflux in patients with oesophageal atresia with a distal

fistula–a systematic clinical, pH-metric, and endoscopic follow-up study. J Pediatr Surg 2007;42(2):370–4.

65. Sistonen SJ, Pakarinen MP, Rintala RJ. Long-term results of esophageal atresia: Helsinki experience and review of literature. Pediatr Surg Int 2011;27(11):1141–9.

66. Sistonen SJ, Koivusalo A, Nieminen U, et al. Esophageal morbidity and function in adults with repaired esophageal atresia with tracheoesophageal fistula: a population-based long-term follow-up. Ann Surg 2010;251(6):1167–73.

67. Friedmacher F, Kroneis B, Huber-Zeyringer A, et al. Postoperative Complications and Functional Outcome after Esophageal Atresia Repair: Results from Longitudinal Single-Center Follow-Up. J Gastrointest Surg 2017;21(6):927–35.

68. Cheng W, Poon KH, Lui VC, et al. Esophageal atresia and achalasialike esophageal dysmotility. J Pediatr Surg 2004;39(10):1581–3.

69. Shawyer AC, D'Souza J, Pemberton J, et al. The management of postoperative reflux in congenital esophageal atresia-tracheoesophageal fistula: a systematic review. Pediatr Surg Int 2014;30(10):987–96.

70. Glen P, Chasse M, Doyle MA, et al. Partial versus complete fundoplication for the correction of pediatric GERD: a systematic review and meta-analysis. PLoS One 2014;9(11):e112417.

71. Schneider A, Michaud L, Gottrand F. Prevalence of Barrett Esophagus in Adolescents and Young Adults With Esophageal Atresia. Ann Surg 2017;266(6):e96.

72. Tullie L, Kelay A, Bethell GS, et al. Barrett's oesophagus and oesophageal cancer following oesophageal atresia repair: a systematic review. BJS Open 2021;5(4):zrab069.

73. Taylor AC, Breen KJ, Auldist A, et al. Gastroesophageal reflux and related pathology in adults who were born with esophageal atresia: a long-term follow-up study. Clin Gastroenterol Hepatol 2007;5(6):702–6.

74. Gibreel W, Zendejas B, Antiel RM, et al. Swallowing Dysfunction and Quality of Life in Adults With Surgically Corrected Esophageal Atresia/Tracheoesophageal Fistula as Infants: Forty Years of Follow-up. Ann Surg 2017;266(2):305–10.

75. Acher CW, Ostlie DJ, Leys CM, et al. Long-Term Outcomes of Patients with Tracheoesophageal Fistula/Esophageal Atresia: Survey Results from Tracheoesophageal Fistula/Esophageal Atresia Online Communities. Eur J Pediatr Surg 2016;26(6):476–80.

76. Shah AR, Lazar EL, Atlas AB. Tracheal diverticula after tracheoesophageal fistula repair: case series and review of the literature. J Pediatr Surg 2009;44(11):2107–11.

77. Mishra PR, Tinawi GK, Stringer MD. Scoliosis after thoracotomy repair of esophageal atresia: a systematic review. Pediatr Surg Int 2020;36(7):755–61.

78. Chetcuti P, Myers NA, Phelan PD, et al. Chest wall deformity in patients with repaired esophageal atresia. J Pediatr Surg 1989;24(3):244–7.

79. Cherup LL, Siewers RD, Futrell JW. Breast and pectoral muscle maldevelopment after anterolateral and posterolateral thoracotomies in children. Ann Thorac Surg 1986;41(5):492–7.

80. Lawal TA, Gosemann JH, Kuebler JF, et al. Thoracoscopy versus thoracotomy improves midterm musculoskeletal status and cosmesis in infants and children. Ann Thorac Surg 2009;87(1):224–8.

81. Laberge JM, Blair GK. Thoracotomy for repair of esophageal atresia: not as bad as they want you to think. Dis Esophagus 2013;26(4):365–71.

82. Rothenberg SS. Thoracoscopic repair of esophageal atresia and tracheoesophageal fistula in neonates, first decade's experience. Dis Esophagus 2013;26(4):359–64.

83. Zhang J, Wu Q, Chen L, et al. Clinical analysis of surgery for type III esophageal atresia via thoracoscopy: a study of a Chinese single-center experience. J Cardiothorac Surg 2020;15(1):55.
84. Spitz L, Kiely EM, Morecroft JA, et al. Oesophageal atresia: at-risk groups for the 1990s. J Pediatr Surg 1994;29(6):723–5.
85. Yamoto M, Nomura A, Fukumoto K, et al. New prognostic classification and managements in infants with esophageal atresia. Pediatr Surg Int 2018;34(10):1019–26.
86. Wang B, Tashiro J, Allan BJ, et al. A nationwide analysis of clinical outcomes among newborns with esophageal atresia and tracheoesophageal fistulas in the United States. J Surg Res 2014;190(2):604–12.
87. Dellenmark-Blom M, Chaplin JE, Gatzinsky V, et al. Health-related quality of life among children, young people and adults with esophageal atresia: a review of the literature and recommendations for future research. Qual Life Res 2015; 24(10):2433–45.

Pediatric Ingestions

Torbjorg Holtestaul, MD[a], Jace Franko, MD[a],
Mauricio A. Escobar Jr, MD[b], Meade Barlow, MD[b],*

KEYWORDS

- Foreign body • Ingestion • Caustic ingestion • Aspiration • Button batteries
- Magnet ingestion

KEY POINTS

- The evaluation and management of foreign body ingestions is determined by the type of object ingested, its location in the gastrointestinal tract, and the presence of symptoms.
- Button batteries are among the most dangerous objects ingested, as mucosal damage can occur in minutes and lead to devastating complications, such as aortoesophageal fistula.
- While an ingested single magnet can be treated like any other blunt object, the ingestion of multiple magnets may require surgical intervention as apposition within the gastrointestinal tract can lead to fistulas, perforation, and peritonitis.
- The management of caustic ingestion is dependent on the extent of mucosal injury and the development of post-ingestion stricture.
- Airway foreign bodies are common and should be removed promptly via rigid bronchoscopy.

PEDIATRIC INGESTIONS

Pediatric ingestions encompass a wide range of diseases, including foreign body ingestions, caustic ingestions, and aspiration. In this article, we will briefly touch on all of these topics, including epidemiology, evaluation, and management of each pathology. Specific topics of interest in the pediatric age group are button batteries and magnets, which have significant morbidity and mortality and require a high index of suspicion to provide timely care. Adult general surgeons may be called upon to assist in the management of these patients in resource-constrained environments. Additional ingestions that will not be covered but deserve mention are superabsorbent objects and food impactions, which are outside the scope of this article.

---

[a] General Surgery, Madigan Army Medical Center, 9040A Jackson Avenue, Joint Base Lewis-McChord, WA 98431, USA; [b] Pediatric Surgery & Pediatric Trauma, Mary Bridge Children's Hospital & Health Network, PO Box 5299, MS: 311-W2-SUR, Tacoma, WA 98415, USA
* Corresponding author. Pediatric Surgery & Pediatric Trauma, Mary Bridge Children's Hospital & Health Network, PO Box 5299, MS: 311-W2-SUR, Tacoma, WA 98415.
E-mail address: meade.barlow@multicare.org

Surg Clin N Am 102 (2022) 779–795
https://doi.org/10.1016/j.suc.2022.07.009
0039-6109/22/© 2022 Elsevier Inc. All rights reserved.

Children who are less than or equal to 5 years make up 42.8% of exposures reported to a poison control center, with ingestion compromising 83% of all human exposure cases.[1] The vast majority of these are accidental, as young children learn to explore their environments with their mouths. Accordingly, 1-year-old children suffer the highest rates of poison exposure. The top five most common substances involved in poison exposures in children less than or equal to 5 years are cosmetics/personal care products (11%), household cleaning substances (11%), analgesics (9%), foreign bodies/toys (7%), and dietary supplements (5%). The top five most common substances involved in fatal exposures in this age group are fumes/gases/vapors (28%), unknown drugs (10%), analgesics (8%), batteries (8%), and anesthetics (5%).[1]

FOREIGN BODY INGESTIONS
Background

As most have witnessed at one point or another, young children will put anything and everything into their mouths. This sensory exploration, while important for development, can lead to potentially dangerous ingestion. A broad spectrum of both blunt and sharp objects can make their way into a child's gastrointestinal (GI) tract, including but not limited to coins, small toys, batteries, magnets, drug packets, safety pins, nails, hairbrush bristles, pine needles, toothpicks, and fish bones, to name a few.[2] The evaluation and management of these ingestions is determined by the type of object ingested, its location in the GI tract, and the presence of symptoms. Throughout the initial evaluation, it is important to distinguish between ingestion and aspiration.

Evaluation and Management

History and physical
When a child presents with a foreign body ingestion, important aspects of the history to elicit include the object ingested, the time since ingestion, and any symptoms the child has experienced. Children may be completely asymptomatic but present with a caretaker-observed ingestion. Blunt foreign bodies can present with vomiting, drooling, fussiness, chest pain, abdominal pain, fever, poor PO intake, dysphagia, odynophagia, cough, stridor, choking, or other respiratory symptoms. Sharp objects may present with similar symptoms, in particular pain, choking, gagging, dysphagia, odynophagia, or drooling.[3,4] This history can also help determine the possible location of the foreign body; for example, esophageal foreign bodies may present with signs of upper GI obstruction, such as vomiting, drooling, dysphagia, a globus sensation, or retrosternal pain.

A focused physical examination should include a close evaluation of the neck, chest, and abdomen. The neck should be inspected for any signs of perforation, including cervical crepitus, pneumomediastinum, or a full neck.[5] The abdomen should be inspected for any signs of peritonitis to suggest obstruction, perforation, or compromised bowel.

Radiographic studies
All children with suspected foreign body ingestion should undergo an X-ray evaluation, even if they are completely asymptomatic.[4] Anteroposterior and lateral radiographs of the neck, chest, abdomen, and pelvis should be obtained and evaluated for location, size, shape, and number of ingested foreign bodies. It is important to distinguish on the radiograph between ingested and aspirated objects. As will be discussed later, it is also imperative to distinguish between coins and button batteries, which can be identified via a double halo and/or step-off sign (**Fig. 1**). A computed tomography (CT) scan may be required to identify radiolucent foreign bodies, such as fish bones,

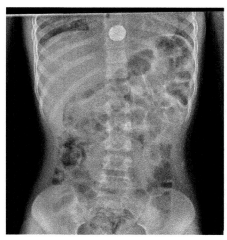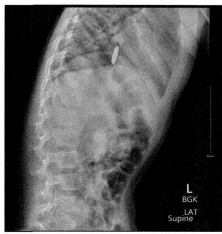

Fig. 1. AP and lateral radiographs of an ingested button battery demonstrating a subtle double-halo sign (AP view) and more obvious step-off sign (lateral view) with the negative anode facing posterior.

wood, plastic, or thin metal objects.[4] In cases where there is a high suspicion of ingestion (eg, a witnessed symptomatic ingestion), it is possible to forego CT for a diagnostic esophagoscopy or to use a lower radiation protocol. It is also critical to evaluate for free or mediastinal air on any acquired imaging. While oral contrast agents can be helpful, the authors recommend against their use in cases of suspected ingestion as they can compromise endoscopy and place the patient at risk for aspiration.[4]

Management
While the majority of foreign bodies (80%) will pass without the need for intervention, there are specific circumstances which require endoscopic or even surgical removal.[4] On initial presentation, it is necessary to ensure the child's airway is protected. For example, if the child is unable to swallow its secretions, then the child is at risk for aspiration and may require intubation. In general, airway protection with endotracheal intubation should be strongly considered during any foreign body removal.

Indications for endoscopy depend on whether the foreign body is blunt or sharp, the location of the ingested object, and the patient's symptoms. In general, endoscopic removal should be performed under general anesthesia in a child-friendly setting. The endoscope type should depend on the child's weight and age; a ≤6 mm endoscope should be used in children less than 10 kg or less than 1 year.[4]

Both the North American Society for Pediatric Gastroenterology, Hepatology and Nutrition (NASPGHAN) and the European Society of Gastrointestinal Endoscopy and European Society for Pediatric Gastroenterology, Hepatology and Nutrition (ESGE/ESPGHAN) have developed excellent guidelines for the endoscopic treatment of ingested foreign bodies in children.[3,4]

Blunt objects. Blunt foreign bodies (including coins and impacted food) in the esophagus should be removed urgently (within 24 hours) even if the child is asymptomatic. If the child is symptomatic, unable to manage its secretions, has respiratory symptoms, or has ingested a button battery, then endoscopic removal should be performed emergently (within 2 hours). The esophagus should be inspected after removal for any signs of mucosal injury.[3,4]

Blunt foreign bodies should be removed from the stomach or duodenum if the child is symptomatic or if the object is greater than 2.5 cm in diameter or greater than 6 cm in length. Long or large objects may have trouble passing through the pylorus, the c-sweep of the duodenum, or the ileocecal valve. If the child is asymptomatic and the object is smaller than the specified dimensions, then the object can be followed with serial X-rays and retrieved if it does not pass after 4 weeks. If at any time the patient becomes symptomatic, then the object should be removed.[3,4] Regardless of location, any sign of obstruction or perforation should prompt surgical consideration for possible exploration.

Sharp objects. The management of sharp ingested objects generally follows Jackson's axiom: "advancing points puncture, trailing do not." (Dr. Chevalier Jackson was a laryngologist and pioneer endoscopist in the late nineteenth and early twentieth centuries who collected over 2000 ingested or aspirated objects retrieved from patients).[6] The most common sharp items requiring removal from children include toothpicks and fish bones.[3] The concern for GI perforation by a sharp foreign body is highest in the ileocecal region, although it has also been reported in the esophagus, pylorus, duodenum, and colon.[3] Complications are highest in patients who are asymptomatic or have a delay in diagnosis of over 48 hours. Those with delayed presentation can suffer from intestinal perforation, extraluminal migration, abscess, peritonitis, or fistula formation.[3]

Any sharp foreign body in the esophagus should be removed urgently. During endoscopy, if the sharp end of the object is positioned cephalad, then one can consider pushing the object into the stomach and subsequently removing the object with the blunt end cephalad. Any sharp object in the stomach should be considered for endoscopic removal unless it is a short object with a heavier blunt end. If the object is distal to the ligament of Treitz and the patient is asymptomatic, the object should be followed clinically with serial X-rays as an inpatient. If the object fails to pass after 3 days or if the patient becomes symptomatic at any time, the object should be removed via enteroscopy or surgical removal.[3]

Button Batteries

Background

One of the most dangerous household items a child can ingest is a button battery, and prompt recognition and management is essential to minimize morbidity and mortality. As soon as the battery is ingested, the clock starts ticking, as mucosal damage can occur in as little as 15 minutes.[7] The most feared complication of button battery ingestion is aortoesophageal fistula (AEF), which results in massive hemorrhage and rapid clinical deterioration with potential demise.

The morbidity and mortality of button battery ingestion have significantly increased in the last 20 years, which has been associated with the larger diameter (>20 mm) and lithium composition of newer batteries. The larger diameter puts the battery at a higher risk of impaction in the esophagus, and the lithium composition allows for greater voltage delivery. Voltage delivery results in injury on impaction when the mucosa bridges the positive and negative terminals of the battery, creating a circuit. This generates hydroxide radicals in the mucosa, causing caustic injury.[3] In one animal model, an implanted esophageal button battery generated a rise in pH from 7 to 13 at the negative pole within 30 minutes of ingestion and was associated with mucosal necrosis with extension to the outer muscular layer.[7] Even old batteries that can no longer power their intended appliances can create a high enough voltage to induce significant mucosal injury.[8] Injury occurrence is not limited to immediately after ingestion and can be present days to weeks later.[3]

Multiple types of injury related to the mucosal damage caused by button batteries have been reported, to include esophageal perforation, stricture, tracheoesophageal fistula, AEF, vocal cord paralysis, and mediastinitis.[3] While all agree that emergent removal of esophageal button batteries is paramount, subsequent management is somewhat controversial, with limited consensus on post-removal imaging and disposition.

Epidemiology

As many as 90,517 button battery ingestions and 33 deaths have been reported to the National Poison Data System between 1985 and 2019, of which 59,751 (66%) ingestions and 30 (91%) deaths occurred in children less than 6 years old.[9] Button battery ingestions and deleterious consequences have been steadily increasing since 2006, and of 3467 ingestions in 2019, 7% had moderate or major effects or death.[9] Accordingly, there has been increasing discussion of button battery ingestion in the literature, with a sharp rise in publication rate in 2010.[10] The Button Battery Task Force, a multidisciplinary national partnership, was established in 2012 to advocate for education and prevention of button battery ingestions.

The most common intended uses of ingested batteries from 2016 to 2018 included hearing aids (36.5%), games/toys (22%), lights (16.5%), and remote controls (5.4%). Of ingested batteries greater than 20 mm in size, the most common intended uses include remote controls (30.5%), games/toys (17.2%), watches (10.9%), and lights (8.6%).[8]

Evaluation and Management

History and physical

When a child presents with a button battery ingestion, the priority should be mobilizing a multidisciplinary team (anesthesia, gastroenterology, and surgery) to get the child to endoscopy for removal as quickly as possible. In the meantime, a thorough history and physical exam and X-rays should be obtained. Risk factors for severe injury include the child's age, the size of the battery, the timing of ingestion, and the current location of the battery.[11] All ingestions should be reported to the National Battery Ingestion Hotline.

Additional components of the history to elicit from the parents include whether the ingestion was witnessed, if any additional objects were ingested (particularly magnets), and the age of the battery (to determine relative voltage). Presentation can vary widely, from completely asymptomatic to a broad range of symptoms, including airway obstruction or wheezing, drooling, vomiting, dysphagia, poor PO intake, coughing, choking, gagging, fever, or sore throat.[8] A particularly high index of suspicion should be maintained when an otherwise healthy toddler presents with an acute onset of severe hematemesis; one should immediately be concerned about button battery impaction and resultant AEF.[11] In the context of a concerning button battery ingestion, some experts have advocated activating a "level 1 trauma" to quickly organize resources to expeditiously evaluate the patient and promptly intervene.[12]

Radiographic studies

Anteroposterior and lateral X-rays should be obtained immediately. Coins and button batteries can be difficult to distinguish on X-ray, therefore, maintaining a high level of suspicion is essential. A button battery will be present with a double halo (or double contour) sign on anteroposterior views and a step-off sign on lateral views (see **Fig. 1**).[3] The direction of the negative pole, or the more narrow side of the battery (the lower step), will sustain the more severe injury due to the elevation in pH caused by the completed circuit. This can be remembered by the 3Ns mnemonic, "negative, narrow, necrotic."[8] If the magnet is located at the level of the aortic arch, then one should be concerned about the impending development of an AEF. There is no role for cross-sectional imaging before endoscopy, and post-removal imaging is discussed in the following sections.

Management

The National Capital Poison Center Button Battery Ingestion Triage and Treatment Guideline is a critical resource for providers treating children with suspected button battery ingestions (**Fig. 2**).[13] When a button battery ingestion is known or suspected, caregivers should advise the child (if under 12-month old) to drink 10 mL of honey every 10 minutes while rushing to the emergency room.[14] Endoscopic management of ingested button batteries is determined by the location of the battery, the age of the patient, the size of the battery, and the patient's symptoms. In their 2015 Clinical Report on Management of Ingested Foreign Bodies in Children, NASPGHAN provided an algorithm for treatment that is summarized in the recommendations later.[3] ESGE/ESPGHAN guidelines recommend similar indications and timelines for endoscopy.[4]

Esophageal button batteries. Any esophageal button battery should be endoscopically removed within 2 hours of ingestion. This emergent timeframe will almost certainly preclude transfer to another facility. Close coordination with anesthesia should occur, and the patient's NPO status should not prolong intervention. Endoscopy should be performed by the most available and experienced provider capable of performing the procedure. When pediatric endoscopists are not available, general surgeons, adult gastroenterologists, or adult otolaryngologists often possess the necessary experience to emergently retrieve the button battery. The authors recommend performing the removal in the operating room (OR) when possible with the rigid esophagoscope available. However, flexible endoscopy is an acceptable option and more readily falls within the skillset of adult providers. In one series of cases, a goal of arrival to endoscopy within 60 minutes of presentation to the facility is recommended.[11] If there has been a prolonged exposure and adequate resources are available, immediate post-removal angiography should be considered to determine the proximity of mucosal injury to the aorta. If there is any evidence of active bleeding or if the patient is clinically unstable, cardiothoracic surgery team should be immediately notified to be on standby in case of AEF.

On endoscopy, the depth and orientation of the impaction should be noted. In particular, the direction of the negative node should be noted as this will likely be the site of greatest mucosal injury and of potential injury to underlying structures. The battery may be closely adhered to the mucosa and can be difficult to remove. A "rat-tooth" forceps can be useful for grasping the step-off of the battery. If removal is not successful with flexible endoscopy, rigid esophagoscopy may be needed for stronger instrumentation. A less desirable, but acceptable maneuver is to push the battery distally into the stomach. Once in the stomach, refer to the discussion later. After removal, the scope should be reinserted to examine the mucosa (**Fig. 3**). Irrigate areas demonstrating mucosal injury with 50 to 150 mL of 0.25% acetic acid to neutralize the pH of the ingested agent. If the anterior esophageal mucosa is involved, then concern should be heightened for possible vascular or tracheal injury. In such a case, bronchoscopy can also be considered to evaluate airway involvement.[5] The stomach and duodenum should also be evaluated when possible for additional foreign bodies or mucosal injury. If severe mucosal injury is evident and the patient will likely need to remain NPO, passage of a feeding tube should be considered. Stable patients being cared for at adult facilities should be considered for transfer to a pediatric center.

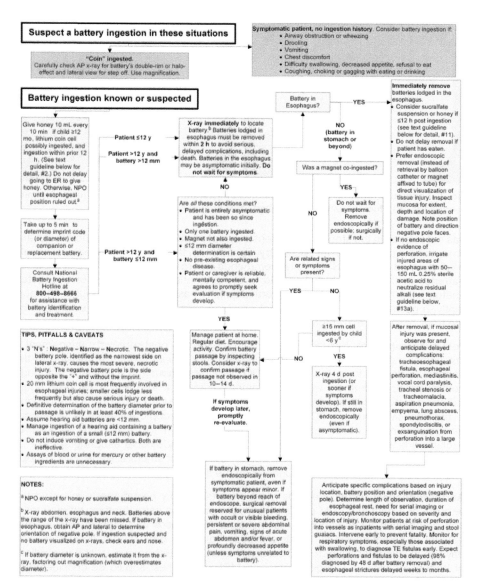

Fig. 2. National capital poison center button battery ingestion triage and treatment guideline.

Gastric button batteries. The removal of button batteries in the stomach is more controversial. NASPGHAN recommends that for any patient who is less than 5 years or with button batteries greater than or equal to 20 mm, endoscopy should be considered for evaluation of any esophageal injury and battery removal. If an asymptomatic patient is more than 5 years of age and/or the ingested battery is less than 20 mm, then outpatient observation can be considered. If outpatient management is elected, then an X-ray should be repeated in 48 hours for a battery greater than or equal to 20 mm. If the battery is less than 20 mm, then an X-ray should be obtained in 10 to 14 days if it

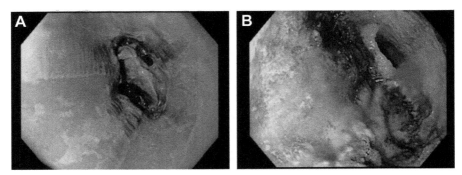

Fig. 3. Endoscopic findings after button battery ingestion. (*A*) Button battery lodged in mid-esophagus. (*B*) Mucosal damage visualized after button battery removal.

has not passed in the stool. If the patient is symptomatic or develops symptoms at any time, or if the battery has not passed by repeat X-ray, then endoscopic removal should be performed.[3] ESGE/ESPGHAN recommends emergent removal (<2 hours) of button batteries in the stomach if the child is symptomatic, has a known or suspected anatomic pathology (eg, Meckel diverticulum), or has swallowed a magnet.[4] Importantly, a gastric foreign body does not preclude esophageal injury, as evidenced by the tragic death of a 16-month-old due to an AEF.[11]

Post-endoscopy care. Similar to gastric button batteries, post-removal management is still somewhat controversial. An esophageal injury should prompt admission to the hospital, orders to keep the patient NPO, and intravenous (IV) antibiotics. Although controversial, the authors would recommend admission for the first 24 to 48 hours following removal with esophageal injury for close monitoring and consider monitoring in the intensive care unit (ICU). In patients with endoscopic evidence of significant mucosal injury, an esophogram should be performed 1 to 7 days after removal to exclude a leak before advancing the child's diet. An additional esophogram in 7 to 14 days should be considered to rule out any evidence of stricture. Repeat endoscopy is generally less useful as it can underestimate the injury to the submucosa.[11]

Aortoesophageal fistula. Perhaps most importantly, any hematemesis following the removal of a battery should prompt the involvement of a cardiothoracic surgery team and preparation for thoracotomy for possible AEF. These can present with a small amount of hematemesis as "sentinel bleeds," and can present in a delayed fashion days to weeks after injury.[11] If esophageal injury is noted on endoscopy (regardless of battery location), CT angiography and MRI of the chest should be considered to exclude aortic injury and determine the proximity of injury to the aorta and airway. If inflammation is noted to extend to the intima of the aorta, pre-emptive surgical management with the involvement of cardiothoracic surgery should be considered. If an injury close to the aorta is found, then an MRI should be performed every 5 to 7 days until the injury is seen to recede.[3] Leinwand et al recommend that it is safe to resume feeding once the esophageal injury is beyond 3 mm from the aorta.

In 1 series of 13 reported pediatric fatalities due to button battery ingestion, 10 were secondary to fatal hemorrhage. The authors of the series designed an algorithm for management of AEFs, both in the scenario of active hemorrhage and a sentinel bleed. For an active hemorrhage, rapid sequence intubation should be performed followed by placement of a Blakemore tube and hemodynamic stabilization with immediate involvement of CT surgery. For a sentinel bleed, large bore IV access should be obtained, CT surgery should be consulted, and a Blakemore brought to the bedside. An X-ray should be obtained to evaluate the location of the battery if it is still present, and if it is not in the esophagus, then a computed tomography angiography should be performed before the child going to the operating room for either endoscopy or thoracotomy if necessary.[15]

MAGNETS
Background

Magnets, in particular neodymium or rare earth magnets, are another example of blunt foreign body ingestion that is an exception to the aforementioned algorithm. Multiple magnet ingestion can be associated with significant morbidity and even mortality as a result of the attraction of two magnets (or a magnet and another metallic foreign body) in distinct locations along the GI tract. This apposition can result in bowel wall necrosis with resultant fistula formation, perforation, obstruction, volvulus, or peritonitis.

The invention and mass distribution of neodymium or rare earth magnets has been associated with an increase in both the incidence and morbidity of magnet ingestion. In 1982, neodymium magnets, which are more than five times stronger than traditional magnets, were invented by General Motors and Sumitomo Special Metals. They have since become ubiquitous in toys, engines, and household appliances.[16] The first reported morbid ingestion of these magnets was in 2002 by McCormick et al.[17] They reported a series of cases of children applying magnets to their nose, penis, and tongue. In the latter case, while trying to emulate a tongue piercing, a 9-year-old girl swallowed the magnets and ultimately suffered from small bowel perforation requiring laparotomy. The advent of desk toys comprised of innumerable small neodymium magnets (such as the buckyball) resulted in the US Consumer Product Safety Commission (CPSC) banning the sale of these products to children in 2009.[16] In 2015, a final rule was published by the CPSC regarding the hazards of these magnets, but this was vacated and remanded by the US Court of Appeals for the Tenth Circuit in 2016.[18] At the time of this article's writing, the topic continues to be debated, with ongoing petitions and responses to and from the CPSC.

Epidemiology

The epidemiology and incidence of magnet ingestion reflect the political turbulence regarding the banning and subsequent reintroduction of these products. A survey of the National Electronic Injury Surveillance System (NEISS) from 2010 to 2015 showed a peak ingestion rate in 2012, with an annual case decrease of 13.3%.[19] In a subsequent review of the NEISS, 23,756 children from 2009 to 2019 presented with suspected magnet ingestion, with an average annual case increase of 6.1%. There was a significant increase in magnet ingestions from 2017 to 2019, following the remanding of the CSPC rule by the federal courts.[20]

Evaluation and Management

The management of a child presenting with magnet ingestion is driven by the presence and acuity of symptoms, the number of foreign bodies ingested, and the location of the magnets within the GI tract. As an increasing number of magnet ingestion cases were reported in the literature, various groups suggested and refined specific algorithms for management.[4,16,21–24] In 2012, NASPGHAN senior leadership developed an algorithm tailored specifically to rare-earth magnet ingestion, which was subsequently incorporated into society's guidelines.[3,16] In 2017, Sola and colleagues published a simplified and elegant algorithm.[23] These are summarized in the management described later.

History and physical

As with all ingestions, the history is a critical portion of the evaluation of a child with an ingested magnet. The critical components include if the ingestion was a witnessed event, the number of suspected ingested foreign bodies (including both magnets and other metallic foreign bodies), the timing of ingestion, and any symptoms the child may have experienced. In one review of children with magnet ingestions, only 39% were symptomatic on presentation, and the most common presenting symptom was abdominal pain. However, 67% of these children had ingested either multiple magnets or a magnet in addition to another metallic foreign body.[23] A physical examination should be performed to rule out peritonitis, which would necessitate immediate surgical intervention. Asymptomatic and minimally symptomatic patients should be transferred to a center with pediatric surgery support. Telephonic consultation with a pediatric surgeon at the receiving facility may help to clarify the need for urgent transfer.

Radiographic studies

All children with suspected ingestion, particularly of magnets, should undergo an abdominal X-ray. If magnets are present in an anteroposterior view, lateral views should be obtained as well. Careful attention should be paid to whether a single magnet or multiple magnets are present.

Treatment

Single magnet. The management of a single magnet ingestion differs significantly from that of multiple magnets or a magnet in the setting of another metallic foreign body. A single magnet can be treated in the same way as any other blunt foreign body ingestion. However, it is hard to be completely sure that the child has only ingested a single magnet. For example, Butterworth and colleagues reported a case of a child who had ingested a magnetic plastic stick from a train set and was discharged for outpatient management. He returned to the hospital in extremis after the plastic coating had eroded and five small magnets were released, ultimately causing jejunal perforation and peritonitis.[22] Children should only be treated in this arm of the algorithm if the magnet ingestion was witnessed, the caregiver is sure that no other objects were ingested, and the radiograph correlates the diagnosis with a single magnet on imaging.

For a single ingested magnet, NASPHAN recommends consulting a pediatric gastroenterologist for consideration of endoscopic removal of magnets within the esophagus or stomach. Alternatively, the patient can be followed with serial X-rays as an outpatient with education of the parents to ensure no further magnetic or metallic objects are nearby for ingestion. Passage should be confirmed on X-ray.[3,16] Sola and colleagues have a similar algorithm: they recommend nonurgent removal of any magnet in the esophagus and otherwise outpatient management of a single ingested magnet with a follow-up abdominal X-ray in 14 days if the magnet has not passed.[23] If the magnet does not progress as expected, a high index of suspicion for undiagnosed multiple magnets should be maintained. Some recommend laxatives or even a colon preparatory solution to encourage passage of the magnet, although there is little evidence to support this practice.

Multiple magnets. The management of multiple magnets (or a single magnet and concomitant ingestion of a metallic foreign body) is more complex given the risk of intestinal complications as discussed earlier. Multiple case series of magnet ingestions have been reported with various rates of endoscopic and surgical intervention.[21,23–25] In one series, the most common location for magnets to be identified was the small intestine or colon (45%), followed by the stomach (42%).

If all foreign bodies are within the stomach or esophagus, a pediatric gastroenterologist should be consulted for removal if the ingestion occurred within 12 hours. If more than 12 hours have passed since ingestion, pediatric surgery should be consulted before endoscopic removal. If the magnets are beyond the stomach and the patient is symptomatic, then surgical removal is indicated. If the patient is asymptomatic and there are no signs of obstruction or perforation on X-ray, then they may be closely followed with serial X-rays for progression. Importantly, children, particularly if they are nonverbal, may have subtle symptoms, and a high index of suspicion for bowel compromise should be maintained. Asymptomatic children may be given a bowel regimen and followed as inpatients with serial X-rays for progression every 8 to 12 hours. If the magnets do not progress within 48 hours, then colonoscopic (if possible) or laparoscopic removal should be performed.[16,21,23]

Surgical procedures. As in most abdominal pathologies, evidence of perforation or peritonitis on examination should prompt surgical exploration. Consequently, most children are safe to undergo transfer to a center with pediatric surgical coverage. However, pediatric patients who present in extremis, evidence of diffuse peritonitis, or free air on imaging studies may not be stable for transfer and necessitate emergent exploration by an available general surgeon. As discussed earlier, a symptomatic child with multiple magnets distal to the stomach or an asymptomatic child with failure of radiographic magnet progression within 48 hours should also undergo surgical removal.

A laparoscopic approach has been described in multiple series, although ultimately the authors recommend that the surgeon proceed with the approach with which they are most comfortable.[23–25] Several techniques of foreign body removal and intestinal repair have been described, including enterotomy with removal and primary repair, small bowel enterectomy with primary anastomosis, wedge resection of the involved stomach, and trans-appendiceal exploration with subsequent appendectomy.[21,23,25] Of note, regardless of the approach to exploration, the bowel should be carefully examined for any areas of necrosis without perforation, which can be subtle but dangerous. The authors recommend that in each of these cases, the entirety of the bowel be inspected carefully as in a trauma patient.

The approach to repair depends on the intraoperative findings; for example, multiple complex fistulas or perforations necessitate a different approach than magnets that have failed to progress but have not compromised the bowel integrity. In the latter case, the trans-appendiceal technique is a particular favorite of the authors. With this technique, the magnets can be brought to the appendix with the assistance of metallic laparoscopic instruments for apposition. Once they are intraluminal, an appendectomy is performed, obviating the need for additional enterotomy or enterectomy (**Fig. 4**). If the magnets are difficult to localize, then fluoroscopy can be a useful intraoperative adjunct.

Caustic Ingestions

Background

Ingestion of caustic agents is a major concern for pediatric emergency room providers with a majority of patients between 1 and 3 years of age. Unfortunately, ingestion of both alkaline and acidic products can result in severe injury with long-term complications. Fortunately, most ingestions by young children are accidental, with the ingested amount being small. Common caustic ingestion products include household cleaning products, most commonly bleach. However, the opposite case is true when caring for adolescents and adults when the ingested volume is large, more commonly

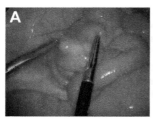
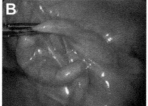
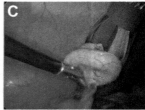

Fig. 4. Laparoscopic removal of multiple magnets via appendectomy. (*A*) Extraluminal manipulation of intraluminal magnets with metal tipped graspers. (*B*) Successful localization of all magnets within appendix. (*C*) Post-appendectomy extraction.

deliberate, and related to suicide attempts. Regardless, appropriate evaluation, workup, treatment, and surveillance are crucial as injury to the oropharynx, esophagus, and stomach can be severe.

Alkali products are more commonly ingested and typically found in household cleaning products, such as drain cleaners and bleach products. They cause liquefactive necrosis as a result of the pH > 11.5.[26,27] Alkali ingestion is generally considered worse as liquefactive necrosis causes transmural damage that may result in esophageal perforation. Acidic compounds are less frequently ingested and are found in some cleaning agents and battery fluids. The mechanism of injury is via coagulative necrosis when the pH is less than 2 and causes more notable injury to the oropharynx as opposed to the esophagus.[28] Most home products have a pH of between 2 and 11, which avoids serious injury to mucosal surfaces.

History and Physical

The initial evaluation is crucial when evaluating patients following ingestions. Questions should seek to obtain information on the timing of exposure, approximate volume ingested, and whether this ingestion was witnessed by a caregiver, as well as the exact brand and substance that was ingested. Often, a caregiver will bring in the container of the ingested solution. The label will provide critical information such as the pH of the ingested substance as well as additional details for when calling the poison control center, which should be performed immediately after initial evaluation of the patient. Presentation varies from completely asymptomatic to drooling, vomiting, chest or abdominal pain, dysphagia, odynophagia, stridor, hoarseness, visible burn injuries to the oral mucosa with erythema, edema, or ulcers, to florid sepsis.

Management

The principles of ATLS should be applied such that if there are concerns for airway protection (eg, stridor, oropharyngeal edema, or hoarseness), early endotracheal intubation for airway protection should be performed. Chemical burn injuries within the GI tract tend to progress and can lead to worsening edema. If the patient is symptomatic, consider a sepsis protocol with bilateral large bore intravenous access, fluid resuscitation, antibiotics and antifungals, proton pump inhibitors, and antiemetics. Neutralizing agents should be avoided, as should blind nasogastric tube placement or agents that could potentially induce vomiting, as this can worsen injuries. Assuming the airway is controlled, most of these children should be stable and undergo transfer to a pediatric center with intensive care, gastroenterology, and surgical support.

The timing of ingestion and patient presentation influence evaluation, but asymptomatic patients without evidence of oropharyngeal injury can be monitored in the emergency department for a short period of time, given an oral diet challenge, and discharged home with close supervision and strict return precautions regarding new or worsening symptoms as damage peaks at 7 to 10 days post-injury.[29,30] However, symptomatic patients should be evaluated with further imaging. Chest radiographs should be the first imaging modality. This can help with assessing for esophageal perforation, but additional abdominal or cervical radiographs may assist with localizing the injury. Even if radiographs are normal, to evaluate for esophageal injury in a patient with high clinical suspicion, a fluoroscopic esophogram with an iso-osmolar water soluble contrast agent should be performed.[31] A proximally placed nasoesophageal tube under fluoroscopy by a trained radiologist may be used for the instillation of contrast if the patient cannot follow instructions. If no leak is identified, immediately repeating the study with thin barium may be considered to increase the sensitivity, but should be weighed against the risk of barium leakage associated with mediastinitis.

If the esophogram is concerning for injury, the patient should undergo upper endoscopy to evaluate the true extent of the injury, which also provides important prognostic information.[32] If only superficial erythema, edema, and/or ulceration are visualized and there is no sepsis, then the patient may be allowed slow diet progression with liquids while monitored in the hospital. If circumferential injury or transmural ulceration with necrosis is present, then the patient should remain NPO with ICU level care before possible diet advancement. Nasogastric tube placement under direct endoscopic vision should be considered as it allows for nutritional support and stents to open the esophagus during the healing phase.[33] Other forms of esophageal stents are not supported in the literature. In patients with severe extensive burns, one may consider gastrostomy tube placement immediately or shortly after initial endoscopy. This tube may be used for feeding and for retrograde dilations of future strictures. If a perforation is identified and the patient is unstable, then operative intervention is required.

The operative approach in unstable patients is similar to that in adults. Key principles include opening the muscle layer to adequately expose the mucosal injury, debriding devitalized tissue, repairing the injury in two layers, buttressing the repair, laying drains, and obtaining distal feeding access. In a high esophageal injury, proximal diversion with cervical esophagostomy may be required. Rarely, esophagogastrectomy may be required, but definitive repair is avoided in the acute setting due to patient instability.

The most common complication is stricture formation, occurring in just over 50% of patients with "deep" or circumferential injuries. Patients should be evaluated for stricture with an esophogram approximately 2 to 3 weeks after ingestion or when obstructive symptoms begin. Most will have symptoms within 2 months.[34–37] Many clinicians wait for 3 to 6 weeks after the initial injury before beginning dilations, as caustic strictures appear to perforate more easily.[38–40] Many different dilators can be used, including standard balloon dilation, but if a gastrostomy tube is present, a Tucker dilator, including a nasogastric string to facilitate passage, can be used for retrograde dilations. This is considered the safest method for esophageal dilation.[33]

The risk of carcinoma after caustic esophageal injury is approximately 2% of the squamous cell type.[41] The American Society for Gastrointestinal Endoscopy recommends beginning endoscopy surveillance 15 to 20 years after ingestion. Any late-onset dysphagia should be promptly evaluated and considered carcinoma until proven otherwise.[31]

Pediatric Aspirations

Background
Foreign body aspiration is a rather common problem, representing 17,500 emergency room visits annually in the United States.[42] It typically presents in patients less than

4 years old with a mortality rate of up to 1.8% and a combined anoxic brain injury/mortality rate of 4%.[42] As such, it is an entity that warrants significant concern by practitioners.

Evaluation and management

Classically, children present with a choking episode, typically after eating or playing, followed by respiratory symptoms such as a cough, stridor, wheezing, or tachypnea. However, the presentation can range from asymptomatic to respiratory collapse, and prompt identification and management are paramount. A focused pulmonary examination should be performed in a setting with ready access to airway management if an aspirated foreign body is suspected.

Typically, the next steps are AP and lateral X-rays of the neck and chest, ideally with inspiratory and expiratory films. Radiopaque foreign bodies are easily identified with this approach, but radiolucent ones can be more subtle. Hyperexpansion on one side of the chest is a frequent finding, but unilateral atelectasis, mediastinal shift, or, not uncommonly, normal films can be seen, and a normal X-ray does not exclude the diagnosis.[43] Scoring systems have been attempted to minimize the incidence of negative bronchoscopy, and recent data have emerged in the utilization of low-dose noncontrast CT to evaluate for radiolucent airway foreign body.[44] In a recent study, CT demonstrated a sensitivity of 100% and a specificity of 98%.[45] The authors recommend this approach in any case of a suspected airway foreign body with diagnostic uncertainty.

Once an airway foreign body has been diagnosed, the patient should be promptly brought to the OR for rigid bronchoscopy for retrieval. In hospitals without pediatric subspecialists, stable patients can be transferred to institutions with pediatric otolaryngology and/or pediatric surgical support. The authors recommend considering use of preoperative inhaled racemic epinephrine in the setting of stridor or IV dexamethasone to manage reactive edema, but the data for this are limited.[46,47] Because of the inherent risks of rigid bronchoscopy (bleeding, laryngospasm, or hypoxia), this should only be performed by a surgeon with adequate experience in these procedures. In addition to pediatric general surgeons and pediatric otolaryngologists, adult cardiothoracic surgeons and adult otolaryngologists often have experience with rigid bronchoscopy. A ventilating bronchoscope should be utilized with spontaneous patient ventilation to avoid propagating the foreign body more distally in the tracheobronchial tree. McGill forceps should be available in the OR. After removal of the offending foreign body, we routinely perform a completion bronchoscopy to confirm there are no additional foreign bodies or pieces to retrieve. For difficult to remove foreign bodies, a Fogarty balloon can be utilized to attempt to retrieve more distally displaced foreign bodies, and a second bronchoscopy can be performed the following day for partially removed foreign bodies.[48] Fluoroscopy can be a useful adjunct for difficult to see foreign bodies, such as sewing needles, to aid in localization and grasping. Chronically impacted distal foreign bodies represent a particular challenge and may require lung resection for removal.

SUMMARY

Pediatric ingestions and aspirations represent a wide variety of challenges to the practitioner. Evaluation and management of these cases should be tailored to the offending agent and managed at an appropriate pediatric center. However, certain emergency situations exist that might preclude transfer and require adult general surgeons to act quickly to rescue a child.

CLINICS CARE POINTS

- The evaluation and management of foreign body ingestions is must be considered against the type of object ingested, the location in the gastrointestinal tract, and the presence of symptoms. Certain ingestions are notoriously dangerous and warrant special consideration.

- Button batteries are among the most dangerous objects ingested, as mucosal damage can occur in minutes and lead to devastating complications such as aortoesophageal fistula. Immediate evaluation with prompt removal should be carried out without delay.

- While a single ingested magnet can be treated like any other blunt object, the ingestion of multiple magnets may need surgical intervention as apposition within the GI tract can lead to fistulas, perforation, and peritonitis.

- The management of caustic ingestions is dependent on the extent of mucosal injury and development of post-ingestion stricture.

- Airway foreign bodies are common and should be removed promptly via rigid bronchoscopy.

DISCLOSURE

The authors have nothing to disclose.

REFERENCES

1. Gummin DD, Mowry JB, Beuhler MC, et al. 2019 Annual report of the American Association of poison control centers' national poison data system (NPDS): 37th annual report. Clin Toxicol Phila Pa 2020;58(12):1360–541.

2. Gurevich Y, Sahn B, Weinstein T. Foreign body ingestion in pediatric patients. Curr Opin Pediatr 2018;30(5):677–82.

3. Kramer RE, Lerner DG, Lin T, et al. Management of ingested foreign bodies in children: a clinical report of the NASPGHAN Endoscopy Committee. J Pediatr Gastroenterol Nutr 2015;60(4):562–74.

4. Thomson M, Tringali A, Dumonceau JM, et al. Paediatric gastrointestinal endoscopy: European society for paediatric gastroenterology hepatology and nutrition and european society of gastrointestinal endoscopy guidelines. J Pediatr Gastroenterol Nutr 2017;64(1):133–53.

5. Esophageal Foreign Bodies | Pediatric Surgery NaT. Available at. https://www.pedsurglibrary.com/apsa/view/Pediatric-Surgery-NaT/829610/all/Esophageal_Foreign_Bodies?refer=true. Accessed January 9, 2022.

6. Schaffer A. Down the hatch and straight into medical history. The New York Times; 2011. Available at: https://www.nytimes.com/2011/01/11/health/11swallow.html. Accessed January 12, 2022.

7. Tanaka J, Yamashita M, Yamashita M, et al. Esophageal electrochemical burns due to button type lithium batteries in dogs. Vet Hum Toxicol 1998;40(4):193–6.

8. Jatana KR, Litovitz T, Reilly JS, et al. Pediatric button battery injuries: 2013 task force update. Int J Pediatr Otorhinolaryngol 2013;77(9):1392–9. https://doi.org/10.1016/j.ijporl.2013.06.006.

9. Button Battery Ingestion Statistics. Available at. https://www.poison.org/battery/stats. Accessed January 11, 2022.

10. Haddad N, Wilson JD, Fard D, et al. Pediatric button battery ingestion: Publication trends in the literature. Am J Otolaryngol 2020;41(3):102401. https://doi.org/10.1016/j.amjoto.2020.102401.

11. Leinwand K, Brumbaugh DE, Kramer RE. Button Battery Ingestion in Children: A Paradigm for Management of Severe Pediatric Foreign Body Ingestions. Gastrointest Endosc Clin N Am 2016;26(1):99–118. https://doi.org/10.1016/j.giec.2015.08.003.

12. Button Battery Ingestion - GlobalCastMD Video Library. Available at. https://videolibrary.globalcastmd.com/button-battery-ingestion. Accessed January 27, 2022.

13. National capital poison center button battery ingestion triage and treatment guidelines. Available at. https://www.poison.org/battery/guideline. Accessed January 12, 2022.

14. Anfang RR, Jatana KR, Linn RL, et al. pH-neutralizing esophageal irrigations as a novel mitigation strategy for button battery injury. Laryngoscope 2019;129(1):49–57. https://doi.org/10.1002/lary.27312.

15. Brumbaugh DE, Colson SB, Sandoval JA, et al. Management of button battery-induced hemorrhage in children. J Pediatr Gastroenterol Nutr 2011;52(5):585–9. https://doi.org/10.1097/MPG.0b013e3181f98916.

16. Hussain SZ, Bousvaros A, Gilger M, et al. Management of ingested magnets in children. J Pediatr Gastroenterol Nutr 2012;55(3):239–42.

17. McCormick S, Brennan P, Yassa J, et al. Children and mini-magnets: an almost fatal attraction. Emerg Med J EMJ 2002;19(1):71–3.

18. Informational briefing package regarding magnet sets.pdf. Available at. https://www.cpsc.gov/s3fs-public/Informational%20Briefing%20Package%20Regarding%20Magnet%20Sets.pdf?FKVcZpHmPKWCZNb7JEl6lr0a31WV72PI. Accessed January 10, 2022.

19. Reeves PT, Nylund CM, Krishnamurthy J, et al. Trends of magnet ingestion in children, an ironic attraction. J Pediatr Gastroenterol Nutr 2018;66(5):e116–21.

20. Reeves PT, Rudolph B, Nylund CM. Magnet ingestions in children presenting to emergency departments in the united states 2009-2019: a problem in flux. J Pediatr Gastroenterol Nutr 2020;71(6):699–703.

21. Han Y, Youn JK, Oh C, et al. Ingestion of multiple magnets in children. J Pediatr Surg 2020;55(10):2201–5.

22. Butterworth J, Feltis B. Toy magnet ingestion in children: revising the algorithm. J Pediatr Surg 2007;42(12):e3–5.

23. Sola R, Rosenfeld EH, Yu YR, et al. Magnet foreign body ingestion: rare occurrence but big consequences. J Pediatr Surg 2018;53(9):1815–9.

24. Waters AM, Teitelbaum DH, Thorne V, et al. Surgical management and morbidity of pediatric magnet ingestions. J Surg Res 2015;199(1):137–40.

25. Strickland M, Rosenfield D, Fecteau A. Magnetic foreign body injuries: a large pediatric hospital experience. J Pediatr 2014;165(2):332–5.

26. Harley EH, Collins MD. Liquid household bleach ingestion in children: a retrospective review. Laryngoscope 1997;107(1):122–5. https://doi.org/10.1097/00005537-199701000-00023.

27. Einhorn A, Horton L, Altieri M, et al. Serious respiratory consequences of detergent ingestions in children. Pediatrics 1989;84(3):472–4.

28. Friedman EM. Caustic ingestions and foreign bodies in the aerodigestive tract of children. Pediatr Clin North Am 1989;36(6):1403–10.

29. Dafoe CS, Ross CA. Acute corrosive oesophagitis. Thorax 1969;24(3):291–4.

30. Johnson EE. A study of corrosive esophagitis. Laryngoscope 1963;73:1651–96.

31. Millar AJW, Cox SG. Caustic injury of the oesophagus. Pediatr Surg Int 2015;31(2):111–21. https://doi.org/10.1007/s00383-014-3642-3.

32. De Lusong MAA, Timbol ABG, Tuazon DJS. Management of esophageal caustic injury. World J Gastrointest Pharmacol Ther 2017;8(2):90–8.
33. Hawkins DB. Dilation of esophageal strictures: comparative morbidity of antegrade and retrograde methods. Ann Otol Rhinol Laryngol 1988;97(5 Pt 1):460–5.
34. Gaudreault P, Parent M, McGuigan MA, et al. Predictability of esophageal injury from signs and symptoms: a study of caustic ingestion in 378 children. Pediatrics 1983;71(5):767–70.
35. Moazam F, Talbert JL, Miller D, et al. Caustic ingestion and its sequelae in children. South Med J 1987;80(2):187–90.
36. Adam JS, Birck HG. Pediatric caustic ingestion. Ann Otol Rhinol Laryngol 1982; 91(6 Pt 1):656–8.
37. Anderson KD, Rouse TM, Randolph JG. A controlled trial of corticosteroids in children with corrosive injury of the esophagus. N Engl J Med 1990;323(10): 637–40.
38. Gumaste VV, Dave PB. Ingestion of corrosive substances by adults. Am J Gastroenterol 1992;87(1):1–5.
39. Keh SM, Onyekwelu N, McManus K, et al. Corrosive injury to upper gastrointestinal tract: Still a major surgical dilemma. World J Gastroenterol 2006;12(32): 5223–8.
40. Karnak I, Tanyel FC, Büyükpamukçu N, et al. Combined use of steroid, antibiotics and early bougienage against stricture formation following caustic esophageal burns. J Cardiovasc Surg (Torino) 1999;40(2):307–10.
41. Kirsh MM, Ritter F. Caustic ingestion and subsequent damage to the oropharyngeal and digestive passages. Ann Thorac Surg 1976;21(1):74–82.
42. Kim IA, Shapiro N, Bhattacharyya N. The national cost burden of bronchial foreign body aspiration in children. Laryngoscope 2015;125(5):1221–4.
43. Gang W, Zhengxia P, Hongbo L, et al. Diagnosis and treatment of tracheobronchial foreign bodies in 1024 children. J Pediatr Surg 2012;47(11):2004–10.
44. Özyüksel G, Arslan UE, Boybeyi-Türer Ö, et al. New scoring system to predict foreign body aspiration in children. J Pediatr Surg 2020;55(8):1663–6. https:// doi.org/10.1016/j.jpedsurg.2019.12.015.
45. Gibbons AT, Casar Berazaluce AM, Hanke RE, et al. Avoiding unnecessary bronchoscopy in children with suspected foreign body aspiration using computed tomography. J Pediatr Surg 2020;55(1):176–81.
46. AuBuchon J, Krucylak C, Murray DJ. Subglottic airway foreign body: a near miss. Anesthesiology 2011;115(6):1300.
47. Tan HK, Tan SS. Inhaled foreign bodies in children–anaesthetic considerations. Singapore Med J 2000;41(10):506–10.
48. Morrow SE, Bickler SW, Kennedy AP, et al. Balloon extraction of esophageal foreign bodies in children. J Pediatr Surg 1998;33(2):266–70.

Common Conditions II
Acute Appendicitis, Intussusception, and Gastrointestinal Bleeding

Patrick N. Nguyen, MD[a], Adam Petchers, MD[a], Sarah Choksi, MD[a],
Mary J. Edwards, MD[b],*

KEYWORDS

- Appendicitis • Intussusception • Gastrointestinal bleeding • Pediatric

APPENDICITIS
Introduction/Background/Prevalence

Acute appendicitis is a common cause of abdominal pain in children. The lifetime risk is estimated to be 8% to 9%, with a peak incidence of 10 to 14 years.[1] As much as 20% to 30% of children presenting with abdominal pain will have acute appendicitis, and about 20% of children with acute appendicitis will present with perforation.[2] Children younger than 4 years have a relatively low incidence of appendicitis, but present rates of perforation in excess of 85%.[3,4] Adult general surgeons usually have the skill set necessary to care for pediatric appendicitis patients. However, institutional experience, anesthesia support, and nursing capability should be considered when adult surgeons consider operating on pediatric patients with appendicitis. There is certainly a host of studies in the literature demonstrating similar outcomes for adult general surgeons when compared with pediatric surgeons in patients with acute appendicitis.

Clinical Evaluation

The classic history of fever, migratory abdominal pain, nausea, vomiting, and anorexia is not sensitive or specific to the disease. Physical examination findings are often nonspecific; therefore, laboratory testing and imaging are frequently required.[5,6] A neutrophil-to-lymphocyte ratio of greater than 3.5 can be suggestive of acute appendicitis. A normal C reactive protein (CRP) is helpful in excluding the diagnosis of appendicitis.[7]

Appendicitis scoring systems integrate clinical and laboratory findings and are helpful in predicting the likelihood of acute appendicitis and identifying which patients benefit from imaging. The Pediatric Appendicitis Score (available at https://www.

[a] General Surgery Division, Albany Medical College, 6th Floor, 50 New Scotland Avenue, Albany, NY 12008, USA; [b] Pediatric Surgery Division, Albany Medical College, 2nd Floor, 50 New Scotland Avenue, Albany, NY 12008, USA
* Corresponding author.
E-mail address: edwardm2@amc.edu

Surg Clin N Am 102 (2022) 797–808
https://doi.org/10.1016/j.suc.2022.07.010
0039-6109/22/© 2022 Elsevier Inc. All rights reserved.
surgical.theclinics.com

mdcalc.com/pediatric-appendicitis-score-pas) is the most established.[8,9] However, utility is limited to preschool children (age <4).[9-11]

Imaging

Computed tomography (CT) scans of the abdomen have long been considered the gold standard for imaging the appendix, with reported sensitivity and specificity of 92% to 97% and 94% to 97%, respectively.[12] CT findings of appendicitis include appendiceal distention greater than 6 mm, appendiceal wall thickening, and peri-appendiceal fat stranding. Intravenous contrast is typically given. Modern scanners acquire images rapidly, so sedation is rarely needed. However, the speed and accuracy of CT must be weighed against the risks of ionizing radiation.

Numerous studies link CT exposure in childhood to malignancy later in life. A recent large cohort study demonstrated a significant increase in leukemia risk for patients who underwent CT scanning before appendectomy as opposed to those who did not.[13] Although increased risk was seen at all ages, it was most significant for patients who were 0 to 15 years old. There was no increased risk of solid organ malignancies, but the study was limited by a follow-up of only 2 to 10 years.

Ultrasound has emerged as the initial imaging modality of choice for children with abdominal pain. Ultrasound findings suggestive of acute appendicitis include an enlarged appendix greater than 6 mm, wall thickening, and noncompressibility. Secondary signs of appendicitis, such as echogenic fat, free fluid, or right lower quadrant phlegmon, can improve sensitivity.[14] Specificity is typically reported to be around 90%, with sensitivity ranging from 85% to 90%.[15] Body habitus, variable anatomy, and sonographer experience significantly impact the sensitivity of ultrasound.[12] Unfortunately, the study can frequently fail to identify the appendix or be interpreted as equivocal in up to 64% of pediatric patients.[16] Often, failure to see the appendix on ultrasound is because of the fact that it is normal. In such cases, clinical observation or cross-sectional imaging with CT or MRI should be considered.

MRI is becoming increasingly useful in the evaluation of pediatric appendicitis. It is a relatively rapid study that offers three-dimensional anatomic detail without radiation or the need for intravenous contrast.[17] Findings suggestive of acute appendicitis are similar to those of CT and ultrasound. However, peri-appendiceal edema on MRI is particularly sensitive and specific for appendicitis.[18] Unfortunately, many institutions lack immediate access to a scanner, which can delay diagnosis.[16] This, and expense, limits its utility as a primary imaging modality. However it has utility in cases where ultrasound is equivocal.[19] A recent study demonstrated that MRI utilized in this capacity provided a sensitivity and specificity of 96% and 98.9%, respectively.[16,20]

Uncomplicated Acute Appendicitis

Operative management

For children with uncomplicated appendicitis, laparoscopic appendectomy is the most expeditious and effective treatment. A 12 to 36 hour delay to appendectomy will not increase rates of surgical site infections, early obstruction, mortality, or perforation as long as the patient receives antibiotics at the time of diagnosis.[21,22] Rates of wound infection and postoperative ileus are lower with laparoscopy compared with open appendectomy.[23,24] Postoperative antibiotics are not indicated. Preoperative antibiotics should be given within 18 to 70 minutes before incision.[25] Institutions adopting protocols for discharge home from the recovery room have not seen increased rates of readmission, clinic visits, or surgical site infections.[26-28] Opioids are rarely required postoperatively and children are discharged on non steroidal anti-inflammatory drugs (NSAIDs) alone.[29,30]

Nonoperative management

Nonoperative management (NOM) of uncomplicated appendicitis is an alternate treatment option. The prospective Non-Operative Treatment for Acute Appendicitis trial proved the short-term feasibility of NOM of uncomplicated appendicitis in patients 14 years and older. This was followed up with several smaller randomized trials in younger children.[31–34] All demonstrate NOM to be safe and 90% effective in most children with rare progression to perforation.[35] Retrospective studies suggest the presence of an appendicolith (fecalith) increases the likelihood of recurrent disease, leading some to consider it a relative contraindication to NOM. Long-term outcomes of NOM are complicated by variable rates of recurrent appendicitis. In one study, 49% of children treated nonoperatively had undergone appendectomy at a 5-year follow-up, most within the first year. Of these, only 17% had histologically confirmed appendicitis,[36] suggesting that patient and parent anxiety regarding potential recurrence plays a significant role in long-term failure.

Complicated Acute Appendicitis

Operative versus nonoperative management

Optimal management of pediatric complicated acute appendicitis is debated. In patients presenting with sepsis and generalized peritonitis, immediate antibiotic administration, fluid resuscitation, and early surgery for source control are indicated. In stable patients with well-localized infection and prolonged symptom duration, NOM, with or without interval appendectomy, may be preferable.[36,37]

Numerous studies suggest early operative management benefits patients when symptom duration is less than 5 days.[38,39] However, these patients are at high risk for postoperative complications, particularly ileus and abscess formation, which complicate treatment in up to 20% of children.[40] Of note, large volume intraoperative peritoneal irrigation has not demonstrated a reduction in this risk.[41]

The optimal duration and spectrum of postoperative antibiotic coverage balances surgical site infection and postoperative abscess prevention with antibiotic stewardship and side effect risk. Limiting intravenous antibiotics to 1 to 2 days, even in patients who recover rapidly, demonstrates an increased rate of skin and surgical site infection (SSI).[25] Discharge on oral antibiotics has not proven beneficial in most studies.[42–44] Most institution-specific pathways integrate clinical data and interval imaging for abscesses to determine antibiotic duration, as opposed to a predetermined duration of days. Such practices have proven safe and effective with regard to infection prevention and readmission rates.[45,46] The ideal period for interval imaging seems to be on postoperative days 6 to 7, since early CT scans (before days 6 and 7) can lead to recurrent CT scans, more radiation exposure, and nontherapeutic drainage procedures.[47,48]

Early small bowel obstructions complicate 1.2% of cases of perforated appendicitis and may be difficult to distinguish from prolonged ileus. Timing of intervention is controversial and must balance the success of NOM with the complications of parenteral nutrition and prolonged length of stay.[49]

Nonoperative management

NOM of appendicitis with intravenous antibiotics and, when needed, image-guided percutaneous abscess drainage can avoid early surgery and its potential complications. However, it can result in higher rates of imaging and, when combined with interval appendectomy, longer cumulative days in the hospital.[37,38,50,51]

The need for interval appendectomy in pediatric patients is controversial. The incidence of recurrent appendicitis after NOM in complicated appendicitis is not well quantified. Given a 3% complication rate of interval appendectomy, further study is needed to determine if it should routinely be offered. Nonetheless, it is often performed.[37,38,50]

Antibiotic Choice

Multiple studies show that narrow-spectrum antibiotic regimens (eg, ceftriaxone and flagyl) have the same SSI rates as broad-spectrum antibiotics in both simple and complicated appendicitis.[46,52,53] However, a recent multi-institutional study suggests monotherapy with piperacillin/tazobactam may be superior.[54] Local antimicrobiograms should be referenced when selecting antibiotics for institutional protocols because resistance can shift first-line antibiotic choices.[55]

INTUSSUSCEPTION
Introduction

Intussusception is the invagination of a segment of bowel into adjacent bowel. Intussusception of the terminal ileum into the ascending colon usually results in obstruction and requires intervention. Overall, the prevalence of ileocolic intussusception is 0.3 to 0.5 per 1000 and most commonly occurs between 6 months and 2 years old.[56] Patients over the age of 5 years or patients with more than two episodes of intussusception should be evaluated for a pathologic lead point.[57,58]

Clinical evaluation

The classic triad of currant jelly stools, abdominal pain, and vomiting is present in less than 20% of children with intussusception. As abdominal pain and vomiting alone are nonspecific symptoms, early ultrasound should be considered in patients in the appropriate age group.[59,60] Ultrasound has a sensitivity and specificity of more than 97% for detecting ileocolic intussusception.[61]

Nonsurgical treatment

Initial management should include intravenous fluid resuscitation and prompt referral for image-guided reduction. In the absence of peritonitis, prophylactic antibiotics are not indicated.[62] Reduction is most commonly done with air under fluoroscopic guidance, although ultrasound guided hydrostatic reduction is becoming more common as it avoids radiation.[63] In select centers, ultrasound guided pneumatic reduction is also done.[64]

If image-guided reduction fails, it is safe to reattempt at least three times as long as progress is demonstrated with each attempt and the child is stable. The failure rate is nearly 100% after four unsuccessful attempts.[65] A delay of 30 minutes to 4 hours between reduction attempts may improve the likelihood of success of subsequent attempts.[62] Perforation is a rare complication, but when this occurs, rapid needle decompression of the abdomen is often needed to evacuate insufflated air.[66] This simple maneuver can typically be done by a pediatric radiologist. Therefore, routine surgeon presence at reductions is not necessary.[62] Reduction under sedation does not increase the risk of perforation and may increase the chance of successful reduction.[67] However, this practice carries the inherent risks of sedation in the face of bowel obstruction, and due to equipment and personnel requirements, may delay reduction attempts.[68]

Most well appearing children can be discharged home after a brief period of observation (4 hours) following successful reduction. Oral intake may be given without confirmatory imaging to prove reduction.[62,69] Recurrence rates within 48 hours are approximately 2.5%, and therefore, routine admission is not necessary in most cases.[70]

Surgical treatment

Children with evidence of bowel perforation or necrosis require immediate surgery. If a pathologic lead point is identified on imaging, then surgery is also required. Finally, if repeated attempts at radiologic reduction are unsuccessful, then operative treatment is indicated.

Laparoscopy is usually the preferred operative approach, with less pain and a shorter hospital stay when compared with an open surgery.[71] The small bowel is reduced through the application of continuous pressure on the distal end intussusceptible within the colon. Traction on the small bowel should be avoided. Indications to convert to an open procedure include inadequate visualization, unsuccessful reduction, evidence of ischemia, perforation, or a pathologic lead point requiring resection.[72] If the bowel cannot be reduced with an open manual attempt, then resection should be done. In the case of successful operative reduction, appendectomy should not be routinely performed if the appendix seems healthy.[62] Ileopexy or cecopexy are not routinely recommended.[73]

Small bowel and small bowel intussusceptions are frequent incidental findings on ultrasound.[74] These are usually transient and spontaneously reduced. If less than 2.5 cm, without proximal dilation, lead point or colon involvement, small bowel-small bowel intussusception should be viewed as a benign, self-limiting entity, and patients should not undergo further imaging or workup for a pathologic lead point.[75] Patients with persistent obstruction, polyposis syndromes, or Henoch–Schönlein purpura may require surgical reduction.

Evaluation of outcome and/or long-term recommendations

Thirty-day recurrence with nonoperative reduction is 2.5%, and 0.7% with operative reduction without bowel resection. This increases by another 3.7% and 2.3%, respectively, at 1 year. Recurrence is 0% with bowel resection.[70,76] Recurrence is typically idiopathic and further workup for a pathologic lead point is not typically considered until the third recurrence. The most common pathologic lead point is a Meckel's diverticulum. In older children, lymphoma should also be considered.[58]

GASTROINTESTINAL BLEED

Gastrointestinal (GI) bleeding in children has a variety of causes and an overall incidence of about 6%.[77] Symptoms are usually mild. About 11% of these patients require hospitalization.[78]

As with all bleeding patients, the first step is clinical evaluation and, if needed, stabilization and resuscitation. A complete history and physical examination will typically generate a diagnosis. Important aspects of the history include the duration, amount, and color of bleeding. A physical examination should include an evaluation of the nose and mouth for a source of swallowed blood, an abdominal examination assessing for pain, masses, and peritonitis, and a rectal examination looking for fissures or polyps. A general skin examination should also be performed to look for other signs of coagulopathy, including petechiae or bruising.

Although the differential diagnosis for GI bleed is broad, the most common conditions are as follows (**Table 1**):

Neonates

In the neonate, swallowed maternal blood is common and rapidly diagnosed with an Apt test. Midgut volvulus occurs when the bowel twists around the root of its mesentery, causing ischemia.[79] This can occasionally be associated with lower GI bleeding. The diagnosis is made by an upper GI contrast study showing abnormal rotation. This

Table 1 Differential Diagonsis for Pediatric Gastrointestinal Bleeding	
Neonatal	Swallowed maternal blood, fissures, necrotizing enterocolitis, midgut volvulus
Infant	Foreign body, peptic ulcer, anal fissure, intussusception, Meckel's diverticulum, infectious, allergic colitis, juvenile polyps
School age	Peptic ulcer, juvenile polyps, inflammatory bowel disease, Henoch–Schönlein purpura, hemolytic uremic syndrome, malignancy, infectious

is a surgical emergency. Necrotizing enterocolitis can also cause GI bleeding in a neonate. Treatment is typically medical, but surgery may be required.

Peptic ulcer disease

Peptic ulcer disease is unusual in children, and is rarely seen in the absence of a predisposing condition, such as chronic NSAID use, *Helicobacter pylori*, corticosteroid use, or stress from trauma/surgery/burns.[80]

Diagnosis of upper GI bleeding from peptic ulcer disease is made endoscopically. Treatment is medical with resuscitation, administration of a proton pump inhibitor, and antibiotics for *H pylori*. For active bleeding, endoscopic control is typically successful. Percutaneous embolization and, finally, surgery are options in refractory cases. Surgical ligation of the bleeding source, local ulcer closure or resection is enough. Formal acid suppressing surgeries should not be routinely done.[81]

Meckel's diverticulum

Meckel's diverticulum is the most common cause of profuse, painless lower GI bleeding in toddlers. Gastric heterotopia leads to acid secretion and mucosal ulceration in the adjacent small intestine. The overall incidence of Meckel's diverticulum is about 2% with ~20% of them containing gastric mucosa.[82]

A diagnosis of a bleeding Meckel's diverticulum can be confirmed with a Technetium 99 scan. While sensitivity is low in adults, in children it is 85% to 98% with very high specificity.[82,83] The sensitivity is improved with the administration of famotidine. In clinically suspicious cases, a negative scan should not preclude laparoscopy for definitive diagnosis.

Bleeding Meckel's diverticulum requires surgical excision to remove gastric heterotopic tissue. A retrospective review in 2017 found diverticulectomy alone eradicates gastric heterotopic mucosa, stops bleeding, and shortens hospital stay compared with segmental small bowel resection.[84] A multi-institution retrospective review in 2018 also demonstrated that diverticulectomy, either open or laparoscopic, is an adequate treatment for bleeding Meckel's diverticulum.[85]

Anal fissure

As with adults, an anal fissure is a tear in the epithelium of the anal canal, usually in the posterior or anterior midline. Children and infants present with painful defecation and rectal bleeding.[86] The diagnosis is easily confirmed by physical examination. There may be an associated skin tag with hypertrophied papilla on the external aspect of the fissure.[86]

Medical treatment alone is sufficient, even in chronic cases, starting with treatment of constipation. In newborns, this may involve formula change; in older children, adequate fluid intake and fiber. Stool softeners, such as polyethylene glycol or lactulose, are often given.[86] In refractory cases, topical 2.5% glyceryl trinitrate (GTN) may be used. In randomized trials, GTN decreases the resting pressure of the anal sphincter and promotes healing.[86,87] Topical calcium channel blockers have not shown similar efficacy in children but are also utilized.[88] Headaches are a common side effect.

The final option, in severe cases, is botulinum toxin injection into the internal sphincter. The toxin works by acting as an inhibitory neurotransmitter to relax the anal sphincter for 2 to 3 months to allow healing. There are limited studies looking at its effectiveness in children in the last 5 years.[86] Although lateral internal sphincterotomy is used regularly to treat chronic anal fissures in adults, it is rarely used in the pediatric population.

Juvenile polyps

Intermittent lower GI bleeding in children can be secondary to juvenile polyps. These are hamartomas typically located in the sigmoid and rectum.[89] Solitary juvenile polyps are benign and can be removed endoscopically without requiring follow-up. However, the autosomal dominant juvenile polyposis syndrome presents with hamartomatous lesions throughout the GI tract and carries an increased risk of developing colon and gastric cancer.[90] Therefore, if two or three juvenile polyps are found on endoscopy, a repeat colonoscopy should be performed within 5 years, or sooner for recurrent bleeding. For juvenile polyposis syndrome, polyps greater than 10 mm should be removed with polypectomy and colonoscopy should be repeated every 1 to 5 years.[90]

CLINICS CARE POINTS

- Ultrasound should be the initial imaging study for pediatric appendicitis. Cross-sectional imaging (computed tomography and MRI) is indicated when ultrasound is nondiagnostic.

- Surgery for uncomplicated appendicitis is typically straightforward and most patients can be discharged from the recovery room safely.

- Optimal treatment of perforated appendicitis may be surgical or medical depending on the clinical presentation of the patient and findings on imaging.

- Ultrasound is the imaging study of choice for suspected intussusception.

- If radiologic reduction of intussusception fails, then additional attempts can be considered before surgery.

- Anal fissures are a common cause of minor lower gastrointestinal (GI) bleeding in infants and toddlers. Treatment of constipation is typically all that is needed.

- Painless, profuse lower GI bleeding in a toddler is a Meckel's diverticulum until proven otherwise. This can usually be diagnosed by technetium scintigraphy, but if not, laparoscopy should be considered. Diverticulectomy is all that is typically required.

DISCLOSURE

The authors have nothing to disclose.

REFERENCES

1. Rentea RM, Peter SDSt, Snyder CL. Pediatric appendicitis: state of the art review. Pediatr Surg Int 2017;33(3):269–83.
2. Cheong LHA, Emil S. Outcomes of Pediatric Appendicitis: An International Comparison of the United States and Canada. JAMA Surg 2014;149(1):50.

3. Addiss DG, Shaffer N, Fowler BS, et al. THE EPIDEMIOLOGY OF APPENDICITIS AND APPENDECTOMY IN THE UNITED STATES. Am J Epidemiol 1990;132(5): 910–25.

4. Levin DE, Pegoli W. Abscess After Appendectomy. Adv Surg 2015;49(1):263–80.

5. Bundy DG, Byerley JS, Liles EA, et al. Does This Child Have Appendicitis? JAMA 2007;298(4):438–51.

6. Benabbas R, Hanna M, Shah J, et al. Diagnostic Accuracy of History, Physical Examination, Laboratory Tests, and Point-of-care Ultrasound for Pediatric Acute Appendicitis in the Emergency Department: A Systematic Review and Meta-analysis. Acad Emerg Med 2017;24(5):523–51.

7. Zouari M, Jallouli M, Louati H, et al. Predictive value of C-reactive protein, ultrasound and Alvarado score in acute appendicitis: a prospective pediatric cohort. Am J Emerg Med 2016;34(2):189–92.

8. Samuel M. Pediatric appendicitis score. J Pediatr Surg 2002;37(6):877–81.

9. Gudjonsdottir J, Marklund E, Hagander L, et al. Clinical Prediction Scores for Pediatric Appendicitis. Eur J Pediatr Surg 2021;31(03):252–60.

10. Glass CC, Rangel SJ. Overview and diagnosis of acute appendicitis in children. Semin Pediatr Surg 2016;25(4):198–203.

11. Rassi R, Muse F, Sánchez-Martínez J, et al. Diagnostic Value of Clinical Prediction Scores for Acute Appendicitis in Children Younger than 4 Years. Eur J Pediatr Surg 2022;32(2):198–205.

12. Covelli JD, Madireddi SP, May LA, et al. MRI for Pediatric Appendicitis in an Adult-Focused General Hospital: A Clinical Effectiveness Study—Challenges and Lessons Learned. Am J Roentgenol 2019;212(1):180–7.

13. Lee KH, Lee S, Park JH, et al. Risk of Hematologic Malignant Neoplasms From Abdominopelvic Computed Tomographic Radiation in Patients Who Underwent Appendectomy. JAMA Surg 2021;156(4):343.

14. Reddan T, Corness J, Harden F, et al. Improving the value of ultrasound in children with suspected appendicitis: a prospective study integrating secondary sonographic signs. Ultrasonography 2019;38(1):67–75.

15. Dhatt S, Sabhaney V, Bray H, et al. Improving the diagnostic accuracy of appendicitis using a multidisciplinary pathway. J Pediatr Surg 2020;55(5):889–92.

16. Swenson DW, Ayyala RS, Sams C, et al. Practical Imaging Strategies for Acute Appendicitis in Children. Am J Roentgenol 2018;211(4):901–9.

17. Kim JR, Suh CH, Yoon HM, et al. Performance of MRI for suspected appendicitis in pediatric patients and negative appendectomy rate: A systematic review and meta-analysis. J Magn Reson Imaging 2018;47(3):767–78.

18. Tung EL, Baird GL, Ayyala RS, et al. Comparison of MRI appendix biometrics in children with and without acute appendicitis. Eur Radiol 2022;32(2):1024–33.

19. Komanchuk J, Martin DA, Killam R, et al. Magnetic Resonance Imaging Provides Useful Diagnostic Information Following Equivocal Ultrasound in Children With Suspected Appendicitis. Can Assoc Radiol J 2021;72(4):797–805.

20. Hwang ME. Sonography and Computed Tomography in Diagnosing Acute Appendicitis. Radiol Technol 2018;89(3):224–37.

21. Gurien LA, Wyrick DL, Smith SD, et al. Optimal timing of appendectomy in the pediatric population. J Surg Res 2016;202(1):126–31.

22. Almström M, Svensson JF, Patkova B, et al. In-hospital Surgical Delay Does Not Increase the Risk for Perforated Appendicitis in Children: A Single-center Retrospective Cohort Study. Ann Surg 2017;265(3):616–21.

23. Aziz O, Athanasiou T, Tekkis PP, et al. Laparoscopic Versus Open Appendectomy in Children: A Meta-Analysis. Ann Surg 2006;243(1):17–27.

24. Lee SL, Yaghoubian A, Kaji A. Laparoscopic vs Open Appendectomy in Children: Outcomes Comparison Based on Age, Sex, and Perforation Status. Arch Surg 2011;146(10):1118–21.
25. Somers KK, Eastwood D, Liu Y, et al. Splitting hairs and challenging guidelines: Defining the role of perioperative antibiotics in pediatric appendicitis patients. J Pediatr Surg 2020;55(3):406–13.
26. Benedict LA, Sujka J, Sobrino J, et al. Same-Day Discharge for Nonperforated Appendicitis in Children: An Updated Institutional Protocol. J Surg Res 2018; 232:346–50.
27. Gee KM, Ngo S, Burkhalter L, et al. Same-day discharge vs . observation after laparoscopic pediatric appendectomy: a prospective cohort study. Transl Gastroenterol Hepatol 2021;6:45.
28. Cairo SB, Raval MV, Browne M, et al. Association of Same-Day Discharge With Hospital Readmission After Appendectomy in Pediatric Patients. JAMA Surg 2017;152(12):1106–12.
29. Anderson KT, Bartz-Kurycki MA, Ferguson DM, et al. Too much of a bad thing: Discharge opioid prescriptions in pediatric appendectomy patients. J Pediatr Surg 2018;53(12):2374–7.
30. Farr BJ, Ranstrom L, Mooney DP. Eliminating Opiate Prescribing for Children after Non-Perforated Appendectomy. J Am Coll Surg 2020;230(6):944–6.
31. Svensson JF, Patkova B, Almström M, et al. Nonoperative Treatment With Antibiotics Versus Surgery for Acute Nonperforated Appendicitis in Children: A Pilot Randomized Controlled Trial. Ann Surg 2015;261(1):67–71.
32. Steiner Z, Buklan G, Stackievicz R, et al. A role for conservative antibiotic treatment in early appendicitis in children. J Pediatr Surg 2015;50(9):1566–8.
33. Minneci PC, Sulkowski JP, Nacion KM, et al. Feasibility of a Nonoperative Management Strategy for Uncomplicated Acute Appendicitis in Children. J Am Coll Surg 2014;219(2):272–9.
34. Minneci PC, Mahida JB, Lodwick DL, et al. Effectiveness of Patient Choice in Nonoperative vs Surgical Management of Pediatric Uncomplicated Acute Appendicitis. JAMA Surg 2016;151(5):408–15.
35. Mikami T. Perforation in pediatric non-complicated appendicitis treated by antibiotics: the real incidence. Pediatr Surg Int 2020;36(1):69–74.
36. Fugazzola P, Coccolini F, Tomasoni M, et al. Early appendectomy vs. conservative management in complicated acute appendicitis in children: A meta-analysis. J Pediatr Surg 2019;54(11):2234–41.
37. St. Peter SD, Aguayo P, Fraser JD, et al. Initial laparoscopic appendectomy versus initial nonoperative management and interval appendectomy for perforated appendicitis with abscess: a prospective, randomized trial. J Pediatr Surg 2010;45(1):236–40.
38. Howell EC, Dubina ED, Lee SL. Perforation risk in pediatric appendicitis: assessment and management. Pediatr Health Med Ther 2018;9:135–45.
39. Saluja S, Sun T, Mao J, et al. Early versus late surgical management of complicated appendicitis in children: A statewide database analysis with one-year follow-up. J Pediatr Surg 2018;53(7):1339–44.
40. Inagaki K, Blackshear C, Morris MW, et al. Pediatric Appendicitis–Factors Associated With Surgical Approach, Complications, and Readmission. J Surg Res 2020;246:395–402.
41. Bi LW, Yan BL, Yang QY, et al. Peritoneal irrigation vs suction alone during pediatric appendectomy for perforated appendicitis: A meta-analysis. Medicine (Baltimore) 2019;98(50):e18047.

42. Desai AA, Alemayehu H, Holcomb GW, et al. Safety of a new protocol decreasing antibiotic utilization after laparoscopic appendectomy for perforated appendicitis in children: A prospective observational study. J Pediatr Surg 2015;50(6):912–4.
43. Gordon AJ, Choi JH, Ginsburg H, et al. Oral Antibiotics and Abscess Formation After Appendectomy for Perforated Appendicitis in Children. J Surg Res 2020; 256:56–60.
44. van Rossem CC, Schreinemacher MHF, van Geloven AAW, et al, for the Snapshot Appendicitis Collaborative Study Group. Antibiotic Duration After Laparoscopic Appendectomy for Acute Complicated Appendicitis. JAMA Surg 2016;151(4): 323–9.
45. Cunningham ME, Zhu H, Hoch CT, et al. Effectiveness of a clinical pathway for pediatric complex appendicitis based on antibiotic stewardship principles. J Pediatr Surg 2020;55(6):1026–31.
46. Seddik TB, Rabsatt LA, Mueller C, et al. Reducing Piperacillin and Tazobactam Use for Pediatric Perforated Appendicitis. J Surg Res 2021;260:141–8.
47. Nielsen JW, Kurtovic KJ, Kenney BD, et al. Postoperative timing of computed tomography scans for abscess in pediatric appendicitis. J Surg Res 2016; 200(1):1–7.
48. Baumann LM, Williams K, Oyetunji TA, et al. Optimal Timing of Postoperative Imaging for Complicated Appendicitis. J Laparoendosc Adv Surg Tech 2018; 28(10):1248–52.
49. Linnaus ME, Ostlie DJ. Complications in common general pediatric surgery procedures. Semin Pediatr Surg 2016;25(6):404–11.
50. Gonzalez DO, Deans KJ, Minneci PC. Role of non-operative management in pediatric appendicitis. Semin Pediatr Surg 2016;25(4):204–7.
51. St. Peter SD, Snyder CL. Operative management of appendicitis. Semin Pediatr Surg 2016;25(4):208–11.
52. Cameron DB, Melvin P, Graham DA, et al. Extended Versus Narrow-spectrum Antibiotics in the Management of Uncomplicated Appendicitis in Children: A Propensity-matched Comparative Effectiveness Study. Ann Surg 2018;268(1): 186–92.
53. Kronman MP, Oron AP, Ross RK, et al. Extended- Versus Narrower-Spectrum Antibiotics for Appendicitis. Pediatrics 2016;138(1):e20154547.
54. Lee J, Garvey EM, Bundrant N, et al. IMPPACT (Intravenous Monotherapy for Postoperative Perforated Appendicitis in Children Trial): Randomized Clinical Trial of Monotherapy Versus Multi-drug Antibiotic Therapy. Ann Surg 2021;274(3): 406–10.
55. Fallon SC, Brandt ML, Hassan SF, et al. Evaluating the effectiveness of a discharge protocol for children with advanced appendicitis. J Surg Res 2013; 184(1):347–51.
56. Blanch AJ, Perel SB, Acworth JP. Paediatric intussusception: epidemiology and outcome. Emerg Med Australas 2007;19(1):45–50.
57. Cho MJ, Nam CW, Choi SH, et al. Management of recurrent ileocolic intussusception. J Pediatr Surg 2020;55(10):2150–3.
58. Fiegel H, Gfroerer S, Rolle U. Systematic review shows that pathological lead points are important and frequent in intussusception and are not limited to infants. Acta Paediatr 2016;105(11):1275–9.
59. Hom J, Kaplan C, Fowler S, et al. Evidence-Based Diagnostic Test Accuracy of History, Physical Examination, and Imaging for Intussusception: A Systematic Review and Meta-analysis. Pediatr Emerg Care 2022;38(1):e225–30.

60. Guo WL, Hu ZC, Tan YL, et al. Risk factors for recurrent intussusception in children: a retrospective cohort study. BMJ Open 2017;7(11):e018604.
61. Plut D, Phillips GS, Johnston PR, et al. Practical Imaging Strategies for Intussusception in Children. AJR Am J Roentgenol 2020;215(6):1449–63.
62. Kelley-Quon LI, Arthur LG, Williams RF, et al. Management of intussusception in children: A systematic review. J Pediatr Surg 2021;56(3):587–96.
63. Liu ST, Tang XB, Li H, et al. Ultrasound-guided hydrostatic reduction versus fluoroscopy-guided air reduction for pediatric intussusception: a multi-center, prospective, cohort study. World J Emerg Surg 2021;16(1):3.
64. Yoon CH, Kim HJ, Goo HW. Intussusception in children: US-guided pneumatic reduction–initial experience. Radiology 2001;218(1):85–8.
65. Hutchason A, Sura A, Vettikattu N, et al. Clinical management and recommendations for children with more than four episodes of recurrent intussusception following successful reduction of each: an institutional review. Clin Radiol 2020; 75(11):864–7.
66. Parikh RS, Weiner T, Dehmer J. Tension Pneumoperitoneum Following Attempted Pneumatic Reduction of Intussusception. Am Surg 2022;88(3):534–5.
67. Feldman O, Weiser G, Hanna M, et al. Success rate of pneumatic reduction of intussusception with and without sedation. Paediatr Anaesth 2017;27(2):190–5.
68. Gal M, Gamsu S, Jacob R, et al. Reduction of ileocolic intussusception under sedation or anaesthesia: a systematic review of complications. Arch Dis Child 2022;107(4):335–40.
69. Delgado-Miguel C, Garcia A, Delgado B, et al. Routine Ultrasound Control after Successful Intussusception Reduction in Children: Is It Really Necessary? Eur J Pediatr Surg 2021;31(1):115–9.
70. Ferrantella A, Quinn K, Parreco J, et al. Incidence of recurrent intussusception in young children: A nationwide readmissions analysis. J Pediatr Surg 2020;55(6): 1023–5.
71. Wei CH, Fu YW, Wang NL, et al. Laparoscopy versus open surgery for idiopathic intussusception in children. Surg Endosc 2015;29(3):668–72.
72. Jamshidi M, Rahimi B, Gilani N. Laparoscopic and open surgery methods in managing surgical intussusceptions: A randomized clinical trial of postoperative complications. Asian J Endosc Surg 2022;15(1):56–62.
73. Zhang Y, Wang Y, Zhang Y, et al. Laparoscopic Ileopexy Versus Laparoscopic Simple Reduction in Children with Multiple Recurrences of Ileocolic Intussusception: A Single-Institution Retrospective Cohort Study. J Laparoendosc Adv Surg Tech A 2020;30(5):576–80.
74. Zhang M, Zhou X, Hu Q, et al. Accurately distinguishing pediatric ileocolic intussusception from small-bowel intussusception using ultrasonography. J Pediatr Surg 2021;56(4):721–6.
75. Melvin JE, Zuckerbraun NS, Nworgu CR, et al. Management and Outcome of Pediatric Patients With Transient Small Bowel-Small Bowel Intussusception. Pediatr Emerg Care 2021;37(3):e110–5.
76. Thanh Xuan N, Huu Son N, Huu Thien H. Treatment Outcome of Acute Intussusception in Children Under Two Years of Age: A Prospective Cohort Study. Cureus 2020;12(4):e7729.
77. Romano C, Oliva S, Martellossi S, et al. Pediatric gastrointestinal bleeding: Perspectives from the Italian Society of Pediatric Gastroenterology. World J Gastroenterol 2017;23(8):1328–37.

78. Pant C, Olyaee M, Sferra TJ, et al. Emergency department visits for gastrointestinal bleeding in children: results from the Nationwide Emergency Department Sample 2006–2011. Curr Med Res Opin 2015;31(2):347–51.
79. Padilla BE, Moses W. Lower Gastrointestinal Bleeding & Intussusception. Surg Clin North Am 2017;97(1):173–88.
80. Sierra D, Wood M, Kolli S, et al. Pediatric Gastritis, Gastropathy, and Peptic Ulcer Disease. Pediatr Rev 2018;39(11):542–9.
81. Owensby S, Taylor K, Wilkins T. Diagnosis and Management of Upper Gastrointestinal Bleeding in Children. J Am Board Fam Med 2015;28(1):134–45.
82. Jaramillo C, Jensen MK, McClain A, et al. Clinical diagnostic predictive score for Meckel diverticulum. J Pediatr Surg 2021;56(9):1673–7.
83. Sinha CK, Pallewatte A, Easty M, et al. Meckel's scan in children: a review of 183 cases referred to two paediatric surgery specialist centres over 18 years. Pediatr Surg Int 2013;29(5):511–7.
84. Robinson JR, Correa H, Brinkman AS, et al. Optimizing surgical resection of the bleeding Meckel diverticulum in children. J Pediatr Surg 2017;52(10):1610–5.
85. Glenn IC, el-shafy IA, Bruns NE, et al. Simple diverticulectomy is adequate for management of bleeding Meckel diverticulum. Pediatr Surg Int 2018;34(4):451–5.
86. Patkova B, Wester T. Anal Fissure in Children. Eur J Pediatr Surg 2020;30(05):391–4.
87. Joda AE, Al-Mayoof AF. Efficacy of nitroglycerine ointment in the treatment of pediatric anal fissure. J Pediatr Surg 2017;52(11):1782–6.
88. Alshehri A, Barghouthi R, Albanyan S, et al. A prospective, double-blind, randomized, placebo-controlled trial comparing the efficacy of polyethylene glycol versus polyethylene glycol combined with topical diltiazem for treating anal fissure in children. J Pediatr Surg 2020;55(10):2017–21.
89. Kim DY, Bae JY, Ko KO, et al. Juvenile Polyp associated with Hypovolemic Shock Due to Massive Lower Gastrointestinal Bleeding. Pediatr Gastroenterol Hepatol Nutr 2019;22(6):613–8.
90. Cohen S, Hyer W, Mas E, et al. Management of Juvenile Polyposis Syndrome in Children and Adolescents: A Position Paper From the ESPGHAN Polyposis Working Group. J Pediatr Gastroenterol Nutr 2019;68(3):453–62.

Management of Abdominal Wall Defects

Victoriya Staab, MD

KEYWORDS

- Congenital abdominal wall defects • Gastroschisis • Omphalocele
- Prune belly syndrome

KEY POINTS

- Complex congenital abdominal wall defects include gastroschisis, omphalocele, and prune belly syndrome.
- There is a spectrum of associated anomalies that need to be evaluated in the neonatal period in patients with congenital abdominal wall defects.
- Treatment of complex congenital anomalies involves a multidisciplinary approach and often requires various abdominal wall closure techniques.

INTRODUCTION

Abdominal wall defects present in various forms that range from various hernias to more complex pediatric surgical conditions that require advanced surgical considerations. Some of these complex conditions include gastroschisis, omphalocele, and prune belly syndrome (PBS).

Gastroschisis

Epidemiology and embryology

Gastoroschisis is defined as a full thickness defect in the abdominal wall with resultant herniation of viscera to the right of the umbilicus. Incidence is approximately 3 to 4 per 10,000 live births.[1] Known risk factors include young maternal age, recreational drug use, and cigarette smoking.[2] Normal fetal abdominal wall development is completed by the 12th week of gestation where the intra-abdominal contents return into the abdominal cavity after completing their herniation and rotation. A disruption of the process results in persistent herniation through a defect to the right of the umbilicus. Typically the small intestine is protruding through the defect but other organs such as the large intestine, stomach, liver, and gonads have also been found herniating.[3] The organs are not covered by any membrane and are therefore exposed to amniotic fluid.

Jersey Shore University Medical Center, Hackensack Meridian Health, 19 Davis Avenue 4th floor, Neptune City, NJ 07753, USA
E-mail address: victoriya1213@gmail.com

Surg Clin N Am 102 (2022) 809–820
https://doi.org/10.1016/j.suc.2022.07.011
surgical.theclinics.com
0039-6109/22/© 2022 Elsevier Inc. All rights reserved.

Although the exact etiology of the congenital defect has not been identified, vascular insult and environmental factors have been suspected. The resultant exposure leads to thickened and edematous bowels and an association with intestinal atresias.

Antenatal course

Most cases are diagnosed antenatally by ultrasound by 20 weeks gestation and then monitored closely with serial ultrasounds. Maternal serum alpha-fetoprotein (AFP) will frequently be elevated. Development of complex gastroschisis should be monitored which included bowel and gastric dilation, polyhydramnios, and intrauterine growth retardation (IUGR).[4] Intestinal stenosis and atresia occurs in approximately 10% of cases and is often associated with polyhydramnios.[5,6] Vanishing or closed gastroschisis results from spontaneous closure of the fascia with resultant compromise to the eviscerated bowel which can lead to ischemia and volvulus and resultant short bowel syndrome or even fetal demise.[7] There has not been any proven role of fetal interventions in improving outcomes.[8] Multidisciplinary team approach to perinatal care with maternal-fetal medicine physicians, obstetricians, pediatric surgeons, and neonatologists is recommended.

Delivery

Optimal time and mode of delivery have been studied and currently the recommendation is induction of labor after 37 weeks is advised.[9] Surgical team evaluation is needed at the time of delivery. After assessment and stabilization of respiratory effort, the herniated viscera should be inspected. The size of the fascial defect should be noted which is usually to the right of the umbilical cord. The length of the umbilical cord should be preserved and umbilical venous and arterial lines avoided. The severity of bowel matting should be noted and separating of bowel loops should not be attempted. A thick inflammatory peel is often identified but removal should not be attempted. The bowel should be inspected for any obvious atresias, ischemia, or signs of perforation such a meconium staining (**Fig. 1**).

It is crucial to be cognizant of evaporative heat losses by keeping the bowel warm and moist. The viscera should be covered with warm moist gauze and blood supply supported either by laying the patient on their right side or creating a cylinder above the abdomen supported by kerlix. The bowel should then be covered in plastic wrap or the baby placed in a bowel bag up to their axillary level. The perfusion to the bowel should be monitored to prevent ischemia during transport to either the operating room or the neonatal intensive care unit.

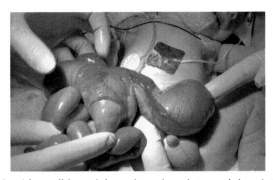

Fig. 1. Gastroschisis with small bowel, large bowel, and stomach herniated.

Neonatal management

Stabilization in the NICU includes obtaining intravenous access and fluid resuscitation and initiating broad-spectrum antibiotics. Historic volume resuscitation of 150% maintenance fluids is no longer recommended but titrated to adequate urine output monitored via foley catheter. Excessive hydration can lead to prolonged ventilator requirements and bowel edema.[10] An orogastric tube should be placed to decompress the stomach. Intubation or sedation is often performed to allow relaxation of the abdominal wall to allow for bedside reduction.

Surgical management

Several options are available to address the exteriorized viscera. If the defect is small and there is a concern for ischemia to the herniated bowel (vanishing/closing gastroschisis), emergent fascial defect extension should be performed laterally away from the defect toward the patient's right. Otherwise in the majority of cases, a bedside immediate or delayed reduction using a silastic silo appliance can be performed (**Fig. 2**). The silo appliance can be placed bedside in the NICU and gentle pressure applied from the distal end until the contents of the bag are fully reduced (**Fig. 3**). Once reduced, standard fascial suture closure or sutureless plastics closure using an onlay of the umbilical cord can be performed.[11,12] If there are any gonads present outside the body, they should be reduced in toward the pelvis. Most testicles will continue to descend into the groin, but some will eventually require an orchiopexy.[13,14] Ladd's procedure for malrotation is not indicated as the rotational anomaly is rarely associated with future volvulus.

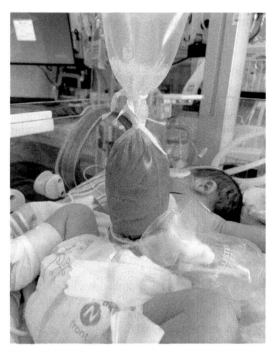

Fig. 2. Bowel placed in a silo appliance.

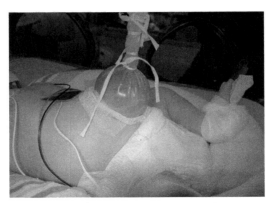

Fig. 3. Ongoing daily reduction of bowel into the abdominal cavity.

Post-reduction

Monitoring for signs of abdominal compartment syndrome from the increased intra-abdominal pressure should be closely monitored including observation of decreased lower extremity perfusion or venous return, increased peak airway pressures, and decreased urine output. Replacement of the silo appliance to allow for decompression and delayed closure is occasionally necessary if any of those signs develop.

Peripherally inserted central catheter (PICC) is ideally placed in the first several days after the neonate is well resuscitated. Prolonged ileus secondary to dysmotility is often the leading cause of prolonged length of stay. Failure to progress on feeds after three weeks should prompt contrast studies for atresia evaluation.[15] Typically a contrast enema is recommended first to evaluate for a microcolon and when that contrast passes, an upper gastrointestinal study with follow-through should be performed to evaluate for atresias.

Long-term sequelae

Most patients with a history of gastroschisis have few long-term sequelae. Dysmotility is common in the first few years of life but is usually self-limited. Persistent gastrointestinal reflux is however very common.[16] As the bowel in patients with gastroschisis is malrotated, bilious emesis should always warrant an emergent evaluation with an upper gastrointestinal series but bowel obstruction is more commonly secondary to adhesions. Otherwise these patients are appropriate for reaching development milestones. Psychologically the biggest concern is an abnormal or absent umbilicus.[17] Complex gastroschisis that results in short bowel syndrome has a significantly higher morbidity and mortality due to intestinal failure and the potential sequelae from line sepsis, parenteral-induced cholestasis, and subsequent liver disease. Liver and small bowel transplant are often needed in severe cases and carry a significant morbidity and mortality risk.[18]

Omphalocele

Epidemiology and embryology

Omphalocele is defined as a midline abdominal wall defect with herniated viscera covered by a membrane sac. They are classified as epigastric, umbilical, or hypogastric. Cranial fold defects result in epigastric omphaloceles.[19,20] Extreme epigastric fusion defects are known as Pentalogy of Cantrell. This is defined as defects of the epigastric abdominal wall, diaphragmatic defects, sternal clefts, pericardial, and cardiac defects.[21] Extreme caudal defects are associated with cloacal exstrophy (**Fig. 4**).

Incidence is approximately 1 per 10,000 live births. These numbers take into account stillbirths, miscarriages, and termination of pregnancy. Known risk factors include older maternal age and obesity. There is a suspected genetic component but no proven gene has yet been discovered.

Associated anomalies

Unlike gastroschisis, patients with omphaloceles frequently have associated anomalies. Common anomalies include chromosomal anomalies such as trisomy 13, 18, and 21. Cardiac anomalies are seen frequently, whereas neurological anomalies are less common.[22] There can be an association between pulmonary hypoplasia and subsequent chest wall developmental problems with large omphaloceles. There is an increased frequency of associated genetic syndromes in patients with omphaloceles, the most common being Beckwith–Wiedemann syndrome. The condition often presents with large for gestational age newborns, organomegaly, macroglossia, omphalocele, hypoglycemia, and increased risk for Wilms tumors, hepatoblastoma, and neuroblastoma.[23]

Antenatal course

Most cases are diagnosed antenatally by ultrasound by 20 weeks gestation and then monitored closely with serial ultrasounds. Most cases are sporadic. Nuchal translucency is associated with omphaloceles and maternal serum AFP is often elevated.[24] Chromosomal anomalies and associated anomalies should be evaluated as they have a high association with fetal demise. Karyotyping via chorionic villus sampling should be performed and families counseled on options for termination especially if major chromosomal anomalies are discovered. The distinction between gastroschisis and omphalocele is the presence of a sac with insertion of the umbilical cord centrally. Occasionally rupture of the sac might occur and the finding could be confused with gastroschisis. In those cases, the insertion of the umbilical cord should be thoroughly

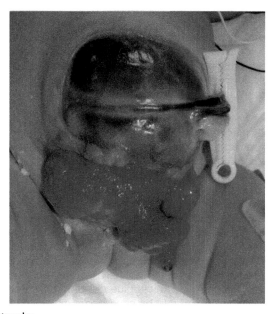

Fig. 4. Cloacal exstrophy.

evaluated using Doppler to distinguish between the two conditions.[19] The size of the omphalocele is often a prognostic indicator with giant omphaloceles and the associated pulmonary hypoplasia.[20] Giant omphalocele can be defined as >5 cm, containing a significant portion of the liver, or greater than 50% of the surface area of the abdominal wall.[25] Lung volume ratios can be evaluated with fetal MRI as a prognostic indicator of pulmonary development. Similar to gastroschisis, there has not been any proven role of fetal interventions in improving outcomes. Multidisciplinary team approach to perinatal care with maternal-fetal medicine physicians, obstetricians, pediatric surgeons, and neonatologists is recommended.

Delivery
Optimal time has been studied and currently the recommendation is to continue the pregnancy to term if no other fetal or maternal variables would preclude safe progression of pregnancy. There is currently no specific contraindication to proceeding with vaginal delivery in these cases.[26] At the time of delivery, standard assessment and stabilization of respiratory effort should be performed. Inspection of the sac should look for any violation of its integrity and then be covered with warm moist gauze. Kinking of the vasculature of the herniated liver should be avoided by supporting the sac or placing the infant on its side.

Neonatal management
Stabilization in the NICU includes obtaining intravenous access and fluid resuscitation. Broad spectrum antibiotics should be initiated. Umbilical lines are typically avoided due to the abnormal locations of the umbilical vein and arteries and challenges with insertion with their trajectory and as well as their interference with surgical management. Gastric decompression can be helpful to facilitate decreasing intra-abdominal pressure. The infant should be examined for any physical findings to suggest any associated syndromes. Chromosomal studies should be performed. Serial serum glucose levels should be obtained if there is any suspicion for Beckwith–Wiedemann syndrome or in infants with IUGR. Pulmonary status and evaluation for associated diaphragmatic hernia should be evaluated with arterial blood gas and a chest radiograph. An echocardiogram and pediatric cardiology consultation should also be obtained to evaluate for any associated congenital cardiac anomalies. Stabilization of cardiac and respiratory status should always be obtained before surgical closure and typically account for a significant delay in patients with cardiac anomalies and pulmonary hypoplasia.[4,27]

Surgical management
A PICC line is ideally placed in the first several days after the neonate is well resuscitated. Decision on surgical closure or medical management depends on the clinical status of the newborn and the size of the defect. Small omphalocele can present as a herniation within the umbilical cord (**Fig. 5**). Large omphaloceles or patients who are not medically stable to undergo surgical correction are treated with the "paint and wait" approach. This technique involves applying a daily topical agent to the sac and allowing eschar formation with the goal of forming a ventral hernia after initial epithelization that can be addressed later in childhood. Agents that are typically used include silver sulfadiazine, bacitracin, and iodine solutions. Nonadhesive dressing is then applied and eventually compression dressings can be added. It typically takes approximately four to ten weeks to fully epithelialize the sac. Small tears in the sac can be repaired with suturing or surgical glue closure.[28] Occasionally bowel or an omphalomesenteric duct remnant can be seen perforating through the sac and that warrants emergent surgical intervention (**Fig. 6**).

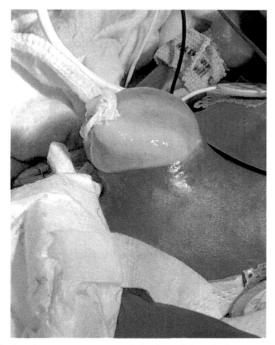

Fig. 5. Small omphalocele presenting as umbilical cord herniation.

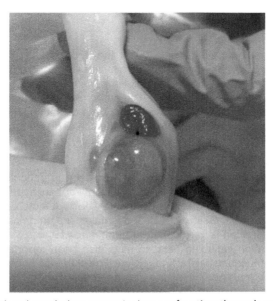

Fig. 6. Small bowel and omphalomesenteric duct perforating through an omphalocele sac.

If the defect is small and the patient's clinical status allows for surgical correction, primary repair can be considered in the neonatal period. Attempts at primary closure should follow principles of monitoring for abdominal compartment syndrome. Bladder or gastric pressures can be monitored as well as airway pressures after closure are important. Urine output and end-organ signs of perfusion should be closely followed. Surgical correction involves removal of the sac and fascial closure which sometimes cannot be easily achieved especially in the epigastric defects. Special care should be taken with the superior aspect of the closure as the hepatic veins often are intimately involved with the sac and are located centrally right under the edge of the defect.

Bridging the fascial gap can be facilitated by several techniques. Silastic sheet can be sewn circumferentially to the fascia for a staged closure. Various mesh products can be used using both biological and synthetic mesh.[29] Component separation and tissue expanders have also been described to achieve closure.[30] If the skin cannot reach to cover the defect, vacuum-assisted closure has also been described.[31]

Feeding can be initiated with return of bowel function. Length of hospitalization is often determined by respiratory support needs. Complications besides compartment syndrome sequelae that have been described include wound infections and dehiscence, mesh complications, enterocutaneous fistulas, and cholestasis.[32]

Long-term sequelae

The outcomes of patients with a history of omphalocele depend on the other associated conditions. Common challenges that face these patients include failure to thrive, gastroesophageal reflux disease, and pulmonary complications.[33] As the bowel in patients with omphalocele is malrotated, bilious emesis should always warrant an emergent evaluation with an upper gastrointestinal series. Psychologically the biggest concern is an abnormal or absent umbilicus and there are neuropsychological development delays that can occur.[17,34] Abdominal wall reconstruction and ventral hernia repair often need to be considered as the child grows. Other associated anomalies often influence long-term outcomes but without them, patients can expect a normal quality of life.

Prune Belly Syndrome

Epidemiology and embryology

Characterized by a congenital deficiency of the abdominal wall musculature with resultant skin having a wrinkled appearance similar to that of a prune. It is associated with hydroureteronephrosis and cryptorchidism. The incidence is approximately 3 in 100,000 and is found mostly in males.[35] The embryology is thought to have resulted from urethral obstruction which leads to urinary tract dilatation. This therefore affects abdominal wall musculature development and testicular descent.[36] There are reports of a potential genetic component as there are multiple reports of familial cases.[37]

Associated anomalies

There are multiple associated anomalies that are seen in patients with PBS, which include pulmonary and cardiac anomalies such as pulmonary hypoplasia, patent ductus arteriosus, reactive airway disease, ventricular septal defects, atrial septal defects, and patent foramen ovale. Gastrointestinal anomalies are commonly associated with PBS as well. Constipation is very common but gastrointestinal atresias, malrotation, anorectal malformation including cloacas have also been reported. Other common anomalies include musculoskeletal findings such as club foot, scoliosis, pectus deformities, sacral and spinal anomalies have also been described.[38,39] Urological anomalies are a main characteristic of PBS. These include dilated, tortuous ureters, severely enlarged bladder, patent urachus, and megalourethra. The severity of the renal dysfunction can vary from normal to severe typically associated with the variable degree of renal dysplasia.[40]

Antenatal course
Urogenital anomalies are often the first signs of PBS in utero that can be seen by the second trimester of fetal development. Oligohydramnios, urethral dilation, hydroureteronephrosis, and enlarged bladder can be detected.[41] Chromosomal anomalies should be checked if PBS is suspected. There have not yet been any significant improved outcomes described with any fetal interventions.[42] Fetal mortality is linked with the severity of disease, especially in those with the earlier detection of anomalies.

Neonatal management
Respiratory stabilization is one of the mainstays of support provided at birth as these newborns often require intubation.[43,44] Prophylactic antibiotics and foley catheter placement is needed for bladder drainage. Monitoring for urinary tract infections is critical. Echocardiograms should be performed to look for cardiac anomalies. Multidisciplinary treatment approach with neonatology, pediatric urology, pediatric surgery, and pediatric nephrology is imperative.

Surgical management
Urological reconstruction is critical for severe urologic anomalies to preserve renal function and the timing of surgery depends on the spectrum of the anatomic concerns. Cutaneous vesicostomy is occasionally needed in the neonatal period if the bladder cannot be decompressed via the urethra. Appendicovesicostomy can be used in older children for intermittent catheterizations. Percutaneous nephrostomy and pyeloplasty are performed when indicated. Abdominal wall reconstruction is performed not only for cosmetic concerns but also for improvement in pulmonary function. Several techniques have been described which describe muscle and fascial mobilization and closure and excessive skin excision.[45,46] Orchiopexy should be performed for the same indications as any patients with cryptorchidism.[47–49]

Long-term sequelae
Mortality in the neonatal period is typically related to pulmonary hypoplasia.[43] Progression to renal failure is linked to degree of obstruction and renal dysplasia. Those patients will progress to requiring renal transplantation in their first two decades of life.[39] Long-term renal function monitoring is critical. Patients with urinary reflux need to be maintained on prophylactic antibiotics. Many will be restricted in their self-assessment of quality of life.[50] It is imperative to have a multidisciplinary approach that is tailored to the severity of the presentation.[51]

CLINICS CARE POINTS

- When evaluating a patient born with gastroschisis, evaluation for adequate perfusion to the bowel and avoiding kinking of the mesentery is critical
- Avoid "running the bowel" by separating matted loops of herniated bowel in gastroschisis, which can result in bowel injury
- Large omphaloceles or those with significant comorbidities should not undergo surgery but rather use the "paint and wait" approach
- It is important to monitor patients with prune belly syndrome for pulmonary hypoplasia and renal

DISCLOSURE

The author has no financial disclosures and no commercial conflicts of interest as related to anything discussed in the following article.

REFERENCES

1. Parker SE, Mai CT, Canfield MA, et al. Updated National Birth Prevalence estimates for selected birth defects in the United States, 2004-2006. Birth Defects Res A Clin Mol Teratol 2010;88(12):1008–16.
2. Draper ES, Rankin J, Tonks AM, et al. Recreational drug use: a major risk factor for gastroschisis? Am J Epidemiol 2008;167(4):485–9.
3. Islam S. Advances in surgery for abdominal wall defects: gastroschisis and omphalocele. Clin Perinatol 2012;39(2):375–86.
4. Gamba P, Midrio P. Abdominal wall defects: prenatal diagnosis, newborn management, and long-term outcomes. Semin Pediatr Surg 2014;23(5):283–90.
5. D'Antonio F, Virgone C, Rizzo G, et al. Prenatal risk factors and outcomes in gastroschisis: a meta-analysis. Pediatrics 2015;136(1):e159–69.
6. Ferreira RG, Mendonça CR, de Moraes CL, et al. Ultrasound markers for complex gastroschisis: a systematic review and meta-analysis. J Clin Med 2021;10(22): 5215.
7. Houben C, Davenport M, Ade-Ajayi N, et al. Closing gastroschisis: diagnosis, management, and outcomes. J Pediatr Surg 2009;44(2):343–7.
8. Luton D, Mitanchez D, Winer N, et al. A randomised controlled trial of amnioexchange for fetal gastroschisis. BJOG 2019;126(10):1233–41.
9. Harper LM, Goetzinger KR, Biggio JR, et al. Timing of elective delivery in gastroschisis: a decision and cost-effectiveness analysis. Ultrasound Obstet Gynecol 2015;46(2):227–32.
10. Jansen LA, Safavi A, Lin Y, et al. Preclosure fluid resuscitation influences outcome in gastroschisis. Am J Perinatol 2012;29(4):307–12.
11. Sandler A, Lawrence J, Meehan J, et al. "Plastic" sutureless abdominal wall closure in gastroschisis. J Pediatr Surg 2004;39:738–41.
12. Joharifard S, Trudeau MO, Miyata S, et al. Canadian Pediatric Surgery Network (CAPSNet). Implementing a standardized gastroschisis protocol significantly increases the rate of primary sutureless closure without compromising closure success or early clinical outcomes. J Pediatr Surg 2022;57(1):12–7.
13. Hill SJ, Durham MM. Management of cryptorchidism and gastroschisis. J Pediatr Surg 2011;46(9):1798–803.
14. Ceccanti S, Migliara G, De Vito C, et al. Prevalence, management and outcome of cryptorchidism associated with gastroschisis: A systematic review and meta-analysis. J Pediatr Surg 2021;13. S0022-3468(21)00494-2.
15. Riddle S, Haberman B, Miquel-Verges F, et al. Gastroschisis with intestinal atresia leads to longer hospitalization and poor feeding outcomes. J Perinatol 2022; 42(2):254–9.
16. van Manen M, Hendson L, Wiley M, et al. Early childhood outcomes of infants born with gastroschisis. J Pediatr Surg 2013;48(8):1682–7.
17. Islam S. Clinical care outcomes in abdominal wall defects. Curr Opin Pediatr 2008;20(3):305–10.
18. Bergholz R, Boettcher M, Reinshagen K, et al. Complex gastroschisis is a different entity to simple gastroschisis affecting morbidity and mortality-a systematic review and meta-analysis. J Pediatr Surg 2014;49(10):1527–32.

19. Victoria T, Andronikou S, Bowen D, et al. Fetal anterior abdominal wall defects: prenatal imaging by magnetic resonance imaging. Pediatr Radiol 2018;48(4): 499–512.

20. Verla MA, Style CC, Olutoye OO. Prenatal diagnosis and management of omphalocele. Semin Pediatr Surg 2019;28(2):84–8.

21. Mallula KK, Sosnowski C, Awad S. Spectrum of Cantrell's pentalogy: case series from a single tertiary care center and review of the literature. Pediatr Cardiol 2013;34(7):1703–10.

22. Ayub SS, Taylor JA. Cardiac anomalies associated with omphalocele. Semin Pediatr Surg 2019;28(2):111–4.

23. NIH. https://rarediseases.info.nih.gov/diseases/3343/beckwith-wiedemann-syndrome.

24. Verla MA, Style CC, Olutoye OO. Prenatal diagnosis and management of omphalocele. Semin Pediatr Surg 2019;28(2):84–8.

25. Klein MD. Congenital defects of the abdominal wall. In: Coran AG, Adzick NS, Krummel TM, et al, editors. Pediatric surgery. 7th edition. Philadelphia: Elsevier; 2012. p. 973–84.

26. Segel SY, Marder SJ, Parry S, et al. Fetal abdominal wall defects and mode of delivery: a systematic review. Obstet Gynecol 2001;98(5 Pt 1):867–73.

27. Christison-Lagay ER, Kelleher CM, Langer JC. Neonatal abdominal wall defects. Semin Fetal Neonatal Med 2011;16(3):164–72.

28. van Eijck FC, Aronson DA, Hoogeveen YL, et al. Past and current surgical treatment of giant omphalocele: outcome of a questionnaire sent to authors. J Pediatr Surg 2011;46(3):482–8.

29. Mortellaro VE, St Peter SD, Fike FB, et al. Review of the evidence on the closure of abdominal wall defects. Pediatr Surg Int 2011;27(4):391–7.

30. van Eijck FC, de Blaauw I, Bleichrodt RP, et al. Closure of giant omphaloceles by the abdominal wall component separation technique in infants. J Pediatr Surg 2008;43(1):246–50.

31. Binet A, Gelas T, Jochault-Ritz S, et al. VAC® therapy a therapeutic alternative in giant omphalocele treatment: a multicenter study. J Plast Reconstr Aesthet Surg 2013;66(12):e373–5.

32. Islam S, St Peter SD, Downard CD, et al. Omphalocele. Contemporary Outcomes from a Multicenter Registry. Abstract presents at the American Academy of Pediatrics Section on Surgery, October 27, 2013, Orlando, FL.

33. Lunzer H, Menardi G, Brezinka C. Long-term follow-up of children with prenatally diagnosed omphalocele and gastroschisis. J Matern Fetal Med 2001;10(6): 385–92.

34. Ginn-Pease ME, King DR, Tarnowski KJ, et al. Psychosocial adjustment and physical growth in children with imperforate anus or abdominal wall defects. J Pediatr Surg 1991;26(9):1129–35.

35. Routh JC, Huang L, Retik AB, et al. Contemporary epidemiology and characterization of newborn males with prune belly syndrome. Urology 2010;76(1):44–8.

36. Stephens FD, Gupta D. Pathogenesis of the prune belly syndrome. J Urol 1994; 152(6 Pt 2):2328–31.

37. Ramasamy R, Haviland M, Woodard JR, et al. Patterns of inheritance in familial prune belly syndrome. Urology 2005;65(6):1227.

38. Geary DF, MacLusky IB, Churchill BM, et al. A broader spectrum of abnormalities in the prune belly syndrome. J Urol 1986;135(2):324–6.

39. Seidel NE, Arlen AM, Smith EA, et al. Clinical manifestations and management of prune-belly syndrome in a large contemporary pediatric population. Urology 2015;85(1):211–5.

40. Woodard JR. The prune belly syndrome. Urol Clin North Am 1978;5(1):75–93.

41. Yamamoto H, Nishikawa S, Hayashi T, et al. Antenatal diagnosis of prune belly syndrome at 11 weeks of gestation. J Obstet Gynaecol Res 2001;27(1):37–40.

42. Leeners B, Sauer I, Schefels J, et al. Prune-belly syndrome: therapeutic options including in utero placement of a vesicoamniotic shunt. J Clin Ultrasound 2000; 28(9):500–7.

43. Routh JC, Huang L, Retik AB, et al. Contemporary epidemiology and characterization of newborn males with prune belly syndrome. Urology 2010;76(1):44–8.

44. Apostel HJCL, Duval ELIM, De Dooy J, et al. Respiratory support in the absence of abdominal muscles: a case study of ventilatory management in prune belly syndrome. Paediatr Respir Rev 2021;37:44–7.

45. Ehrlich RM, Lesavoy MA, Fine RN. Total abdominal wall reconstruction in the prune belly syndrome. J Urol 1986;136(1 Pt 2):282–5.

46. Monfort G, Guys JM, Bocciardi A, et al. A novel technique for reconstruction of the abdominal wall in the prune belly syndrome. J Urol 1991;146(Pt 2):639–40.

47. Woodard JR. Lessons learned in 3 decades of managing the prune-belly syndrome. J Urol 1998;159(5):1680.

48. Patil KK, Duffy PG, Woodhouse CR, et al. Long-term outcome of Fowler-Stephens orchiopexy in boys with prune-belly syndrome. J Urol 2004;171(4):1666–9.

49. Fernández-Bautista B, Angulo JM, Burgos L, et al. Surgical approach to prune-belly syndrome: a review of our series and novel surgical technique. J Pediatr Urol 2021;17(5):704.e1–6.

50. Grimsby GM, Harrison SM, Granberg CF, et al. Impact and frequency of extra-genitourinary manifestations of prune belly syndrome. J Pediatr Urol 2015; 11(5):280.e1-6.

51. Lopes RI, Baker LA, Dénes FT. Modern management of and update on prune belly syndrome. J Pediatr Urol 2021;17(4):548–54.

Small Bowel Congenital Anomalies: A Review and Update

Grant Morris, MD, MPH[a],*, Alfred Kennedy Jr, MD[b]

KEYWORDS

- Congenital • Omphalomesenteric duct • Meckel • Web • Atresia • Duplication

KEY POINTS

- There are several congenital anomalies that occur and present most commonly in infancy; however, some may not present until adulthood.
- Definitive therapy for these congenital anomalies is surgical in nature and require surgery to be performed urgently.
- The overall prognosis of congenital anomalies of the small intestine is very good and has improved with improved medical management and the advent of newer surgical modalities.

INTRODUCTION

Congenital anomalies of the gastrointestinal (GI) tract can affect any portion of the GI tract from the esophagus to the anus. These include intestinal atresias, intestinal duplications, and disorders of the omphalomesenteric duct. Many of these will present in the neonatal period, usually with obstruction. Presentation can also occur into adulthood. Some of these entities can be life threatening, making it imperative to rapidly diagnose and provide appropriate therapy. It is important to realize that many of these anomalies of the small intestine are also associated with other congenital anomalies. Some of these anomalies were associated with high mortalities in the first half the 1900s, but now, owing to improved medical therapy, including total parenteral nutrition (TPN) and newer surgical modalities, the prognosis of congenital anomalies of the small intestine is very good. This article reviews anomalies of the small intestine, including disorders of the omphalomesenteric (vitelline) duct, duodenal web, duodenal atresia, jejunoileal atresia, and intestinal duplications.

OMPHALOMESENTERIC (VITELLINE) DUCT DISORDERS

Disorders of the omphalomesenteric duct include Meckel diverticulum, umbilicoileal fistula, umbilical sinus, fibrous cord, and vitelline cyst. These various entities represent

[a] Department of Pediatric Gastroenterology, Geisinger Health System, 100 North Academy Avenue, Danville, PA 17822, USA; [b] Department of Pediatric Surgery, Geisinger Health System, 100 North Academy Avenue, Danville, PA 17822, USA
* Corresponding author.
E-mail address: gamorris@geisinger.edu

Surg Clin N Am 102 (2022) 821–835
https://doi.org/10.1016/j.suc.2022.07.012
0039-6109/22/© 2022 Elsevier Inc. All rights reserved.

failure of portions of the omphalomesenteric duct to involve in early gestation (**Fig. 1**). Meckel diverticulum is the most common congenital anomaly of the GI tract. This is named after Johann Meckel, who first described its embryonic origin in the 1800s.[1] It is found in approximately 2% of the population with a male-to-female ratio of 2–4:1.[2] Meckel diverticulum is a true diverticulum, containing all 3 layers of the bowel wall: mucosa, muscularis, and serosa. The diverticula may contain ectopic mucosa, with gastric mucosa being the most common, present in 50% to 60% of the cases. They may also contain pancreatic, duodenal, or rarely, colonic or hepatobiliary mucosa.[3] Ectopic gastric mucosa secretes acid that can lead to ulceration of adjacent ileal mucosa with subsequent hemorrhage. The "rule of 2's" has been associated with Meckel diverticulum: it occurs in 2% of the population; it is located about 2 feet from the ileocecal valve (in adults); it is typically about 2 inches long and presents in those less than 2 years of age 50% of the time.

The majority, 85% to 95%, of patients with a Meckel diverticulum are asymptomatic.[4] The most common presentation of a Meckel in children is painless rectal bleeding that can be acute or chronic.[3] Typically, the bleeding consists of dark red or maroon blood, but melena is also possible.

Small bowel obstruction is the second most common presentation of a child born with Meckel diverticulum.[4] There are 5 sources of obstruction: (1) A Meckel diverticulum may be the lead point for ileocolic intussusception. In fact, Meckel diverticulum is the most common anatomic lead point for such intussusception and may lead to recurrent obstruction following successful hydrostatic reduction; (2) Prolapse of the diverticulum through a persistent omphalomesenteric effect may result in complete intestinal obstruction; (3) Volvulus may occur involving the associated ileum around a persistent fibrous band emanating from the tip of the diverticulum and ending at the umbilicus, following the path of the omphalomesenteric duct; (4) A loop of small intestine may become involved within an internal hernia produced by an aberrant right vitelline artery or fibrous band arising from the associated mesentery; (5) Last, a Meckel diverticulum may become incarcerated within an inguinal hernia (Littre hernia). All of these entities require prompt diagnosis and surgical repair, including resection of the diverticulum and possibly the associate small intestine should there be vascular compromise. Meckel diverticulitis can also perforate resulting in peritonitis and may mimic an acute appendicitis, usually presenting later in life. Children with trisomy 18 are at higher risk for this.[5]

Persistence of the omphalomesenteric duct may present with umbilical drainage (succus) owing to a fistula between the ileum and umbilicus early in life. The diagnosis

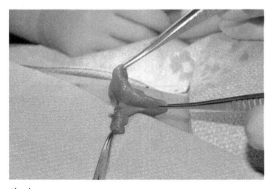

Fig. 1. Meckel diverticulum.

is usually self-evident but may be confirmed with sonography. Other sources of persistent drainage in the newborn period include patent urachal anomalies. The urachus is a remnant of the allantois and forms the median umbilical ligament. Drainage of clear urine may be noted if patency includes a fistula to the dome of the bladder. Sonography may also assist with diagnosis.

The diagnostic approach depends on the presenting symptoms. For the patient presenting with bleeding, the most sensitive test to diagnose a Meckel diverticulum is a technetium-99m pertechnetate scintigraphy, Meckel scan. This test has an 85% to 95% sensitivity and specificity in children.[6] The sensitivity and specificity appear to be lower in adults.[7] Technetium-99m pertechnetate is administered intravenously, and serial abdominal images are obtained using a gamma camera over 60 minutes (**Fig. 2**). Parietal cells of the gastric mucosa take up technetium-99m pertechnetate, revealing ectopic gastric mucosa in the right lower quadrant. There is excretion of technetium-99m pertechnetate by the kidneys resulting in ureters and bladder being visualized as well. Administration of histamine-2 receptor antagonists increases the uptake and retention of the pertechnetate by the gastric mucosa enhancing the detection of a Meckel diverticulum.[8,9] This pharmacologic enhancement may be beneficial for patients with an initial negative scan with a high index of clinical suspicion. False positive results have been noted in patients with intussusception, hydronephrosis, arteriovenous malformation, inflammatory bowel disease, and intestinal duplication owing to heterotopic gastric mucosa. False negative scans can be due to suboptimal examination technique, impaired blood supply to the bowel, or insufficient mass of ectopic gastric tissue to take up the isotope. Patients with a Meckel who do not have ectopic gastric mucosa will have a negative scan.

Additional alternatives to investigate GI bleeding include capsule endoscopy and double-balloon enteroscopy. Capsule endoscopy has identified a Meckel in patients with unexplained GI bleeding,[10,11] although 1 case did report retention of the capsule with cooccurring enteroliths.[12] Retrograde and prograde double-balloon enteroscopy has been described as a means of visualizing a Meckel diverticulum in patients with GI bleeding. In addition, this has also aided in therapy.[13,14] Double-balloon enteroscopy has been demonstrated to be relatively safe in the hands of experienced professionals and can be considered if other diagnostic procedures have failed to reveal a suspected Meckel.[15] A retrospective study found diagnostic yield for double-balloon

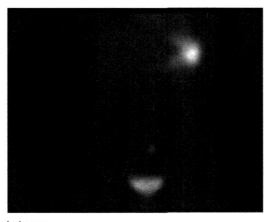

Fig. 2. Positive Meckel scan.

enteroscopy to be significantly greater than capsule endoscopy.[16] Arteriography can be used to identify the source of bleeding if the Meckel scan is negative, but it requires fairly brisk bleeding, 1 mL per minute. The upper GI and small bowel follow-through series is typically not very helpful in this situation. Finally, in the setting of a negative workup and a high clinical suspicion, some patients may be considered for a diagnostic laparoscopy given that this is minimally invasive and safe in the hands of an experienced surgeon. In those presenting with obstructive symptoms, a conventional radiographic approach is undertaken.

Once a symptomatic Meckel diverticulum has been identified, the standard of care is laparoscopic removal. Conventional laparoscopy is often used, but reports of single-incision laparoscopic surgery are emerging.[17] If a Meckel is found incidentally, the management is controversial. In asymptomatic patients in whom it is noted radiographically, many would recommend close follow-up without surgical intervention.[18] If there is discovery of an incidental Meckel during an operative procedure for another condition, some would recommend its removal owing to low risk of complications and future risk of complications.[19] Others, however, recommend leaving it in.[20] The macroscopic appearance of a Meckel does not indicate if heterotopic gastric mucosa is present or not and thus does not aid in the decision to remove it.[21]

The treatment of an incidentally found Meckel diverticulum in the adult population is also controversial. Proponents of resection cite outdated literature related to a conservative approach and increased risk of complications in adulthood, including malignancy as well as a relatively low morbidity particularly when performed with a minimally invasive approach.[22] Consideration for diverticulectomy should be given to patients younger than 50 years, those with ectopic tissue, or those with a broad base.[23]

DUODENAL WEB (STENOSIS)

Duodenal webs occur when there is incomplete bowel lumen recanalization during the 8th to 10th week of gestation. This results in a thin web (windsock) of the mucosa and submucosa layers causing some degree of obstruction.[24] The web is located in the second portion of the duodenum 85% to 90% of the time.[25] Much less frequently, they are located in the third or fourth portion of the duodenum.[26] The incidence of duodenal web is estimated to be 1 in 10,000 to 1 in 40,000 live births.[27] Duodenal webs are most often congenital; however, it has been described that they may be a rare complication of long-term nonsteroidal anti-inflammatory use.[28,29] This is frequently associated with other congenital anomalies, including Down syndrome, malrotation, congenital heart disease, and annular pancreas.[24,30]

Duodenal webs can present prenatally with in utero growth failure and/or polyhydramnios. Most other cases present in infancy with bilious emesis, food refusal, or failure to thrive.[31] In addition, duodenal web has been reported to cause upper GI bleeding in infants.[32,33] Webs are not exclusive to children, as they can also present at older ages.[31,34,35]

Duodenal webs are often more difficult to diagnose than atresias owing to the partial nature of obstruction. The diagnosis of a duodenal web can be considered prenatally by noting polyhydramnios and a dilated stomach on ultrasound. A plain abdominal radiograph may be normal or reveal a "double-bubble" sign from a dilated proximal duodenum and stomach. Distal air within the GI tract will be noted owing to the incomplete nature of the obstruction. An upper GI series may reveal the classic windsock sign.[26,36]

Therapeutic options are duodenoduodenostomy or duodenotomy with excision/lysis of the web. In cases whereby there is an enlarged proximal duodenum (duodenal diameter ≥5 cm), imbrications (the operative overlapping of layers of tissue in the closure of wounds or the repair of defects) or tapering duodenoplasty may be required.[37] During any attempt at resection of a duodenal web, care should be given to identify the ampulla of Vater, as it may be injured because of its proximity to the obstructing web. The ampulla may be identified by gentle compression of the gallbladder while viewing within the medial wall of the duodenal lumen for expression of bile. Surgery can be performed as an open procedure or laparoscopically. Some have noted that either approach was equally effective with no significant differences in outcome.[38] Some have noted that the laparoscopic approach was associated with a shorter length of stay and more rapid advancement to full feeding,[39] whereas others thought that the open procedure was preferable.[40] Ultimately, larger studies are needed to provide better evidence. More recently, there are reports of advanced endoscopy using several techniques to treat duodenal webs.[27,30,41–47] To date, there have not been any studies published comparing surgical versus endoscopic approaches. Both approaches are associated with complications, including bleeding and pancreatitis, whereas endoscopic approaches may be associated with incomplete obliteration of the web.[42] For patients that have prolonged duodenal ileus, there may be a benefit to using TPN or a transanastomotic tube for enteral nutrition.[48] If malrotation is present, a Ladd procedure should be performed. Long-term prognosis is very good and is primarily dependent on any associated congenital anomalies.[49]

DUODENAL ATRESIA

Duodenal atresia has a reported incidence of approximately 1 in 5000 to 10,000 live births,[50,51] with the most recent data at 0.9 per 10,000.[52] There are 4 major types of duodenal atresia[53] (**Fig. 3**). Type 1 is complete mucosal membrane or diaphragm with the muscularis and serosa remaining intact such that there is no discontinuity of the bowel (as above). Type 2 consists of a fibrous cord connecting the 2 segments of duodenum that are discontinuous. This differs from type 3, where there is no fibrous connection between the proximal and distal segments of duodenum (most common). Type 4 consists of several atretic segments such that it appears like a string of sausages. Duodenal atresia results from failure of recanalization of the duodenum after the seventh week of gestation, perhaps from an ischemic event, or genetic factors may also play a role.[54] Duodenal atresia, unlike other intestinal atresias, is commonly

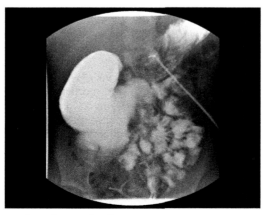

Fig. 3. Long-term sequelae of megaduodenum.

associated with other congenital anomalies, such as Down syndrome, which is present in 25% to 40% of cases.[55] Other associated anomalies include VATER (vertebral defects, anal anomalies, esophageal atresia, and renal abnormalities), malrotation, annular pancreas, biliary tract abnormalities, cardiac, and mandibulofacial anomalies.[52]

The initial manifestation of duodenal atresia or other intestinal atresia may be maternal polyhydramnios owing to the infant's inability to swallow and absorb the amniotic fluid. The postnatal presentation is typically within the first day or 2 of life with obstructive symptoms, such as persistent emesis, bilious emesis, gastric distention, or feeding difficulties.[54] The physical examination differs from jejunal or ileal atresia in that the abdomen is typically not distended owing to the proximal obstruction in duodenal atresia.

Perinatal ultrasound may be the first diagnostic test in the evaluation of duodenal atresia. One should consider intestinal atresia in an infant with maternal polyhydramnios because about 15% of infants with this will have GI tract abnormalities,[56] and up to 80% of duodenal atresia cases will have polyhydramnios.[3] Other ultrasonic findings may include a "double-bubble" sign. This also is the classic finding on a plain radiograph because of the dilated proximal duodenum and stomach associated with lack of bowel gas in the distal intestine.[57] If the double-bubble sign is noted, most think that no other radiographic studies are required. Administration of contrast into the upper GI tract could lead to aspiration. As the double-bubble sign may occur in instances of malrotation, some investigators recommend performing contrast studies looking for a malpositioned colon and cecum as may be present in malrotation.[58]

Once duodenal atresia is identified, a nasogastric or orogastric tube should be placed to decompress the stomach and minimize aspiration along with routine supportive management, such as intravenous fluids. Echocardiography should be considered in infants displaying features of trisomy 21 to exclude endocardial cushion defects. Once clinically stable, surgical repair via laparotomy or laparoscopy is indicated. Options for surgical therapy include a side-to-side or end-to-side duodenoduodenostomy or duodenojejunostomy. Before performing the anastomosis, a small rubber catheter should be passed distally to investigate for any additional intraluminal obstruction.[48] As with duodenal web, there is some controversy regarding performing surgery as an open procedure or laparoscopically.[38-40,48] One review concluded duodenal atresia should only undergo laparoscopic repair at designated centers of expertise.[59] Delayed transition to full enteral nutrition is more likely to occur in patients with comorbid congenital heart disease or malrotation and prematurity[60]; however, most of these cases were repaired via laparotomy. Intraoperatively, it is important to exclude any associated malrotation, other small bowel atresia, or annular pancreas.

Long-term prognosis for duodenal atresia is very favorable with approximately 90% survival.[49] The major causes of morbidity and mortality from duodenal atresia are related to associated anomalies, such as trisomy 21 or congenital heart disease. Infants with a birth weight of less than 2 kg are also at higher risk of mortality.[61]

Long-term complications include megaduodenum, duodenogastric reflux, gastritis, blind-loop syndrome, and gastroesophageal reflux disease. Megaduodenum may result from anastomotic obstruction or from the inherent dysmotility of the proximal duodenum.[62] Kimura and colleagues[63] reported no instances of megaduodenum in patients undergoing the "diamond-shaped" anastomosis. Blind-loop syndrome occurs more commonly in children undergoing duodenojejunostomy and may improve after conversion to standard duodenoduodenostomy.[64]

JEJUNOILEAL ATRESIA

Jejunoileal atresias are discussed separately from duodenal atresia owing to differences in cause, associated anomalies as well as treatment and outcome. Jejunoileal atresias occur as a result of an in utero vascular accident.[65] Maternal smoking and cocaine use have been associated with intestinal atresia.[66] There is an estimated incidence of approximately 1 to 3 per 10,000 live births.[52] This disorder affects both sexes equally. Jejunoileal atresias are equally distributed between the jejunum and ileum. Associated congenital anomalies are less common with jejunoileal atresia than duodenal atresia. The most commonly associated conditions are cystic fibrosis, malrotation, and gastroschisis, all of which are present in about 10% of cases.[67] Intestinal atresia is associated with low birth weight and multiparity.

There is a rare disorder of multiple intestinal atresias that can occur anywhere in the GI tract and is almost always fatal.[68] Hereditary multiple intestinal atresia is an autosomal recessive disorder that consists of multiple atretic segments that occurs most commonly in French Canadians and may be associated with combined immune deficiency. This is due to mutations of tetratricopeptide repeat domain–7A (TTC7A) gene. The TTC7A protein is important for the development and function of the thymus and intestinal epithelium.[69] This mutation has also been associated with very early onset inflammatory bowel disease.[70]

There are 4 types of intestinal atresia based on the anatomic characteristics[53] (**Fig. 4**). Type I is an intraluminal web consisting of mucosa and submucosa with continuity of the proximal and distal muscular layers without a mesenteric defect. Type II atresia is when the bowel is discontinuous but without a mesenteric defect. Type III has 2 subtypes. In type IIIA, the bowel is discontinuous, and there is also a mesenteric defect. Type IIIB has discontinuous bowel but with an extensive mesenteric defect with the bowel wrapped around a single artery such that it looks like a Christmas tree or apple peel (**Fig. 5**). Type IV consists of multiple atretic segments that appear like a string of sausage.

The typical presentation is an infant in the first 1 to 2 days of life with bilious vomiting, a history of maternal polyhydramnios, and abdominal distention depending on the level of atresia with more distal lesions having more distention. The infant may also have feeding difficulties and hyperbilirubinemia. With more distal lesions, there may be failure to pass meconium. Infants with more proximal lesions may pass meconium owing to the generation of succus entericus.

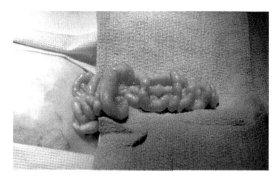

Fig. 4. Type IIIB jejunal atresia with associated "apple-peel" or "Christmas-tree" deformity of the mesentery. Note the single vessel within the center of the coils of bowel responsible for perfusion of the distal intestinal segment.

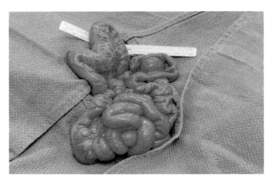

Fig. 5. Intestinal duplication cyst.

The diagnosis of jejunoileal atresia may be detected by prenatal ultrasound. Findings suggestive of atresia include dilated, echogenic bowel, and maternal polyhydramnios that is seen in about one-third of cases. These findings, however, have a poor predictive value for bowel abnormalities, and when questionable, fetal MRI can be considered.[71] Postnatally, the first step in the workup is a plain abdominal radiograph that often reveals multiple dilated loops of intestine with air fluid levels and at times a triple-bubble sign: dilated stomach, duodenum, and proximal jejunum.[72] Peritoneal calcifications suggest the presence of meconium peritonitis, which is a sign of intrauterine intestinal perforation and can be seen in about 12% of cases.[71] The presence of meconium peritonitis should raise suspicion of a meconium ileus and cystic fibrosis. The obstructive findings noted above can also be seen in other disorders, such as Hirschsprung disease. A barium enema may help to distinguish atresia from other obstructive disorders. Infants with jejunoileal atresia typically have a microcolon. If meconium ileus is present, one may consider meglumine diatrizoate (Gastrografin) enema that is hypertonic and can help evacuate the meconium as well as make a diagnosis.

Once diagnosed, surgical therapy should be undertaken expeditiously. Preoperatively, the neonate needs to be stabilized and have fluid and electrolyte abnormalities corrected. A nasogastric tube should be placed to decompress the stomach and minimize aspiration. Broad-spectrum antibiotics are indicated to help decrease risk of infection, which is a major cause of mortality. Surgery can be done via an open approach or laparoscopically, but the latter can be challenging.[73,74] Intraoperatively, the entire bowel is closely examined for sites of obstruction and the presence of other atresias. It is also important to assess patency of the colon either by preoperative contrast study or by intraoperative irrigation of the distal atretic limb. If malrotation or gastroschisis is present, they must also be corrected.

Postoperative mortality is related to prematurity, associated anomalies, infection, and short gut syndrome. Postoperative complications include anastomotic leak, stenosis at the site of anastomosis, and short gut syndrome. In addition, these patients may have oral feeding intolerance, which is more likely if any of the following are present: meconium peritonitis, luminal discrepancy, number of anastomoses, presence of immature ganglion, and short bowel syndrome.[75] The complexity of jejunoileal atresia (based on Grosfeld classification), when there are not any other congenital malformations, is not associated with a worse prognosis in terms of initiation of enteral nutrition, postoperative complications, duration of postoperative TPN, and percentage of short bowel syndrome.[76]

The prognosis for infants with jejunoileal atresia is very good with more than 90% survival.[67] The prognosis for those with short gut syndrome is dependent on the length of the remaining small bowel, the presence of the ileocecal valve, and the dependence on long-term parenteral nutrition.[77] Wilmore,[78] in 1972, published data on prognosis of short gut syndrome in infants. Those with greater than 40 cm of small bowel had a 95% survival rate. This decreased to 50% in those with 15 to 40 cm and an intact ileocecal valve. Those with less than 40 cm and no ileocecal valve, and those with less than 15 cm with the ileocecal valve did not survive. Things have improved since then because of newer surgical techniques, including bowel lengthening procedures (STEP procedure), improved medical care, and the ability to perform small bowel transplantation.[79] There are case reports of infants surviving with only 10 cm.[80] For those with short bowel syndrome, the overall prognosis is that 47% will wean from TPN, 26% will have a small bowel transplant, and 27% will not survive.[81] Small bowel dilation may be seen in short- and long-term survivors secondary to dysmotility or anastomotic strictures. Normalizing small bowel caliber may improve peristalsis through either plication, tapering, or anastomotic revision.[82] Reoperation may also be required for adhesive obstruction.[83]

SMALL BOWEL DUPLICATIONS

GI duplications are rare, estimated to occur in 1 per 100,000 births.[84] Calder is given credit for the first report of intestinal duplications in 1733. These were known by several terms, such as giant diverticula, enteric cysts, intestinal duplex, and "unusual Meckel diverticulum," until Ladd popularized the term intestinal duplication in the 1930s.[85] Males appear to be more commonly affected, 60% to 80% of cases, and about one-third have associated congenital anomalies.[86,87] It is estimated that 2% to 12% are found in the duodenum, about 44% in the ileum, and about 50% in the jejunum.[88] Multiple duplications are noted in 15% to 20% of cases.

The cause of duplications is unknown.[89] Theories include abnormalities in recanalization, a vascular insult, persistence of embryonic diverticula, and partial twining. Duplications can be cystic or tubular, depending on their length.[90] They consist of an epithelial lining from some portion of the GI track and a smooth muscle wall that are located on the mesenteric side of the intestine. Most duplications do not communicate with the adjacent bowel.[87]

Duplications can present at any age; however, 60% to 80% present in the first 2 years of life.[86,91,92] The presentation depends on the size and the epithelial type of the duplication. Small cystic duplications can be the lead point of an intussusception. Larger tubular duplications can accumulate secretions, dilate, and cause obstructive type symptoms. Those that are lined with gastric epithelium will secrete acid, which can result in ulceration and present with bleeding or perforation. Other modes of presentation include chronic abdominal pain, nausea and vomiting, jaundice, pancreatitis, or abdominal mass.[90,93,94]

Small bowel duplications may be detected by prenatal sonography.[87,95–97] Ultrasound is commonly used as part of the evaluation of an acute abdomen or a mass and may detect a duplication. Enteric duplications on ultrasonography often have an inner hyperechoic rim with an outer surrounding hypoechoic layer ("double-wall" sign) along with peristalsis being present.[95] Other diagnostic imaging considerations include computed tomographic scan, MRI, contrast studies and radionuclide scans.[88,92,98] Contrast studies can be helpful in those cases whereby there is communication of the duplication with the native GI track or by demonstrating a mass effect. Technetium-99m pertechnetate scanning can be useful in those duplications containing ectopic gastric mucosa, but this is the case in only 15% to 25% of cases.[90]

Endoscopic ultrasound has been used more recently to diagnose duplications in the upper GI tract, including the duodenum.[88] Many duplications are detected incidentally during surgery for another reason.

Treatment of duplication cysts, in general, is excision of the lesion to avoid or correct complications, including bleeding, volvulus, intestinal necrosis, and malignant degeneration.[90,99] The adjacent normal bowel frequently requires concomitant resection because of the common blood supply. The surgery can be performed via open or laparoscopic approach.[95] Duplications near the ampulla of Vater pose a challenge and may not be able to be removed. Those that cannot be excised should be drained and the mucosa stripped. The cyst may then be drained into the adjacent intestine to prevent recurrent collection of fluid. For proximal lesions, an endoscopic approach can be considered when a skilled advanced endoscopist is available.[93,94] For lesions with gastric mucosa that cannot be removed, one can use acid suppressants to minimize bleeding. In cases of enteric duplications being detected prenatally, prenatal surgery is not required; however, serial ultrasound surveillance is recommended to monitor size.[87] Complex tubular duplications present technical challenges and require individual reconstruction. Long-term complication of excision relates to the amount of intestine resected as well as the possibility of adhesive small bowel obstruction.

SUMMARY

Congenital anomalies of the small bowel are varied in type, most of which present with intestinal obstruction. Although manifestation of these is typically in the child, initial presentation and complications of therapy may present well into adulthood. Meckel diverticulum typically presents as painless GI bleeding in children. Other manifestations may present later. Duplications can also present as GI bleeding or as a mass or obstruction. Again, these anomalies present more commonly early in life, but they may not present until adulthood. Radiographic studies are the mainstay in the diagnosis of congenital anomalies of the small intestine. Upon making the diagnosis of a congenital anomaly of the small intestine, one also needs to assess for the presence of associated disorders. Once diagnosed, operative therapy is required for most congenital anomalies of the small intestine. The overall prognosis of these disorders is favorable owing to improved medical and surgical therapies. As mortality for these anomalies has decreased, remote complications of their repair will likely present to the general surgeon later in life.

CLINICS CARE POINTS

- Many children with congenital lesions of the gastrointestinal tract are surviving to adulthood and may require additional surgical intervention related to their original anomaly.
- Children are not just small adults; ergo, adults are not just large children. Consult with a pediatric surgeon, if possible, should surgical intervention be required in an adult surviving congenital-based surgery.
- Review all the pertinent anatomy and pathophysiology as it relates to the congenital lesion before intervening.
- Obtain any operative reports or pathology and imaging reports preoperatively to use as a "roadmap."
- Involve other consultants familiar with childhood diseases, as is necessary for optimal outcomes.

REFERENCES

1. Opitz JM, Schultka R, Gobbel L. Meckel on developmental pathology. Am J Med Genet A 2006;140(2):115–28.
2. Sagar J, Kumar V, Shah DK. Meckel's diverticulum: a systematic review. J R Soc Med 2006;99(10):501–5.
3. St-Vil D, Brandt ML, Panic S, et al. Meckel's diverticulum in children: a 20-year review. J Pediatr Surg 1991;26(11):1289–92.
4. Elsayes KM, Menias CO, Harvin HJ, et al. Imaging manifestations of Meckel's diverticulum. AJR Am J Roentgenol 2007;189(1):81–8.
5. Hayashi A, Kumada T, Furukawa O, et al. Severe acute abdomen caused by symptomatic Meckel's diverticulum in three children with trisomy 18. Am J Med Genet A 2015;167A(10):2447–50.
6. Sinha CK, Pallewatte A, Easty M, et al. Meckel's scan in children: a review of 183 cases referred to two paediatric surgery specialist centres over 18 years. Pediatr Surg Int 2013;29(5):511–7.
7. Lin S, Suhocki PV, Ludwig KA, et al. Gastrointestinal bleeding in adult patients with Meckel's diverticulum: the role of technetium 99m pertechnetate scan. South Med J 2002;95(11):1338–41.
8. Petrokubi RJ, Baum S, Rohrer GV. Cimetidine administration resulting in improved pertechnetate imaging of Meckel's diverticulum. Clin Nucl Med 1978;3(10):385–8.
9. Rerksuppaphol S, Hutson JM, Oliver MR. Ranitidine-enhanced 99mtechnetium pertechnetate imaging in children improves the sensitivity of identifying heterotopic gastric mucosa in Meckel's diverticulum. Pediatr Surg Int 2004;20(5):323–5.
10. Xinias I, Mavroudi A, Fotoulaki M, et al. Wireless capsule endoscopy detects Meckel's diverticulum in a child with unexplained intestinal blood loss. Case Rep Gastroenterol 2012;6(3):650–9.
11. Desai SS, Alkhouri R, Baker SS. Identification of Meckel diverticulum by capsule endoscopy. J Pediatr Gastroenterol Nutr 2012;54(2):161.
12. Courcoutsakis N, Pitiakoudis M, Mimidis K, et al. Capsule retention in a giant Meckel's diverticulum containing multiple enteroliths. Endoscopy 2011;43:E308–9.
13. Qi S, Huang H, Wei D, et al. Diagnosis and minimally invasive surgical treatment of bleeding Meckel's diverticulum in children using double-balloon enteroscopy. J Pediatr Surg 2015;50(9):1610–2.
14. Fukushima M, Kawanami C, Inoue S, et al. A case series of Meckel's diverticulum: usefulness of double-balloon enteroscopy for diagnosis. BMC Gastroenterol 2014;14:155.
15. Zheng CF, Huang Y, Tang ZF, et al. Double-balloon enteroscopy for the diagnosis of Meckel's diverticulum in pediatric patients with obscure GI bleeding. Gastrointest Endosc 2014;79(2):354–8.
16. He Q, Zhang Y, Xiao B, et al. Double-balloon enteroscopy for diagnosis of Meckel's diverticulum: comparison with operative findings and capsule endoscopy. Surgery 2013;153(4):549–54.
17. Chan KW, Lee KH, Wong HY, et al. Laparoscopic excision of Meckel's diverticulum in children: what is the current evidence? World J Gastroenterol 2014;20(41):15158–62.
18. Zani A, Eaton S, Rees CM, et al. Incidentally detected Meckel diverticulum: to resect or not to resect? Ann Surg 2008;247(2):276–81.

19. Bani-Hani KE, Shatnawi NJ. Meckel's diverticulum: comparison of incidental and symptomatic cases. World J Surg 2004;28(9):917–20.
20. Soltero MJ, Bill AH. The natural history of Meckel's diverticulum and its relation to incidental removal. A study of 202 cases of diseased Meckel's diverticulum found in King County, Washington, over a fifteen-year period. Ann J Surg 1976;132(2): 168–73.
21. Gezer HO, Temiz A, Ince E, et al. Meckel diverticulum in children: evaluation of macroscopic appearance for guidance in subsequent surgery. J Pediatr Surg 2015;51(7):1177–80 [Epub ahead of print].
22. Zani A, Eaton S, Rees CM, et al. Incidentally detected Meckel's diverticulum: To resect or not to resect? Ann Surg 2008;247:275–81.
23. Park JJ, Wolff BG, Tollefson MK, et al. Meckel diverticulum: The Mayo Clinic experience with 1476 patients (1950-2002). Ann Surg 2005;241(3):529–33.
24. Eksarko P, Nazir S, Kessler E, et al. Duodenal web associated with malrotation and review of literature. J Surg Case Rep 2013;2013(12).
25. Melek M, Edirne YE. Two cases of duodenal obstruction due to a congenital web. World J Gastroenterol 2008;14(8):1305–7.
26. Materne R. The duodenal windsock sign. Radiology 2001;218(3):749–50.
27. Beeks A, Gosche J, Giles H, et al. Endoscopic dilation and partial resection of a duodenal web in an infant. J Pediatr Gastroenterol Nutr 2009;48(3):378–81.
28. Serracino-Inglott F, Smith GH, Anderson DN. Duodenal webs–no age limit. HBO (Oxford) 2003;5(3):186–7.
29. Rha SE, Lee JH, Lee SY, et al. Duodenal diaphragm associated with long-term use of nonsteroidal anti-inflammatory drugs: a rare cause of duodenal obstruction in an adult. AJR Am J Roentgenol 2000;175(3):920–1.
30. Lee SS, Hwang ST, Jang NG, et al. A case of congenital duodenal web causing duodenal stenosis in a down syndrome child: endoscopic resection with an insulated-tip knife. Gut Liver 2011;5(1):105–9.
31. Karnsakul W, Gillespie S, Cannon ML, et al. Food refusal as an unusual presentation in a toddler with duodenal web. Clin Pediatr (Phila) 2009;48(1):81–3.
32. Nagpal R, Schnaufer L, Altschuler SM. Duodenal web presenting with gastrointestinal bleeding in a seven-month-old infant. J Pediatr Gastroenterol Nutri 1993;16(1):90–2.
33. Al Shahwani N, Mandhan P, Elkadhi A, et al. Congenital duodenal obstruction associated with Down's syndrome presenting with hematemesis. J Surg Case Rep 2013;2013(12).
34. Ladd AP, Madura JA. Congenital duodenal anomalies in the adult. Arch Surg 2001;136(5):576–84.
35. Sarkar S, Apte A, Sarkar N, et al. Vomiting and food refusal causing failure to thrive in a 2-year-old: an unusual and late manifestation of congenital duodenal web. BMJ Case Rep 2011.
36. Eisenberg RL, Levine MS. Miscellaneous abnormalities of the stomach and duodenum. In: Gore RM, Levine MS, editors. Textbook of gastrointestinal Radiology. 4th edition. Philadelphia, PA: Elsevier Saunders; 2015. Available at: https://www.clinicalkey.com/#!/content/book/3-s2.0-B9781455751174000349. Accessed January 12, 2016.
37. Sarin YK, Sharma A, Sinha S, et al. Duodenal webs: an experience with 18 patients. J Neonatal Surg 2012;1(2):20.
38. Jensen AR, Short SS, Anselmo DM, et al. Laparoscopic versus open treatment of congenital duodenal obstruction: multicenter short-term outcomes analysis. J Laparoendosc Adv Surg Tech A 2013;23(10):876–80.

39. Spilde TL, Peter SD, Keckler SJ, et al. Open vs laparoscopic repair of congenital duodenal obstructions: a concurrent series. J Pediatr Surg 2008;43(6):1002–5.

40. Parmentier B, Peycelon M, Muller CO, et al. Laparoscopic management of congenital duodenal atresia or stenosis. A single-center early experience. J Pediatr Surg 2015;50(11):1833–6.

41. Barabino A, Gandullia P, Arrigo S, et al. Successful endoscopic treatment of a double duodenal web in an infant. Gastrointest Endosc 2011;73(2):401–3.

42. Barabino A, Arrigo S, Gandullia P, et al. Duodenal web: complications and failure of endoscopic treatment. Gastrointest Endosc 2012;75(5):1123–4.

43. Bleve C, Costa L, Bertoncello V, et al. Endoscopic resection of a duodenal web in an 11-month-old infant with multiple malformations. Endoscopy 2015;47(S 01): E210–1.

44. Huang MH, Bian HQ, Liang C, et al. Gastroscopic treatment of membranous duodenal stenosis in infants and children: report of 6 cases. J Pediatr Surg 2015;50(3):413–6.

45. Kay GA, Lobe TE, Custer MD, et al. Endoscopic laser ablation of obstructing congenital duodenal webs in the newborn: a case report of limited success with criteria for patient selection. J Pediatr Surg 1992;27(3):279–81.

46. Kay S, Yoder S, Rothenberg S. Laparoscopic duodenoduodenostomy in the neonate. J Pediatr Surg 2009;44(5):906–8.

47. Torroni F, De Angelis P, Caldaro T, et al. Endoscopic membranectomy of duodenal diaphragm: pediatric experience. Gastrointest Endosc 2006;63(3): 530–1.

48. Son TN, Liem NT, Kien HH. Laparoscopic simple oblique duodenoduodenostomy in management of congenital duodenal obstruction in children. J Laparoendosc Adv Surg Tech A 2015;25(2):163–6.

49. Escobar MA, Ladd AP, Grosfeld JL, et al. Duodenal atresia and stenosis: long-term follow-up over 30 years. J Pediatr Surg 2004;39(6):867–71.

50. Hartman GE. Intestinal Obstruction. In: Stevenson DK, Cohen RS, Sunshine P, editors. Neonatology: clinical Practice and procedures. New York, NY: McGraw-Hill; 2015. Available at: http://accesspediatrics.mhmedical.com/content.aspx?bookid=1462&Sectionid=8559234. Accessed January 12, 2016.

51. Song C, Upperman JS, NiklasV. Structural Anomalies of the gastrointestinal tract. In: Gleason CA, Devaskar SU, editors. Avery's diseases of the newborn. 9th edition. Philadelphia, PA: Elsevier Saunders; 2012. Available at: http//www.clinicalkey.com/#!/content/book/3-s2.0-B9781437701340100691. Accessed January 12, 2016.

52. Best KE, Tennant PW, Addor MC, et al. Epidemiology of small intestinal atresia in Europe: a register-based study. Arch Dis Child Fetal Neonatal Ed 2012;97(5): F353–8.

53. Grosfeld JL, Ballantine TV, Shoemaker R. Operative management of intestinal atresia and stenosis based on pathologic findings. J Pediatr Surg 1979;14(3): 368–75.

54. Lloyd DA, Kenny SE. Congenital anomalies including hernias. In: Kleinman R, Sanderson I, Goulet O, et al, editors. Walker's pediatric gastrointestinal disease. 5th edition. Hamilton, Ontario: B.C. Decker Inc.; 2008. Available at: http://www.r2library.com/Resource/detail/1550093649/ch0013s0509. Accessed January 12, 2016.

55. Freeman SB, Torfs CP, Romitti PA, et al. Congenital gastrointestinal defects in Down syndrome: a report from the Atlanta and National Down Syndrome Projects. Clin Genet 2009;75(2):180–4.

56. Pauer HU, Viereck V, Krauss V, et al. Incidence of fetal malformations in pregnancies complicated by oligo- and polyhydramnios. Arch Gynecol Obstet 2003; 268(1):52–6.
57. Correia-Pinto J, Ribeiro A. Congenital duodenal obstruction and double-bubble sign. N Engl J Med 2014;371(11):e16.
58. Strouse PJ. Malrotation Semin Roentgenol 2008;43(1):7–14.
59. van der Zee DC. Laparoscopic repair of duodenal atresia: revisited. World J Surg 2011;35(8):1781–4.
60. Bairdain S, Yu DC, Lien C, et al. A modern cohort of duodenal obstruction patients: predictors of delayed transition to full enteral nutrition. J Nutr Metab 2014.
61. Piper HG, Alesbury J, Waterford SD, et al. Intestinal atresias: factors affecting clinical outcomes. J Pediatr Surg 2008;43(7):1244–8.
62. Spingland N, Yazbeck s. Complications associated with surgical treatment of congenital intrinsic duodenal obstruction. J Pediatr Surg 1990;25:1127–30.
63. Kimura k, Mokohara N, Nishijimi E, et al. Diamond -shaped anastomosis for duodenal atrsia: an experience with 44 patients over 15 years. J Pediatr Surg 1990;25:977–9.
64. Rescorola FJ, Grosfeld JL. Duodenal atresia in infancy and childhood: improved survival and long-term follow-up. Contemp Surg 1988;33:22–7.
65. Louw JH, Barnard CN. Congenital intestinal atresia; observations on its origin. Lancet 1955;269(6899):1065–7.
66. Werler MM, Sheehan JE, Mitchell AA. Maternal medication use and risks of gastroschisis and small intestinal atresia. Am J Epidemiol 2002;155(1):26–31.
67. Guttman FM, Braun P, Garance PH, et al. Multiple atresias and a new syndrome of hereditary multiple atresias involving the gastrointestinal tract from stomach to rectum. J Pediatr Surg 1973;8(5):633–40.
68. Fernandez I, Patey N, Marchand V, et al. Multiple intestinal atresia with combined immune deficiency related to TTC7A defect is a multiorgan pathology: study of a French Canadian-based cohort. Medicine (Baltimore) 2014;93(29):e327.
69. Dalla Vecchia LK, Grosfeld JL, West KW, et al. Intestinal atresia and stenosis: a 25-year experience with 277 cases. Arch Surg 1998;133(5):490–6.
70. Avitzur Y, Guo C, Mastropaolo LA, et al. Mutations in tetratricopeptide repeat domain 7A result in a severe form of very early onset inflammatory bowel disease. Gastroenterology 2014;146(4):1028–39.
71. Frischer JS, Azizkhan RG. Jejunoileal atresia and stenosis. In: Coran AG, editor. Pediatric surgery. 7th ed. Philadelphia, PA: Elsevier Saunders; 2012. Available at: https://www.clinicalkey.com/#!/content/book/3-s2.0-B9780323072557000829. Accessed January 12, 2016.
72. Vinocur DN, Lee EY, Eisenberg RL. Neonatal Intestinal Obstruction. AJR Am J Roentgenol 2012;198(1):W1–10.
73. Juang D, Snyder CL. Neonatal bowel obstruction. Surg Clin North Am 2012;92(3): 685–711.
74. Tajiri T, Ieiri S, Kinoshita Y, et al. Transumbilical approach for neonatal surgical diseases: woundless operation. Pediatr Surg Int 2008;24(10):1123–6.
75. Wang J, Du L, Cai W, et al. Prolonged feeding difficulties after surgical correction on intestinal atresia: a 13-year experience. J Pediatr Surg 2014;49(11):1593–7.
76. Federici S, Sabatino MD, Domenichelli V, et al. Worst prognosis in the "complex" jejunoileal atresia: is it real? Eur J Pediatr Surg Rep 2015;3(1):7–11.
77. Calisti A, Olivieri C, Coletta R, et al. Jejunoileal atresia: factors affecting the outcome and long-term sequelae. J Clin Neonatol 2012;1(1):38–41.

78. Wilmore DW. Factors correlating with a successful outcome following extensive intestinal resection in newborn infants. J Pediatr 1972;80(1):88–95.
79. Thompson JS, Rochling FA, Weseman RA, et al. Current management of short bowel syndrome. Curr Probl Surg 2012;49(2):52–115.
80. Infantino BJ, Mercer DF, Hobson BD, et al. Successful rehabilitation in pediatric ultrashort small bowel syndrome. J Pediatr 2013;163(5):1361–6.
81. Squires RH, Duggan C, Teitelbaum DH, et al. Natural history of pediatric intestinal failure: initial report from the pediatric intestinal failure consortium. J Pediatr 2012; 161(4):723–8.
82. Weber TR, Dane DW, Grosfeld JL. Tapering enteroplasty in infants with bowel atresia and short gut. Arch Surg 1982;117:684.
83. Wilkins BW, Spitz L. Incidence of postoperative adhesion obstruction following neonatal laparotomy. Br J Surg 1986;73:762–4.
84. Tsai SD, Sopha SC, Fishman EK. Isolated duodenal duplication cyst presenting as a complex solid and cystic mass in the upper abdomen. J Radiol Case Rep 2013;7(11):32–7.
85. Ladd WE. Duplications of the alimentary tract. South Med J 1937;30:363–71.
86. Ildstad ST, Tollerud DJ, Weiss RG, et al. Duplications of the alimentary tract. Clinical characteristics, preferred treatment, and associated malformations. Ann Surg 1988;208(2):184–9.
87. Laje P, Flake AW, Adzick NS. Prenatal diagnosis and postnatal resection of intra-abdominal enteric duplications. J Pediatr Surg 2010;45(7):1554–8.
88. Liu R, Adler DG. Duplication cysts: Diagnosis, management, and the role of endoscopic ultrasound. Endosc Ultrasound 2014;3(3):152–60. This article reviews the literature on duplication cysts and discusses the role of endoscopic ultrasound and fine needle aspiration in management.
89. Stern LE, Warner BW. Gastrointestinal duplications. Semin Pediatr Surg 2000; 9(3):135–40.
90. Niu BB, Bai YZ. Ileal tubular duplication in a 4-year-old girl. Surgery 2015;157(1): 166–7.
91. Karkera PJ, Bendre P, D'souza F, et al. Tubular colonic duplication presenting as rectovestibular fistula. Pediatr Gastroenterol Hepatol Nutr 2015;18(3):197–201.
92. Li BL, Huang X, Zheng CJ, et al. Ileal duplication mimicking intestinal intussusception: a congenital condition rarely reported in adult. World J Gastroenterol 2013;19(38):6500–4.
93. Arantes V, Nery SR, Starling SV, et al. Duodenal duplication cyst causing acute recurrent pancreatitis managed curatively by endoscopic marsupialization. Endoscopy 2012;44(S 02):E117–8.
94. Meier AH, Mellinger JD. Endoscopic management of a duodenal duplication cyst. J Pediatr Surg 2012;47(11):e33–5.
95. Ballehaninna UK, Nguyen T, Burjonrappa SC. Laparoscopic resection of antenataly identified duodenal duplication cyst. JSLS 2013;17(3):454–8.
96. Palacios A, De Vera M, Martinez-Escoriza JC. Prenatal sonographic findings of duodenal duplication: case report. J Clin Ultrasound 2013;41(S 1):1–5.
97. Vivier PH, Beurdeley TH, Bachy S, et al. Ileal duplication. Diagn Interv Imaging 2013;94(1):98–100.
98. Hur J, Yoon CS, Kim MJ, et al. Imaging features of gastrointestinal tract duplications in infants and children: from oesophagus to rectum. Pediatr Radiol 2007; 37(7):691–9.
99. Chen JJ, Lee HC, Yeung CY, et al. Meta-analysis: The clinical features of the duodenal duplication cyst. J Pediatr Surg 2010;45:1598–606.

Malrotation
Management of Disorders of Gut Rotation for the General Surgeon

Woo S. Do, MD*, Craig W. Lillehei, MD

KEYWORDS

- Malrotation • Midgut volvulus • Intestinal rotational abnormality • Ladd procedure

KEY POINTS

- Consider bilious emesis in a newborn malrotation with volvulus until proven otherwise; do not wait until the child is ill-appearing to evaluate and/or operate.
- Detorse in a counterclockwise fashion (turn back the hands of time); following detorsion, make every effort to preserve maximal bowel length.
- Fully Kocherize the duodenum, mobilize the cecum, and broaden the mesentery. In doing so, you will lyse the adhesive bands (Ladd bands) between the cecum and the structures to its right.
- The principles of damage control (including temporary abdominal closure, resuscitation, and planned "second look") that apply to adults can also be applied to children.

INTRODUCTION

Disorders of gut rotation encompass a wide array of clinical presentations, from the incidental imaging finding in an asymptomatic adult to the newborn at risk for catastrophic bowel loss. In the modern era, many of these patients will receive care by dedicated pediatric surgeons and specialists, particularly if there are superimposed conditions outside of the scope of this article (such as heterotaxy or cardiac anomalies). Nonetheless, it is not only possible but probable that the general surgeon may encounter clinical challenges relevant to gut rotation. The purpose of this article is to provide the general surgeon with a clinical blueprint to navigate scenarios relevant to the disorders of gut rotation.

[a] Pediatric Surgery, Boston Children's Hospital, 300 Longwood Avenue, Fegan 3, Boston, MA 02115, USA
* Corresponding author.
E-mail address: Woo.Do@childrens.harvard.edu

Surg Clin N Am 102 (2022) 837–845
https://doi.org/10.1016/j.suc.2022.07.013
0039-6109/22/Published by Elsevier Inc.
surgical.theclinics.com

Embryology

A review of the embryologic steps in normal rotation can help us understand the anatomic basis for the clinical manifestations of malrotation. Early in gestation, the midgut protrudes from the abdominal cavity and elongates as a U-shaped loop around the superior mesenteric vessels. At the completion of physiologic herniation (around week 10 of gestation), the midgut is a long loop of bowel arising from a narrow pedicle (or mesenteric axis). We refer to the proximal part of the loop as the duodenojejunal limb and the distal part as the cecocolic limb.[1]

When the bowel returns to the abdominal cavity, 3 factors directly affect the future risk of volvulus.

- Rotation: First, the midgut rotates 270° counterclockwise. This effectively places the duodenojejunal limb to the left of the mesenteric axis and the cecocolic limb to the right. This event is responsible for the c-loop appearance of the duodenum.
- Mesenteric width: A narrow mesentery is directly related to the risk of volvulus.
- Retroperitoneal fixation: The fixation of the duodenojejunal limb to the left of the axis yields the ligament of Treitz (LOT). The fixation of the cecocolic limb serves as the beginning of the retroperitoneal part of the right colon. Malposition and malfixation of the cecum can result in Ladd bands positioned across the duodenum.

Anomalies in any of the above 3 factors can result in the following variants of gut rotation:

- In classic malrotation, all 3 of the above events fail to occur. The c-loop of the duodenum is absent. The duodenojejunal junction stays to the right of midline and does not become fixed to the retroperitoneum in the expected position of the LOT. The mesentery stays narrow. Ladd bands can be present between the cecum (in the mid-upper abdomen) and the structures to the right of it, including the right lateral abdominal wall, gallbladder, and the duodenum. These adhesive bands can cause extrinsic compression of the duodenum and act as a source of obstruction independent of volvulus.
- In cases of incomplete rotation, the fourth portion of the duodenum or the duodenojejunal junction may fail to completely cross the midline or rise to the level of the pylorus.
- Reverse rotation is a rare variant that occurs when the midgut makes a clockwise turn (typically 90°) during the embryologic development. This results in the duodenum being anterior to the superior mesenteric artery (SMA) and the colon being posterior to the SMA. The part of the colon in the retro-arterial tunnel is at risk of extrinsic compression and partial obstruction. As in cases of classic malrotation, the midgut can still be at risk of volvulus.
- In cases of normal rotation without fixation, paraduodenal, or paracolic hernias can form.

Clinical Presentation

"Bilious emesis in a newborn is malrotation with volvulus until proven otherwise." This dictum remains a good one to stand by. Although the differential for newborn bilious emesis is broad, malrotation with volvulus is the single entity for which delay in intervention will yield a catastrophic outcome. Classic teaching holds that 20% to 50% of newborn bilious emesis consults will truly have an underlying surgical pathologic condition, of which malrotation with volvulus carries particular importance in terms of clinical urgency.[2–4] Most cases of malrotation (>50%) present in the first month of life, 30% in the first week, 15% within the first year. About 95% have bilious emesis.[5,6]

On physical examination, abdominal distension can be variable. It is important not to be falsely reassured by a flat, soft, nontender abdomen. Because the obstruction is high at the level of the duodenum, volvulus can still be present with a "reassuring" abdominal examination, normal laboratories (including white blood cell count and serum lactate), and even a normal appearing abdominal X-ray. **Figs. 1** and **2** highlight the potential differences seen between 2 patients who both had benign abdominal examinations but were found to have malrotation with volvulus; the first was a newborn with radiographic signs of duodenal obstruction and the second showed no such signs.

Ominous findings include bloody emesis/stools,which suggest intestinal ischemia, or peritonitis, which suggests perforation. Operative intervention should not be delayed while awaiting workup for a child *in extremis.*

Preoperative/Preprocedure Planning

Initial assessment of the infant should proceed with a thorough history and physical examination, laboratory tests, and an abdominal radiograph (see **Figs. 1** and **2**). That said, the crux of this diagnosis lies in the upper gastrointestinal (GI) series, which must be obtained expeditiously. Once the surgical consult has been received, it is a standard practice for the surgeon to accompany the infant to the fluoroscopy suite and (if warranted) proceed directly to the operating room. During this process, it is critical for the surgeon to be notified of any key electrolyte derangements, which bear prompt communication to the anesthesiologist.

The upper GI series must meet the following requirements to effectively rule-out malrotation with midgut volvulus. Each of these features coincides with the embryologic events previously described:

- The c-loop of the duodenum must cross over midline.
- The fourth portion of the duodenum (or the duodenojejunal junction) must rise back up to the level of the pylorus.

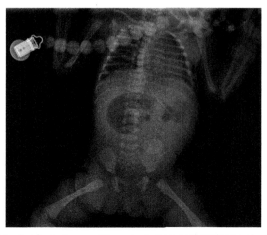

Fig. 1. Plain radiograph of newborn with malrotation and midgut volvulus. Depicted is the "double-bubble" sign of a dilated stomach and duodenum secondary to duodenal obstruction.

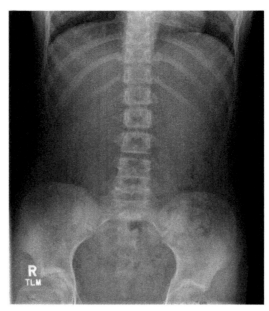

Fig. 2. Plain radiograph of 11-year-old child with malrotation and midgut volvulus. Note the absence of findings suggestive of obstruction.

- On a lateral view, the duodenum must go posteriorly to assume a retroperitoneal position.

In cases of malrotation with midgut volvulus, the upper GI series can show a "corkscrew" pattern of the jejunum. **Fig. 3** demonstrates this finding in the infant depicted in **Fig. 1**. Similarly, **Fig. 4** demonstrates the swirling jejunum in the child depicted in **Fig. 4**.

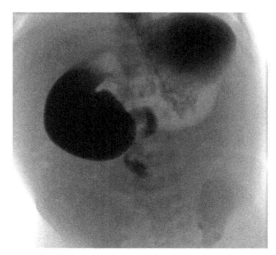

Fig. 3. Upper GI series of newborn with malrotation and midgut volvulus. Depicted is a dilated duodenal bulb with swirling or "corkscrew" pattern of the jejunum, suggestive of volvulus.

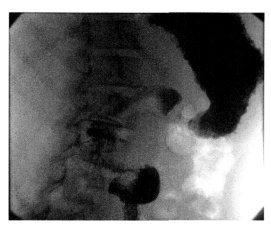

Fig. 4. Upper GI series of 11-year-old child with malrotation and midgut volvulus. Note that the duodenojejunal junction fails to rise to the level of the pylorus. The "corkscrew" pattern of the jejunum is suggestive of volvulus.

Although the characteristic features of volvulus are as depicted above, the upper GI findings for malrotation without volvulus can be subtle. After ruling out an acute volvulus, further investigation may be required.

An abdominal ultrasound can rapidly help clarify the presence of volvulus (**Fig. 5**). Normally, the superior mesenteric vein (SMV) should be to the patient's right of the SMA. Note that the upper GI remains the gold standard for diagnosis. However, we again stress the importance of an expeditious workup; one should not wait until the child is ill to proceed to the OR.

If the child is well-appearing and there is diagnostic uncertainty, it would be reasonable to proceed onto a diagnostic laparoscopy. At time of diagnostic laparoscopy, if malrotation with volvulus is found, immediate detorsion is warranted. Whether that intervention is laparoscopic or open remains a topic of controversy within the pediatric surgical community. We would recommend proceeding in the fashion that allows an expeditious detorsion.

Procedural Approach

First described in the 1930s, the Ladd procedure remains the mainstay of surgical management for malrotation with midgut volvulus.[7,8] The objective of the Ladd procedure is to reduce the risk of future obstruction or volvulus. This goal is achieved in the following steps (highlighted in **Fig. 6**):

1. Transverse laparotomy
   a. As infant abdomens have a characteristically short xiphopubic distance (ie, they are wider than they are tall), a transverse laparotomy is traditionally the approach espoused by pediatric surgeons. In older children and adults, a vertical midline laparotomy is still the incision of choice.
   b. General considerations for infant laparotomy:
      i. The umbilical vein (ligamentum teres) is a midline structure that can be quite large in a newborn. Unlike the adult where this structure is obliterated, this ligament may still be canalized in a newborn. Thus, this structure can and should be ligated prior to division.

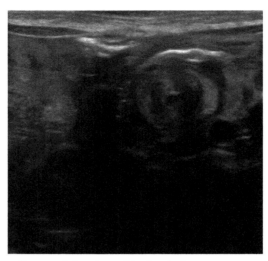

Fig. 5. Swirl sign on ultrasound showing midgut volvulus.

    ii. The liver is relatively large within the abdomen of the newborn and can occupy much of the upper abdomen. Although all tissue handling should be done carefully and thoughtfully, particular caution should be applied to the newborn liver. Dangerous subcapsular hematomas can develop rapidly in the septic, underresuscitated, or premature baby. Recall that the total blood volume is approximately 80 mL/kg, so even 10 mL of blood loss in a 2 kg baby can be substantial.

2. Detorse the bowel in a counterclockwise fashion. A helpful mnemonic is to "turn back the hands of time." Perform as many rotations as are necessary to ensure the mesentery lies flat without any twists.

3. Bowel is prone to torse if there is a narrow mesentery; therefore, a critical portion of this procedure is to broaden the mesentery. This involves scoring the peritoneum overlying the mesentery, so that the mesentery can be stretched broadly.

4. Fully Kocherize the duodenum and mobilize the cecum. In doing so, you will lyse the adhesive bands (Ladd bands) between the cecum and the structures to its right (this can include the duodenum, the gallbladder, and the right lateral abdominal wall). On completion, the duodenum should now have a straight, downward course.

5. Avoid pexies. Instinctively, one might be inclined to secure the bowel in the desired configuration with sutures (ie, pexy sutures). Historically, such efforts had been tried to prevent future recurrence, but this ultimately only yielded higher rates of bowel obstruction. As such,as this practice is no longer advocated.

In the situation that the bowel is questionably viable or frankly necrotic, one should be aware of the harm that can accompany the detorsion of bowel, which can lead to ischemia-reperfusion injury. Communicate with the anesthesiologist before detorsion. Be prepared to administer calcium for cardiac myocyte stabilization. Anticipate potential swings in hemodynamics and have code drugs on hand.

Following detorsion, every effort should be made to preserve maximal bowel length. Detorse and observe. Only frankly necrotic segments of bowel should be resected. If there is any uncertainty regarding viability of bowel, it is better to err on the side of preserving bowel and planning a "second look."

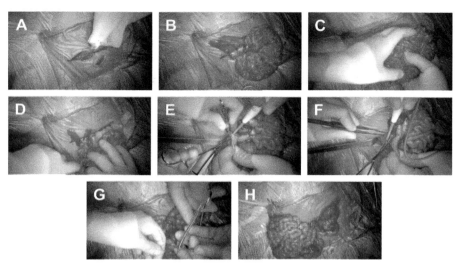

Fig. 6. (*A*) Transverse supraumbilical laparotomy in a newborn. This was done approximately one fingerbreadth above the umbilicus. Note the incision can be extended across midline. (*B*) Midgut volvulus. The bowel was eviscerated to expose the mesenteric root, revealing a narrow mesenteric axis with midgut volvulus. (*C*) Detorsion. "Turn back the hands of time" with a counterclockwise detorsion until the mesentery lies flat without twists. (*D*) Detorsion. "Turn back the hands of time" with a counterclockwise detorsion until the mesentery lies flat without twists. (*E*) Lysis of Ladd bands. It is important to identify any adhesive bands from the cecum, which can drape over the duodenum and act as a source of obstruction independent of volvulus. (*F*) Lysis of Ladd bands. It is important to identify any adhesive bands from the cecum, which can drape over the duodenum and act as a source of obstruction independent of volvulus. (*G*) Incidental appendectomy. Appendectomy at the time of Ladd procedure is recommended to avoid future diagnostic uncertainty. (*H*) Configuration of bowel following Ladd procedure. Note the small bowel to the right and the colon to the left.

The principles of damage control, temporary abdominal closure, resuscitation, and planned "second look," which apply to adults can also be applied to children. Silos are a good option for temporary abdominal closure but any form of temporary abdominal closure will work. The key principle is to allow for reinspection of bowel while avoiding abdominal compartment syndrome.

Although the loss of the midgut was previously fatal, advances in intestinal rehabilitation and small bowel transplantation have meaningfully expanded the options available for patients with short bowel syndrome.[9]

Postprocedure Care

Postoperatively many of these patients will have slow return of bowel function. A nasogastric (NG) tube should be maintained until the return of bowel function. Parenteral nutrition may be required. If the nutritional status was reasonable going into the procedure, we recommend giving the child up to about a week to be able to resume normal feeds. Most children following Ladd procedure will be able to tolerate feeds normally.

Outcomes

Although the likelihood of recurrent volvulus is relatively low after Ladd procedure, it can occur (incidence 1%). The most common reason for recurrent emesis is adhesive

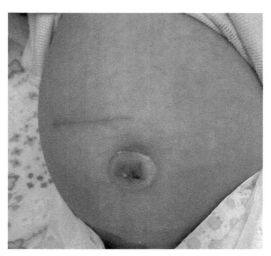

Fig. 7. Cosmetic outcome of transverse laparotomy.

small bowel obstruction (incidence up to 10%–15%).[10,11] Nonetheless, as recurrent volvulus is a worrisome event, patients should be counseled to seek immediate medical attention for recurrent emesis. Recurrent bilious emesis demands immediate attention. The cosmetic outcome of a transverse laparotomy is depicted in **Fig. 7**.

Special Considerations: Incidental Malrotation

In the modern era of imaging technology, variations of malrotation are more commonly being found incidentally in older populations. If truly asymptomatic, we recommend taking an approach of counseling the patient of the risk of volvulus, specifically that any episode of bilious emesis demands immediate medical attention. However, many of these patients will have vague symptoms that prompted the imaging study. Barring other considerations, it is appropriate to do a formal Ladd procedure in a symptomatic patient.[12]

CLINICS CARE POINTS

- Abdominal distension can be variable. Do not be falsely reassured by a flat, soft, nontender abdomen.
- Volvulus can still be present with a "reassuring" abdominal examination, normal laboratories (including WBC and serum lactate) and even a normal-appearing abdominal X-ray.
- Late findings: Bloody emesis or bloody stools suggest intestinal ischemia; peritonitis suggests perforation.
- If the child is well-appearing and there is some diagnostic uncertainty, it is reasonable to proceed onto diagnostic laparoscopy; at that point, if malrotation with volvulus is found, immediate detorsion is warranted.
- Incidental imaging finding of malrotation: if truly asymptomatic, counsel the patient of the risk of volvulus, specifically that any episode of bilious emesis demands immediate attention. However, many of these patients will have vague symptoms that prompted the imaging study. Barring other considerations, it is appropriate to do a formal Ladd procedure in a symptomatic patient.

DISCLOSURE

The views expressed are those of the authors and do not reflect the official policy or position of the Army, the Department of Defense, or the US Government. The authors have no conflicts of interest to disclose.

REFERENCES

1. Emil S. Chapter 28: Malrotation and midgut volvulus. In: Emil S, editor. Clinical pediatric surgery. Wolters Kluwer; 2019. p. 274–80.
2. Cullis PS, Mullan E, Jackson A, et al. An audit of bilious vomiting in term neonates referred for pediatric surgical assessment: can we reduce unnecessary transfers? J Pediatr Surg 2018;53(11):2123–7.
3. Godbole P, Stringer MD. Bilious vomiting in the newborn: How often is it pathologic? J Pediatr Surg 2002;37(6):909–11.
4. Jackson R, Folaranmi SE, Goel N. Approach to the baby with bilious vomiting. Paediatrics Child Health 2021;32(1):1–6.
5. Pursley D, Hansen AR, Puder M. Chapter 7.4: Obstruction. In: Hansen AR, Puder M, editors. Manual of neonatal surgical intensive care. 3rd editiion. Shelton, CT: People's Medical Publishing House; 2016. p. 291–312.
6. Bonasso PC, Dassinger S, Smith SD. Chapter 31: Malrotation. In: Holcomb GW, Murphy JP, St Peter SD, editors. Ashcraft's pediatric surgery. Elsevier; 2019. p. 507–16.
7. Ladd WE. Congenital obstruction of the duodenum in children. N Engl J Med 1932;206:277e283.
8. Ladd WE. Surgical diseases of the alimentary tract in infants. N Engl J Med 1936; 215:705e708.
9. Duggan CP, Jaksic T. Pediatric intestinal failure. N Engl J Med 2017;377(7): 666–75.
10. Langer JC. Intestinal rotation abnormalities and midgut volvulus. Surg Clin 2017; 97(1):147–59.
11. Murphy FL, Sparnon AL. Long-term complications following intestinal malrotation and the Ladd's procedure: a 15 year review. Pediatr Surg Int 2006;22(4):326–9.
12. Malek NM, Burd RS. Surgical treatment of malrotation after infancy: a population-based study. J Pediatr Surg 2005;40:285–9.

Surgical Support of the Developmentally Delayed or Neurologically Impaired Child

Robert L. Ricca, MD[a],*, Edward Penn, MD[b]

KEYWORDS

- Neurologically impaired • Developmental delay • Long-term management
- Shared decision-making

KEY POINTS

- Many children with underlying neurologic or developmental delays may require surgical intervention to provide improved activities of daily living and improved quality of life.
- General surgeons may be called upon to manage patients with chronic medical conditions and may benefit from an understanding of indications for previous surgical interventions and management of long-term complications to improve outcomes.
- Shared decision-making between the family, surgeon, and health care providers is essential to optimize surgical outcomes.
- Indications for tracheostomy tube placement in children have changed over the last several decades. Surgeons must be able to manage unplanned decannulation and complications such as tracheo-innominate artery fistula.
- Gastrostomy tubes are commonly placed in children with underlying neurologic impairment to provide enteral access for medication and nutritional support. Common complications include dislodgement and migration toward the costal margin leading to leakage and pain.
- Anti-reflux surgery in children with developmental delay or neurologic impairment should be predicated upon underlying symptoms to optimize outcomes.
- Laparoscopy is a useful adjunct in the placement of ventriculoperitoneal shunts, especially in the setting of shunt revision.
- Ventriculoperitoneal shunts may be preserved in the setting of a clean or clean-contaminated wound. Consultation with neurosurgery and infectious disease will assist with perioperative management.

[a] Division of Pediatric Surgery, University of South Carolina, Greenville, Prisma Health Upstate, Greenville Memorial Hospital, 48 Cross Park Court, Greenville, SC 29605, USA; [b] Greenville ENT Allergy and Associates, Prisma Upstate, Greenville Memorial Hospital, Greenville, SC, USA
* Corresponding author.
E-mail address: robert.ricca@prismahealth.org

Surg Clin N Am 102 (2022) 847–860
https://doi.org/10.1016/j.suc.2022.07.014
0039-6109/22/© 2022 Elsevier Inc. All rights reserved.

surgical.theclinics.com

INTRODUCTION

Developmental delays and neurologic impairment are not uncommon in the pediatric patient, many of whom will receive care from a pediatric surgeon at some point during their childhood. According to the World Health Organization, approximately 5% of children under the age of 14 years have a moderate-to-severe developmental delay. Furthermore, up to 15% of children under the age of 5 are diagnosed with a developmental delay.[1] These conditions vary greatly from children with underlying chromosomal anomalies including Trisomy 21 or Trisomy 18 to children with cerebral palsy, prematurity, and congenital conditions that predispose a child to a neurologic insult or developmental delay. Advances in medical care and improved treatment options have allowed these patients to live longer with improved quality of life. Despite these advances, children with neurologic disorders have been shown to account for a disproportionate number of intensive care unit (ICU) stays and mortality when compared with children without neurologic disorders.[2]

Many of these patients will reach adulthood and transition care to adult providers. This creates a requirement for adult practitioners to have a baseline understanding of the long-term implication and potential complications of surgical procedures that have been performed. These patients may also require emergent or urgent surgical management by an adult surgeon during childhood in settings where pediatric surgeons may not be readily available. These practitioners will require a thorough understanding of anatomic variances that have been created due to the surgical procedures that have been performed as well as how to manage acute complications of surgical devices.[3] Children with neurologic impairment and developmental delay may require assistance with their airway, enteral access as well as bowel and bladder management. These patients may also have underlying neurologic conditions, such as hydrocephalus, that require long-term management with various ventricular shunts. These children routinely are under the care of a parent, guardian, or other caregiver who is intimately aware of the patient's medical and surgical history. Treatment decisions may have a profound impact on the quality of life of both the patient and the caregiver and thus a shared decision-making model is important to not only obtain a thorough history but to also gain the trust of the patient and the caregiver.[4-6] It is important that the surgeon caring for these patients, at any point in time, has a thorough understanding of the underlying anatomy, and potential consequences to care and interact fully with both the patient and caregiver.

DISCUSSION
Shared Decision-Making

Management of any pediatric patient should include a comprehensive discussion with the parent or caregiver as well as an age-appropriate discussion with the patient themselves.[4-6] If available, child life specialists can serve to assist both the family and the patient cope with stressful and potentially traumatic situations, such as an upcoming surgery or procedure. Utilization of these resources can be invaluable in developing a strong relationship between the provider and patient as well as the provider and the family.[7] Although it is imperative to develop a therapeutic relationship with the patient who is receiving care, it is also important to develop a relationship with the parent or caregiver. This may be even more important when caring for a child with an underlying development delay or neurologic devastation.[8] Decisions regarding the management of tracheostomy tubes, gastrostomy tubes or other feeding devices, and other surgical decisions impact the parents and caregivers of all children. These decisions should be discussed in a detailed fashion with the parent or caregiver to ensure the surgeon understands the impact not only on the patient but also the impact on the parent or caregiver, the ability of the caregiver to continue to help outside of the hospital as well as the impact on other family members including siblings, grandparents, and extended family. The surgeon needs to recognize that the caregivers of children with neurologic impairment or developmental delay tend to have devised a daily routine that allows for maximal care of their child. Surgical decisions may have a significant impact and unintended consequences with regard to this daily routine and the care provided outside of the hospital. Decisions that may seem simple and clear in the patient's best interest from a medical standpoint may have unintended consequences on the ability of the caregiver to help at home or may impact the caregiver negatively regarding work or other requirements. A shared decision-making model is thus recommended when evaluating a child with developmental delay or neurologic impairment to understand what is in the best interest of the patient while taking into consideration the role of the primary caregiver.

Initial Evaluation

Children with underlying neurologic impairment or developmental delay will have a varied ability to participate fully in the evaluation of a surgical issue. This can result in difficulty with both accurate history taking and completing of a physical examination. Underlying reasons may include an inability to communicate with the surgeon, a limited understanding of the medical history, or limitations due to pain, anxiety, or mistrust of the health care provider. The surgical history and the history of the presenting illness may need to be obtained from the patient's guardians or caregivers and the medical records. In an inpatient setting the history may be augmented by input from the primary care team and nursing staff. This should not be a reason to avoid interaction with the patient themselves, but instead the surgeon should take the opportunity to seek out alternative sources for clarification, verification, and amplifying information. Many children with complex medical histories may have received care at various institutions creating a fragmented health care record preventing a thorough review of the prior medical and surgical history. Detailed questioning of the patient and the family member regarding prior surgical history and confirmation of these surgical procedures through physical examination, review of the medical record, and radiographic imaging if available is necessary prior to any further surgical thearpy.

Completion of a thorough physical examination may also be complicated by the underlying neurologic impairment. The patient may be apprehensive regarding examinations especially if they are experiencing pain or discomfort, if the examination requires evaluation of a sensitive area such as the genitalia or perianal region or if the patient has had past experiences that have led to mistrust of health care professionals. Patients with underlying neurologic impairment may also not be able to adequately verbalize pain or discomfort or localize symptoms to a certain region. Surgeons must be able to delineate secondary signs such as involuntary guarding, induration or erythema, and nonverbal cues such as withdrawal during the physical examination to adequately identify peritonitis or other indications for prompt surgical intervention. Discussion with the caregiver or guardian can provide the surgeon with information regarding how the patient typically responds to painful, or other, stimulus. The surgeon may also need to consider the use of sedation or anxiolytics when performing examinations, especially of the genitalia or perianal region to allow for a thorough examination and to avoid physical discomfort while alleviating emotional duress.

It is not uncommon to selectively use radiographic imaging, especially modalities that use ionizing radiation, when evaluating pediatric patients. These same efforts should be used when evaluating the pediatric patient with an underlying neurologic impairment, however, it must be recognized that radiographic evaluation may be necessary due to limited history, difficulty with physical examination and complexity of prior medical care. Ancillary studies may be required to better delineate underlying anatomy that has been modified or augmented in the previous surgery. Although many caregivers and guardians are extremely well-versed in the past medical history of their child, it may be prudent to obtain further imaging for preoperative planning especially if the condition is not emergent or life-threatening. These efforts may prove to be beneficial in avoiding complications from unknown altered anatomy due to surgeries such as bladder augmentation, enteral access, or other procedures.

Tracheostomy

The indications for tracheostomy have changed dramatically around the world in the last several decades. Previously the primary indication was upper airway obstruction because of infectious etiologies. However, with the advent of vaccines and broad-spectrum antibiotics, there is a decrease in the number of tracheostomies performed because of infections. Instead, multiple studies have shown that neurologic impairment with concomitant polyneuropathy or central hypoventilation has become the leading indication for tracheostomy in children.[9–11] Tracheostomy may also be performed for the following reasons:

a. Airway obstruction that may be because of congenital anomalies, tumors, or infectious disease
b. Airway protection due to underlying neurologic conditions or traumatic brain injury
c. Assistance with weaning from the ventilator
d. Prevention of laryngotracheal stenosis
e. Pulmonary toilet[10]

Owing to the permanent nature of some of these underlying conditions along with improved life expectancy with many congenital conditions as children grow, they will require a longer tracheostomy tube size. The size of the tracheostomy tube is important to ensure that is small enough to allow the child to speak yet large enough to prevent an air leak during ventilation and allow for adequate respiration. The child should be followed by an otolaryngologist with plans to increase the tube size as needed. Typically, based on growth, this may be every one to 2 years.[12] The following formulas are helpful in determining the appropriate size of the tracheostomy tube based upon the child's age:

Inner diameter (mm) = (age [years]/3) + 3.5,
Outer diameter (mm) = (age [years]/3) + 5.5.[12]

General surgeons should be aware of the potential long-term complications associated with tracheostomy tube placement. Families are instructed to change the tracheostomy tube approximately every week to prevent infectious complications, prevention of granulation tissue, mucous plugging of the tube and to ensure appropriate hygiene.[13–15] Surgeons should be aware of how to manage a dislodged tracheostomy from inadvertent loss or decannulation as well as an inability of the family to replace the tracheostomy tube during weekly exchange because of bleeding, granulation tissue, or other factors. Parents and caregivers are all trained in cardiopulmonary resuscitation (CPR) before discharge from the hospital after initial tracheostomy placement. Patients in the extremis may be managed with a bag valve mask to the tracheostomy opening rather than the oropharynx if resuscitation efforts are ongoing. Replacement of the tracheostomy tube should be done in a smooth curved motion to account for the angulation that naturally occurs between the native trachea and the established tracheocutaneous fistula. A shoulder roll may be used to assist with alignment of the airway, especially in children who are obese or younger children who have a proportionately larger occiput. If resistance is met due to an inability to align the airway, excess granulation tissue or a cutaneous fistula that has decreased in diameter; the tracheostomy tube should not be forced into the airway to prevent complications.[14,15] Use of a smaller tracheostomy tube if available or use of an endotracheal tube, which should be nearly universally available, will allow for accommodation navigation of a narrow fistula tract. Prompt referral to an otorhinolaryngologist should be made for evaluation of the tracheocutaneous fistula and trachea as well as dilation, if necessary, to replace the initial size tracheostomy.

Granulation tissue may form at the skin incision site, or it can occur distally in the trachea leading to bleeding. Granulation tissue should be treated with silver nitrate when it forms. Prevention using appropriate weekly tracheostomy tube changes is important. If persistent, granulation tissue can form a fibrotic scar that may lead to a stricture and stenosis at the tracheocutaneous fistula or in the airway. Intraluminal granulation tissue may also occur and will typically present as bleeding during tracheostomy tube changes. This may be identified but with bronchoscopy or flexible tracheobronchoscopy during routine surveillance visits. Referral to an otorhinolaryngologist for further evaluation is appropriate, especially in the setting of bleeding with tracheostomy tube change and persistent granulation tissue.[15]

Severe complications may also occur especially in children with inappropriately sized tracheostomy tubes or overinflated cuffs. Tracheoesophageal fistula may occur in pediatric patients who have a tracheostomy tube that is posteriorly displaced or one that has an overinflated balloon. These typically occur in less than 1% of patients with a tracheostomy. This leads to pressure necrosis on the posterior wall of the trachea and development of an abnormal communication between the trachea and esophagus. These patients present with aspiration events and pneumonitis. They should be evaluated with plain radiograph of the chest which may show an air-filled esophagus as well as barium swallow and bronchoscopy. Treatment is surgical for division and closure of the fistula tract.[15–17]

Tracheo-arterial or tracheo-innominate artery fistulae are life-threatening complications of tracheostomy tube placement and can occur in less than 1% of patients with tracheostomy tubes (**Figs. 1 and 2**). Typically this is due to a tracheostomy that is placed too low (toward the carina) or in a patient with an ill-fitting tracheostomy tube that is too long. Bleeding that occurs more than 48 hours after tracheostomy tube placement may herald a fistula and should be referred to an otorhinolaryngologist for further evaluation. These fistulae are associated with a high mortality rate, reported as more than 80%. They can present with a sentinel or herald bleed that is profuse bright red blood from the tracheostomy site. These may present within hours to days of a catastrophic event. Management is surgical to divide the fistula tract and repair the injury. Immediate management of a catastrophic event may include placement of an endotracheal tube which will allow for inflation of the balloon distal to the fistula to allow for airway control as well as potentially tamponade the bleeding. The Utley maneuver may be performed which is the placement of a finger into the tracheostomy site with upward pressure on the distal sternum to apply pressure to the innominate artery. This bleeding should be treated as an emergent surgical event with the initiation of a massive transfusion protocol.[15,18–20]

Enteral Access

Gastrostomy tube placement is one of the more common procedures performed in pediatric patients with developmental delay or neurologic impairment. Along with

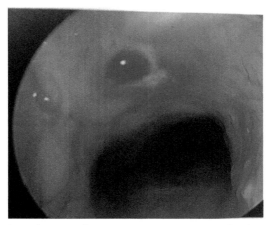

Fig. 1. Bronchoscopic evaluation of tracheo-innominate artery fistula on the anterior wall of the trachea.

tracheostomy tube placement, gastrostomy tubes may be placed due to an inability to protect the airway and an uncoordinated swallow mechanism that increases the risk of aspiration. In addition, these may be placed due to an inability to take in an adequate caloric volume for growth due to multiple reasons. Enteral access may also be required due to an inability to take medication required for underlying medical conditions.[21] Gastrostomy tubes may also be converted to gastrojejunostomy tubes due to persistent reflux or intestinal motility disorders that prevent gastric feeds.[22] Owing to the prevalence of gastrostomy tubes in pediatric patients with developmental delays or neurologic impairment, general surgeons should be comfortable with the management of complications that may arise. Although gastrostomy tubes are meant to function as a permanent source of enteral support, there is a percentage of gastrostomy

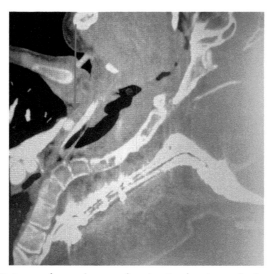

Fig. 2. Computed tomography angiogram showing trachea innominate artery fistula in the same patient. (Arrow points to fistula).

tubes that will require revision. Typically, these are gastrostomy tubes that are put in at a younger age and tubes that have been in place for a prolonged period.[23]

One of the most common complications or management issues that will be faced by any medical provider caring for a child with a gastrostomy tube is a dislodged tube. It should be expected that the gastrocutaneous fistula tract will close over time if the gastrostomy tube is not replaced in an expeditious fashion. Parents should be instructed not only in the care of the gastrostomy tube but also in the replacement of these tubes. However, there may be times when the family is not comfortable replacing the tube, is unable to replace the tube due to stricture of the tract or there may be times when the tube is damaged or unable to be replaced. Children with gastrostomy tubes should have a spare tube at home for replacement as needed. In the event, the patient presents for care of a dislodged gastrostomy tube a similar-sized tube (both in diameter and stem length in the setting of a button-type gastrostomy tube) should be replaced through the tract. If there is resistance because of closure of the tract, dilation may be required. Multiple options are available to dilate the tract. Hegar dilators are metal or plastic dilators, with a blunt end to avoid injury, that can be used to sequentially dilate the gastrostomy tract. I have found foley catheters to be useful as they can also dilate the tract while also serving as a tube with a balloon to maintain patency if one needs to seek out a replacement gastrostomy tube or to provide a break period to the patient between dilation events.[24] After replacement of the gastrostomy tube confirmation of gastric placement should be obtained by return of gastric contents and instillation of water into the stomach. If there is any concern, a contrast study can be obtained to confirm the proper placement of the gastrostomy tube in the stomach.

Gastric erosion, gastric ulceration, or a "buried bumper" syndrome may be seen in patients with longstanding gastrostomy tubes. This has been reported in patients who have undergone percutaneous endoscopic gastrostomy (PEG) tube placement but can be seen in any patient who has a gastrostomy tube for enteral support. This has been described in patients with PEG tubes because of a pressure phenomenon when the external bumper is too tightly adherent to the skin causing internal pressure from the internal bumper on the gastric mucosa.[25] In pediatric patients, we can see this same phenomenon occur as the child grows and gains weight increasing the subcutaneous tissue present. This will require a longer-length gastrostomy tube, especially in the setting of a button-type gastrostomy tube. Pediatric patients should be seen on a regular basis to ensure that the tube fits appropriately. It should not be tight at the skin level and should spin freely. Any tube that is too tight should be lengthened by increasing the stem length of the button-type tube or by allowing the external bumper to be relaxed and pull away from the skin. It is a misconception that a gastrostomy tube needs to be tight to prevent leakage of enteric contents. A tube that is too tight may leak more than a properly fitted gastrostomy tube by causing erosion or changing the shape of the internal bumper or balloon leading to leakage. Children who have erosion of the gastrostomy tube may require surgical closure of the tract and replacement of the gastrostomy tube in a new site.[26]

Migration of the gastrostomy tube fistula site can also occur. Gastrostomy tubes should be placed several centimeters below the costal margin; however, as a child grows the gastrostomy tube site may migrate closer to the costal margin leading to pain and leakage with each breath. This migration is because of a preponderance of growth in the trunk and extremities later in life as well as a downward angulation of the costal margin from the near horizontal alignment as an infant.[24] Children who have a gastrostomy tube placed near the costal margin at a young age can be expected to have migration toward the rib cage and ultimately require relocation of the

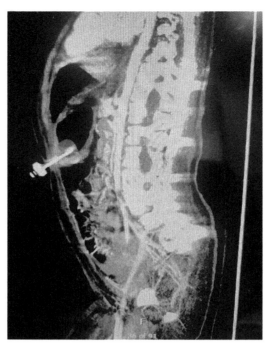

Fig. 3. Computed tomography scan showing downward angulation of gastrostomy tube that has migrated toward the costal margin causing persistent leakage and pain.

gastrostomy tube.**Fig. 3** Initial placement of the gastrostomy tube should be as far from the costal margin as possible to prevent this complication.[27] Some of these children with chronic medical conditions may be lost to follow-up during their adolescent years and present to a general surgeon as a young adult with pain or leakage at the gastrostomy site. Proper surgical planning for revision of the gastrostomy tube to prevent future complications will ensure long-term success and continued enteral support.[28,29]

Anti-Reflux Surgery/Fundoplication

It is worthwhile to mention the use of anti-reflux surgeries in children with underlying neurologic or developmental delays. Many of these children will be prone to gastroesophageal reflux and complications such as recurrent pneumonia or esophagitis. Previously it has been routine to perform an anti-reflux procedure, such as a Nissen fundoplication, at the time of enteral access. Many children who require enteral access have oropharyngeal dysfunction and will have recurrent aspiration events, pulmonary infections, or other life-threatening events.[30] Children with neurologic impairment also have a high incidence of gastroesophageal reflux, reported to be as high as 70%.[30] It can be difficult to determine whether these children are having pulmonary events due to descending aspiration (oropharyngeal dysfunction) or ascending aspiration (gastroesophageal reflux). As such, it is not uncommon to see children undergoing enteral access to also have a concurrent anti-reflux operation.

Concern has been raised due to the associated complication rates of anti-reflux surgery including failure and recurrence of symptoms, bowel obstruction, slipped fundoplication or hiatal hernia, and adhesions as well as mortality in some subsets of patients.[31] Concurrently, the medical treatment of gastroesophageal reflux disease has markedly improved with better understanding of the cause of esophagitis (eosinophilic esophagitis) as well as improved medication such as proton pump inhibitors. Recent literature has focused on the optimal management strategy of gastroesophageal reflux in pediatric patients with underlying neurologic impairment. A recent single-center retrospective review evaluated the outcomes of children with underlying gastroesophageal disease who underwent enteral access. The most common indication for enteral access was neurologic impairment found in 74% of patients. A total of 55 patients out of 96 who had a known diagnosis of gastroesophageal reflux underwent gastrostomy alone. Symptoms improved or stabilized in 64% of these patients. The other 41 patients underwent a combined gastrostomy and fundoplication. Fifteen percent of these patients had worsening reflux symptoms. There were also five reported complications including gastric perforation, dumping, and gastroesophageal stenosis.[32] Yamoto and colleagues[33] further evaluated the underlying risk of dumping syndrome following fundoplication in children and identified age less than 12 months, severe scoliosis (not uncommonly found in children with NI), and microgastria as risk factors. A recent study also evaluated the role of anti-reflux surgery in the treatment of aspiration pneumonia. They noted that fundoplication does decrease the risk but does not prevent further episodes of aspiration.[34]

Clearly, fundoplication does have a role in the management of patients with both gastroesophageal reflux disease (GERD) and neurological impairment (NI) or developmental delay. The optimal treatment strategy continues to evolve. A recent survey was conducted among pediatric gastroenterologists who are members of the European Society of Gastroenterology, Hepatology, and Nutrition. Regarding the question of the best initial management of gastroesophageal reflux disease in the pediatric patient, 77% of respondents felt that proton-pump inhibitors were the optimal first-line treatment. A total of 80% of respondents felt that an anti-reflux operation would be reasonable in the setting of proven failure of medical management. Given the high prevalence of GERD in children with NI and developmental delay, it is expected that surgeons will be consulted for discussion of surgical intervention.[35] A thorough understanding of the risks and benefits along with a shared decision-making approach is important to ensure an appropriate individualized treatment plan. Surgeons should look for documented evidence of the failure of medical management before recommending anti-reflux surgery in this patient population.

Ventriculoperitoneal Shunts

Surgeons should be prepared to encounter patients with ventriculoperitoneal (VP) shunts when caring for patients with neurologic impairment or developmental delay. VP shunts are one of the most common procedures performed for the management of hydrocephalus.[36] Surgeons may need to make decisions regarding the management of the shunt when caring for children who require intra-abdominal surgery for other indications such as appendicitis or bowel obstruction. Surgeons may also be asked to assist a neurosurgeon with the placement or replacement of VP shunts that are nonfunctional. A well-thought-out plan for the management of the VP shunt can ensure the longevity of the shunt and continued management of the underlying hydrocephalus.

Patients with VP shunts may present with intra-abdominal catastrophes that are either because of the persistent shunt material or that are unrelated to the shunt material. Delayed perforation can occur in patients who have VP shunts in place or in patients who have had abandoned shunt material because of encasement and fibrosis.[37] In addition, patients with VP shunts may present with intra-abdominal contamination because of appendicitis, intestinal ischemia, bowel obstruction, or trauma.

Recognizing when to externalize the shunt material to prevent long-term complications is paramount. Recent literature has suggested that in the absence of gross contamination, clean or clean-contaminated wounds, the VP shunt can be left in situ and managed with perioperative antibiotics.[38,39] Patients with gross contamination of enteric contents should be managed with a shunt externalization procedure.[39] This will require removal of the abdominal portion of the shunt at any point distal to the shunt valve and allow it to drain into an external collection system. In most instances, this will require monitoring of the patient in an ICU until the shunt can be replaced. Prompt consultation with neurosurgery is paramount to ensure appropriate management of the shunt material as well as consultation with infectious disease to determine the appropriate course of antibiotics.

Surgeons may also be consulted for assistance with the replacement of nonfunctional VP shunts especially in the setting of a patient with prior abdominal surgeries or in those with known pseudocyst formation. In some instances, there is limited space available for placement of the abdominal portion of the VP shunt and a decision may be made to place the shunt into the pleural cavity or the vascular system to allow for continued management of hydrocephalus. Recent literature has supported the use of the laparoscopic placement of the abdominal portion of the VP shunt to ensure appropriate placement into the peritoneal cavity. Similarly, laparoscopic placement may allow for treatment of intra-peritoneal adhesions or cyst formation to allow for improved longevity of the catheter. Laparoscopy may also improve visualization of the peritoneal cavity to ensure proper placement of the peritoneal portion of the catheter (**Fig. 4**). A recent single-institution review showed that laparoscopic placement of the VP shunt allowed for shorter operative time and longer time to shunt malfunction.[40]

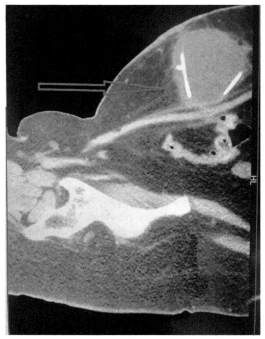

Fig. 4. Computed tomography scan showing extraperitoneal placement of a ventriculoperitoneal shunt in a patient with multiple prior abdominal surgeries.

Bowel and Bladder Management

Children who have a neurologic impairment or developmental delay many times also have underlying constipation or bowel management requirements as well as neurogenic bladders. Children with underlying neurologic impairment may require complex medical and surgical management of bowel function. Surgeons should be aware of the pharmacologic options for long-term management. These children may have undergone surgical procedures to assist with their management programs. Children who require enema therapy to remain clean and avoid accidents may have undergone a cecostomy tube or a Malone antegrade continent enema (MACE) procedure.[41] Similarly, patients with neurogenic bladder or who may otherwise require intermittent bladder catheterization may have undergone an appendicovesicostomy or Mitrofanoff procedure.[42–44] This procedure allows for the connection of the umbilicus to the bladder with the use of the appendix. These patients may have also undergone bladder augmentation or neobladder construction to allow for increased storage capacity and prevent reflux into the ureters. Surgeons should be aware of these procedures and bowel and bladder management during the perioperative period to ensure appropriate pre- and postoperative care. In addition, surgeons should be aware of the anatomic changes that may be present due to these surgeries to prevent unexpected complications or disruption of the bowel and bladder management program.

SUMMARY

General surgeons should be comfortable with the management of children with neurologic impairment or developmental delay. These patients may present in an elective fashion after transitioning care as an adult or may present in an emergent or urgent fashion due to an underlying complication. It is important that surgeons involve the family and caregivers in the management of patients with developmental delays or neurologic impairment using a shared decision-making model. This will build trust with the family and ensure that the management decisions do not have significant adverse effects on the ability of the caregiver to continue to manage the patient in the outpatient setting. Surgeons may routinely see complications arising from tracheostomy tube management, gastrostomy tube management, or may be faced with decisions regarding VP shunt management in the setting of an abdominal infection. Being able to recognize these issues and provide immediate medical management will improve the outcomes for these patients and allow them to have an improved quality of life. General surgeons should have a low threshold to consult pediatric specialists whether they are pediatric surgeons, pediatric ENT surgeons, or pediatricians to ensure the optimal care is provided.

CLINICS CARE POINTS

- A shared decision-making model and involvement of caregivers is vital to the successful management of pediatric patients with neurologic impairment/developmental delay.

- Tracheostomy dislodgement requires emergent management and may require utilization of a smaller tracheostomy tube or endotracheal tube in the setting of stricture.

- Brisk tracheal stomal bleeding should be urgently evaluated to ensure there is no evidence of tracheo-innominate artery fistula as this may represent a herald bleed. Digital manipulation of the stoma applying upward pressure (Utley maneuver) can compress the artery until surgical ligation is performed.

- Gastrostomy tube dislodgement is not uncommon and can be managed through serial dilation of the tract with foley catheters and replacement of the gastrostomy tube in the emergency room.
- Migration of the gastrostomy tube toward the costal margin may occur as the child grows and may lead to angulation of the tract and leakage with skin breakdown or other complications. This may require surgical closure of the tract and subsequent replacement of the gastrostomy tube further away from the costal margin.
- Children with ventriculoperitoneal shunts may present with a need for urgent surgical exploration of the abdomen. Those children with clean or clean-contaminated wounds may be managed without externalization of the shunt. Children with contaminated or dirty wounds will require externalization and consultation with neurosurgery is recommended.

DISCLOSURE

The authors have nothing to disclose.

REFERENCES

1. World Health Organization. The global burden of disease. Geneva: World Health Organization Press; 2008.
2. Moreau JF, Fink EL, Hartman ME, et al. Hospitalizations of children with neurologic disorders in the United States. Pediatr Crit Care Med 2013;14(8):801–10.
3. Callahan ST, Winitzer RF, Keenan P. Transition from pediatric to adult-oriented health care: a challenge for patients with chronic disease. Curr Opin Pediatr 2001;13(4):310–6.
4. Wijngaarde RO, Hein I, Daams J, et al. Chronically ill children's participation and health outcomes in shared decision-making: a scoping review. Eur J Pediatr 2021;180(8):2345–57.
5. Wyatt KD, List B, Brinkman WB, et al. Shared Decision Making in Pediatrics: A Systematic Review and Meta-analysis. Acad Pediatr 2015;15(6):573–83.
6. Madrigal VN, Kelly KP. Supporting Family Decision-making for a Child Who Is Seriously Ill: Creating Synchrony and Connection. Pediatrics 2018;142(Suppl 3):S170–7.
7. Romito B, Jewell J, Jackson M. AAP Committee on Hospital Care: Association of Child Life Professionals. Child Life Services. Pediatrics 2021;147(1). e2020040261.
8. Bogetz JF, Trowbridge A, Lewis H, et al. Forming Clinician-Parent Therapeutic Alliance for Children with Severe Neurologic Impairment. Hosp Pediatr 2022; 12(3):282–92.
9. Ogilvie LN, Kozak JK, Chiu S, et al. Changes in pediatric tracheostomy 1982-2011: a Canadian tertiary children's hospital review. J Pediatr Surg 2014; 49(11):1549–53.
10. Singh A, Zubair A. Pediatric Tracheostomy. In: StatPearls [Internet]. Treasure Island (FL): StatPearls Publishing; 2022 [Updated 2022 Jan 25].
11. Swift AC, Rogers JH. The changing indications for tracheostomy in children. J Laryngol Otol 1987;101(12):1258–62.
12. Behl S, Watt JWH. Prediction of tracheostomy tube size for paediatric long-term ventilation: an audit of children with spinal cord injury. BJA: Br J Anaesth 2005; 94(Issue 1):88–91.
13. Tracheostomy tube changes. Available at: https://www.tracheostomyeducation.com/tracheostomy-tube-changes/on 10 March 2022.

14. Guide to Pediatric Tracheostomy Care at Home. Available at: https://www.ghschildrens.org/wp-content/uploads/2017/12/17-0330-Guide-for-Pediatric-Tracheostomy-Care-Digital.pdf. Accessed date March 10 2022.
15. Watters K. Tracheostomy in Infants and Children. Respir Care 2017;62(6): 799–825.
16. Sanwal MK, Ganjoo P, Tandon MS. Posttracheostomy tracheoesophageal fistula. J Anaesthesiol Clin Pharmacol 2012;28(1):140–1.
17. Birman C, Beckenham E. Acquired tracheo-esophageal fistula in the pediatric population. Int J Pediatr Otorhinolaryngol 1998;44(2):109–13.
18. Saleem T, Anjum F, Baril DT. Tracheo innominate artery fistula. Treasure Island (FL): StatPearls Publishing; 2022 [Updated 2022 Jan 11]. In: StatPearls [Internet].
19. Kondajji A, Dombrowska A, Allemang M, et al. Emergent Management of a Tracheoinnominate Fistula in the Community Hospital Setting. Cureus 2020;12(6): e8403. https://doi.org/10.7759/cureus.840.
20. Reger B, Neu R, Hofmann HS, et al. High mortality in patients with tracheoarterial fistulas: clinical experience and treatment recommendations. Interactive Cardio-Vascular Thorac Surg 2018;26(Issue 1):12–7.
21. Ackroyd R, Saincher M, Cheng S, et al. Gastrostomy tube insertion in children: the Edmonton experience. Can J Gastroenterol 2011;25(5):265–8.
22. DeRaddo JS, Skummer P, Rivera M, et al. Conversion to Gastrojejunostomy Tubes in Developmentally Disabled Children Intolerant to Gastrostomy Tube Feeding. J Pediatr Gastroenterol Nutr 2019;69(3):e75–8.
23. Conlon SJ, Janik TA, Janik JS, et al. Gastrostomy revision: incidence and indications. J Pediatr Surg 2004;39(9):1390–5.
24. Bhambani S, Phan TH, Brown L, et al. Replacement of Dislodged Gastrostomy Tubes After Stoma Dilation in the Pediatric Emergency Department. West J Emerg Med 2017;18(4):770–4.
25. Zouk AN, Batra H. Managing complications of percutaneous tracheostomy and gastrostomy. J Thorac Dis 2021;13(8):5314–30.
26. Soscia J, Friedman JN. A guide to the management of common gastrostomy and gastrojejunostomy tube problems. Paediatr Child Health 2011;16(5):281–7.
27. Siddiqui MM, Griffiths MD. Revision of long-term gastrostomy. J Pediatr Gastroenterol Nutr 2012;55(5):559–61.
28. Rentea R, Svetanoff WJ, Dekonenko C, et al. A simple technique for the management of refractory gastrostomy site complications a technical innovation in gastrostomy tube site revision. J Pediatr Surg Case Rep 2020;52:101335.
29. Koivusalo A, Pakarinen MP, Pyörälä S, et al. Revision of prolapsed feeding gastrostomy with a modified Janeway 'gastric tube. Pediatr Surg Int 2006;22(2):202–4.
30. Romano C, van Winckel M, Hulst J, et al. European Society for Paediatric Gastroenterology, Hepatology and Nutrition Guidelines for the evaluation and treatment of gastrointestinal and nutritional complications in children with neurological impairment. J Pediatr Gastroenterol Nutr 2017;65:242–64.
31. Al Namshan MK, Al Kharashi NM, Crankson SJ, et al. The outcomes of fundoplication and gastrostomy in neurologically impaired children in a tertiary care hospital in Saudi Arabia. Saudi Med J 2019;40(8):810–4.
32. Guillén Redondo P, Espinosa Góngora R, Luis Huertas AL, et al. Routine antireflux surgery combined with gastrostomy in children: is it really necessary? Our single-center experience. Cir Pediatr 2021;34(2):67–73.
33. Yamoto M, Fukumoto K, Takahashi T, et al. Risk factors of dumping syndrome after fundoplication for gastroesophageal reflux in children. Pediatr Surg Int 2021; 37(2):183–9.

34. Maret-Ouda J, Santoni G, Artama M, et al. Aspiration pneumonia after antireflux surgery among neurologically impaired children with GERD. J Pediatr Surg 2020; 55(11):2408–12.

35. Romano C, Dipasquale V, Van Winckel M, et al. Management of Gastrointestinal and Nutritional Problems in Children with Neurological Impairment: A Survey of Practice. J Pediatr Gastroenterol Nutr 2021;72(4):e97–101.

36. Fowler JB, De Jesus O, Mesfin FB. Ventriculoperitoneal Shunt. In: StatPearls [Internet]. Treasure Island (FL): StatPearls Publishing; 2022 [Updated 2021 Sep 9].

37. Bosy HH, Albarnawi BM, Ashour KM, et al. Early Anal Protrusion of Distal Ventriculoperitoneal Catheter Due to Iatrogenic Colonic Perforation: A Case Report and Review of Literature. Cureus 2021;13(12):e20296.

38. Dalfino JC, Adamo MA, Gandhi RH, et al. Conservative management of ventriculoperitoneal shunts in the setting of abdominal and pelvic infections. J Neurosurg Pediatr 2012;9(1):69–72.

39. Li G, Dutta S. Perioperative management of ventriculoperitoneal shunts during abdominal surgery. Surg Neurol 2008;70(5):492–5 ; discussion 495-7.

40. Sykes AG, Sisson WB, Gonda DD, et al. Just Stick a Scope in: Laparoscopic Ventriculoperitoneal Shunt Placement in the Pediatric Reoperative Abdomen. J Surg Res 2022;269:212–7.

41. Mosiello G, Safder S, Marshall D, et al. Neurogenic Bowel Dysfunction in Children and Adolescents. J Clin Med 2021;10(8):1669.

42. Sager C, Barroso U Jr, Bastos JM, et al. Management of neurogenic bladder dysfunction in children update and recommendations on medical treatment. Int Braz J Urol 2022;48(1):31–51.

43. Kim J, Kang SK, Lee YS, et al. Long-term usage pattern and satisfaction survey of continent catheterizable channels. J Pediatr Urol 2021;29. S1477-5131(21) 00512-X.

44. Stein R, Bogaert G, Dogan HS, et al. EAU/ESPU guidelines on the management of neurogenic bladder in children and adolescent part II operative management. Neurourol Urodyn 2020;39(2):498–506.

Medical and Surgical Aspects of Intestinal Failure in the Child

Danielle Wendel, MD, Patrick J. Javid, MD*

KEYWORDS

- Intestinal failure • Short bowel syndrome • Pediatric • Bowel lengthening
- Bowel tapering • Parenteral nutrition • Intestinal adaptation

KEY POINTS

- Children with intestinal failure are surviving well into adolescence and beyond with the evolution of medical, nutritional, and surgical management.
- Intestinal rehabilitation is the priority in children with short bowel syndrome.
- Children may still wean off parenteral nutrition after many years of intestinal rehabilitation.
- Bowel lengthening and tapering is one of many tools used in intestinal rehabilitation although the indications are not fully defined.

INTRODUCTION

The care of children with intestinal failure (IF) has changed significantly over the past two decades. What was once considered a disease process with high risk for early mortality, children with IF now routinely survive long-term well into childhood and beyond. The dramatic change in outcomes is due to advances in medical, surgical, and nutrition therapies that are used together in the practice of pediatric intestinal rehabilitation. Pediatric IF has become a chronic disease that brings about its own challenges of optimizing outcomes and transition to adult care in older children.

HISTORY

Before the 1990s, children with short bowel syndrome who developed complications from long-term parenteral nutrition (PN) or chronic central venous access had a limited life expectancy. In these patients, progressive cholestatic liver disease led to cirrhosis, uncontrolled bleeding, and refractory sepsis. The limited success of intestinal

University of Washington School of Medicine, Seattle Children's Hospital, 4800 Sand Point Way Northeast, Seattle, WA 98105, USA
* Corresponding author. Seattle Children's Hospital, 4800 Sand Point Way Northeast, Ocean A. 9.220, Seattle, WA 98105.
E-mail address: Patrick.javid@seattlechildrens.org

Surg Clin N Am 102 (2022) 861–872
https://doi.org/10.1016/j.suc.2022.07.015
0039-6109/22/© 2022 Elsevier Inc. All rights reserved.

surgical.theclinics.com

transplantation offered some hope for these patients, but it was often a race between progression of disease and the ability to find a suitable and appropriately sized intestinal graft for these small patients.

Contemporary care of infants and children with IF evolved from the established multidisciplinary efforts of the transplantation team.[1] In this way, the wait for an intestinal allograft necessitated the early stages of intestinal rehabilitation as providers attempted various strategies to delay the progression of intestinal failure-associated liver disease (IFALD). This multidisciplinary care, performed by pediatric surgeons and gastroenterologists alike, led to unexpected success and improved survival without transplantation. The early strategy for intestinal rehabilitation in the child—including the safe administration of PN with lipid restriction algorithms, gradual advancement of enteral feeds, and prevention and aggressive treatment of complications such as bacterial overgrowth and central line-associated bloodstream infection—allowed these children to grow and, in many cases, to reach enteral autonomy.

With these changes, the era of pediatric intestinal rehabilitation in the focused multidisciplinary program was born in the late 1990s and early 2000s. Survival of children with IF increased significantly[2,3] and the number of children undergoing or listed for intestinal transplantation dropped. In most cases, children with IF—including children with the shortest bowel lengths—are now referred for intestinal rehabilitation before consultation for intestinal transplantation, and intestinal transplantation is reserved for the older child or in the setting of a younger child with loss of venous access or advanced liver disease.

Data continue to show that intestinal rehabilitation is successful when performed in the setting of a dedicated, multidisciplinary program. A recent multicenter analysis showed that in a cohort of children with IF, the incidence of enteral autonomy was 53%, transplantation 17%, and death 10.5%.[4]

DEFINITION

The best definition of pediatric IF continues to evolve. The most widely used definition is that IF represents "the reduction of functional gut mass below that which can sustain life, resulting in dependence on supplemental parenteral support for a minimum of 60 days within an interval of 74 consecutive days."[5] In this manner, the term IF encompasses short bowel syndrome but also disorders of gastrointestinal motility and congenital enterocyte pathologies such as microvillus inclusion disease and tufting enteropathy. Short bowel syndrome is the most common cause of IF, and this is most often the result of surgical resection of small intestine in infancy. Ultra-short bowel syndrome in the child has been defined as short bowel syndrome in which the remnant small bowel length is less than 20 cm after index surgical management. The most common etiologies of IF secondary to short bowel syndrome in children are necrotizing enterocolitis and gastroschisis.

MEDICAL THERAPY FOR INTESTINAL FAILURE

Intestinal adaptation is the compensatory process of structural and functional changes that occur after intestinal resection that increase the absorption of fluid and nutrients in the remaining bowel.[6] Medical therapy in IF focuses on maximizing adaptation while minimizing the complications associated with long-term PN and IF. Of the many potential complications, small-intestinal bacterial overgrowth (SIBO) and central line-associated bloodstream infections (CLABSI) predominate pediatric IF management, whereas there are new frontiers for medications that promote the process of adaptation.

Small Intestinal Bacterial Overgrowth

Changes in intestinal motility and altered intestinal anatomy put patients with IF at risk for SIBO with mainly anaerobic organisms. Diagnosis is largely clinical with abdominal distention, gassiness, vomiting, weight loss, increased stool output, gastrointestinal bleeding, and malnutrition.[7,8] Symptoms are caused by bacterial fermentation of carbohydrates, deconjugation of bile acids contributing to fat-malabsorption and fat-soluble vitamin deficiency, depletion of nutrients secondary to bacterial consumption, and intestinal inflammation/ulceration.[9,10]

Treatment of SIBO is important as it has been associated with malnutrition, CLABSI secondary to translocation, and progression of IFALD. Medical management focuses on reducing simple carbohydrates and control of the bacterial population with antibiotics and avoidance of acid suppression. The most commonly used antibiotics target gram negative and anaerobic organisms such as metronidazole and rifaximin.[11] Rifaximin is broad spectrum and has low systemic absorption leading to few systemic side effects. There is no consensus on duration of therapy, combination therapy, or cycling of antibiotic therapy for SIBO. Probiotics are used with caution in this population as they can contribute to overgrowth and have been linked to probiotic-associated CLABSI.[12] In cases of medically refractory SIBO, evaluation for anatomic causes of poor intestinal motility, such as intermittent obstruction at an intestinal anastamosis, may be helpful.

Central Line-Associated Bloodstream Infections

Although there have been significant improvements in CLABSI rates, sepsis remains a major source of mortality in patients with IF.[13] Studies have shown a high rate (70%) of bacteremia in patients with IF who present to the emergency department with fever.[14] As a result, all IF patients with fever are brought to the emergency room where central and peripheral blood cultures are obtained, broad-spectrum antibiotics are initiated, and children are admitted to the hospital for observation. Initial antibiotic choice is driven by local susceptibility patterns with fungal coverage typically reserved for ill-appearing patients. With the success of clearing blood cultures and the goal of central access preservation, most CLABSI in IF patients can be treated without central line removal.[15,16]

Antimicrobial lock therapy has become standard in the prevention and treatment of CLABSI in children with IF. Until recently ethanol locks were the preferred option as they have been shown to significantly decrease rates of CLABSI.[17] Unfortunately, due to regulatory issues, use of ethanol locks has become cost-prohibitive resulting in the need for alternative antimicrobial locks. Antibiotic locks are not preferred because of the potential for resistance, narrow spectrum of activity, and ineffectiveness against the biofilm that forms within catheters. Alternative locks have been successfully used outside the United States including sodium EDTA and taurolidine.[18,19]

Hormone Analog Therapy

The focus of IF management has traditionally been on limiting complications while exposing the intestine to nutrients to stimulate adaptation without any treatments that specifically promote this process. This changed with the recent approval of glucagon-like peptide 2 (GLP-2) analog, teduglutide (Takeda). Teduglutide is currently the only approved hormone analog for the treatment of short bowel syndrome in children ≥1 year of age. Native GLP-2 is an enteroendocrine hormone produced in the terminal ilium and proximal colon in response to exposure to luminal nutrients.[20] Teduglutide was developed to have a longer half-life than native GLP-2 so that it can be dosed subcutaneously daily. In adult and pediatric studies, it is been shown to improve fluid absorption and decrease the need for PN support by slowing gastric emptying, increasing villus height and crypt depth.[21,22] As with other hormone replacement medications, and similar to the adult population, cessation of the drug has shown reversal of these effects.

NUTRITIONAL THERAPY FOR INTESTINAL FAILURE

The introduction of PN in the 1960s allowed for the survival of patients with IF. Although lifesaving, there are many risks associated with the central access required for PN and the content of the PN itself requires close management by a team experienced in home PN management. With a focus on reducing these risks, patients can now survive and thrive while receiving long-term PN and allowing the bowel time to adapt. Although there are various aspects of PN management in patients with IF, the role of intravenous lipids in the development of IFALD has been of particular interest.

The traditional soy-based intravenous lipid emulsions contain phytosterols, high levels of pro-inflammatory omega-6 fatty acids, and low levels of antioxidants found in other emulsions.[23] As a result, there were deleterious effects on the liver resulting in frequent issues with cholestatic liver disease and the need for a liver transplant. To decrease these effects, soy-based lipid dosing was minimized (1 g/kg/d) requiring higher doses of dextrose and further strain on the liver. Alternative lipid formulations have been developed to prevent and treat IFALD. Omegaven (Fresenius Kabi) is a fish oil-based omega-3 fatty acid lipid emulsion that has been shown to reverse cholestasis resulting from IFALD, although it is not intended to be the sole long-term lipid provision.[24] To provide a more balanced fatty acid profile, SMOFlipid (Fresenius Kabi) is a mixed lipid emulsion developed with soy (30%), MCT (30%), olive (25%), and fish oil (15%) and has been shown to prevent development and progression of IFALD.[25] Both Omegaven and SMOFlipid contain significant amounts of vitamin E, an antioxidant. Although Omegaven is also typically dosed at 1 g/kg/d, SMOF can be safely dosed at higher levels (2–3 g/kg/d) which allows a better distribution of PN macronutrients.

Enteral nutrition, specifically more complex macronutrients, has been shown to stimulate adaptation in the intestine after resection.[26] In infants with IF, human milk is preferred as it contains growth factors, immunoglobulins, human milk oligosaccharides, and other beneficial components that improve tolerability, stimulate growth/adaptation, and educate the immune system.[27] Historically, infants with IF were started on elemental formula because it was thought to be better tolerated and easier to absorb although this was not based on high-quality evidence. This practice has been challenged more recently by the studies suggesting improved adaptation with more complex nutrients and success with human milk and standard formulas.

Improvements in feed tolerance are often seen when solid foods are introduced into the diet of patients with IF. The same has been shown with blenderized feeds which have become more accessible with the development of commercially available products. Oral aversion is a common, multifactorial issue in patients with IF that often interferes with enteral feed advancement and PN weaning as there is often a limit to the amount of formula IF patients tolerate. Early oral feeding during the developmentally appropriate time is key to developing the skills necessary to prevent oral aversion. As a result, delaying gastrostomy placement in favor of oral feeding may help prevent oral aversion by shifting the focus away from tube feeding and back to oral feeding.[28]

Vitamin and Micronutrient Monitoring and Supplementation

Depending on the remaining intestinal anatomy and complications associated with IF, several nutrient deficiencies occur. These are more common and often difficult to correct when patients are enterally autonomous because their remaining intestine is tasked with absorbing what was previously provided parenterally.[29] Close laboratory monitoring is required to detect and provide treatment for these issues. Although there are numerous deficiencies seen in IF, the most common include iron, fat-soluble vitamins, and vitamin B12 deficiency.

Iron deficiency results from issues with absorption, increased losses through inflammation and bleeding, as well as lack of provision of iron in PN. Monitoring includes iron studies including ferritin and routine CBC monitoring. Enteral and parenteral supplementation is used to treat deficiency, andiron sucrose and increasingly ferric carboxymaltose are used as intravenous options. Iron sucrose is typically given at lower doses more frequently, whereas ferric carboxymaltose is given at a higher dose and has been shown to have longer-lasting effects.[30]

Patients with IF often have multi-factorial issues with fat malabsorption often leading to severe fat-soluble vitamin deficiencies.[31] While receiving PN, fat-soluble vitamins are administered as an additive to the PN although levels of parenteral vitamin D are occasionally insufficient. Although patients are receiving intravenous lipids with either SMOFlipid or Omegaven rarely have vitamin E deficiency secondary to the amount they receive in the lipid emulsion.[32] The doses of fat-soluble vitamins required for enterally autonomous patients can be several-fold higher than standard doses because of intestinal malabsorption.

As a result of the loss of the terminal ileum, many patients with IF will develop vitamin B12 deficiency over time. If untreated, this can lead to megaloblastic anemia and potentially irreversible neurologic consequences.[33] Deficiency does not typically occur until after patients are weaned from PN as it is provided in the parenteral multivitamin supplement. To monitor for deficiency serum B12 and methylmalonic acid (MMA) levels should be checked as serum B12 alone is a poor indicator of total body B12 levels. Although elevated MMA levels are seen in vitamin B12 deficiency, they are also increased in SIBO and renal disease complicating the interpretation of B12 status.[34] Supplementation is best via intramuscular injection. There are also intranasal and sublingual formulations although studies are lacking in their effectiveness.

SURGICAL THERAPY FOR INTESTINAL FAILURE

Children with IF require active surgical evaluation and consultation ideally through a multidisciplinary intestinal rehabilitation center. Surgical care involves important decisions about the indications and timing of stoma closure, autologous intestinal reconstruction, feeding tube access, and advanced surgery for complications of IF.

Restoration of Intestinal Continuity

There is universal consensus in the field of pediatric IF that, when feasible, small bowel stomas should be closed early in the course of IF and usually before hospital discharge. Stomas are created in the neonate and infant for a variety of reasons including diversion in the setting of inflammation (such as in necrotizing enterocolitis), congenital obstruction (intestinal atresia, gastroschisis), and long segment functional dysmotility (Hirschsprung's disease). Stomas are excellent for diverting the fecal stream but serve to negate the full absorptive and digestive capacity of the remnant small and large bowel. Even in the patient who has had a massive intestinal resection, stomas compound short bowel syndrome by decreasing the available intestinal mucosal mass to absorb nutrients, fluid, and electrolytes. This can result in dehydration, electrolyte imbalance, and poor growth. Therefore, there is widespread agreement that stomas should be closed starting 6 weeks after the initial surgical resection. The one exception is in the setting of long-segment Hirschsprung's disease in which there is no distal ganglionated bowel to reconnect the small bowel remnant. The ostomy in these patients will usually remain in place, often for years, until the bowel adapts to allow for an anastamosis to the very distal rectum without copious diarrhea.

Autologous Intestinal Reconstruction

Bowel lengthening and tapering play an important role in the surgical management of children with IF. However, the optimal timing and indications for these procedures have not been fully defined. Bowel lengthening has the benefit of slowing down intestinal transit so that enteric contents may have more time to be absorbed. This is especially important in the patient with short bowel length and significant malabsorption at baseline. Bowel tapering allows for reconstruction of the dilated small bowel so that the smooth muscle is less stretched. This allows for the small bowel lumen to better approximate the diameter of more distal bowel and, in theory, may optimize motility. Tapering can also reduce the risk of small bowel bacterial overgrowth which occurs frequently in chronically dilated bowel and leads to further dysmotility, bacterial translocation, and nutrient malabsorption.

Antimesenteric tapering involves resection of a portion of the antimesenteric wall of the small intestine and then closure using a handsewn or stapled technique. The resection can be performed over a chest tube or large red rubber catheter placed in the bowel lumen to help approximate the appropriate diameter of the intestinal and to avoid resecting too much of the small bowel lumen. Tapering is performed in the setting of dysmotility secondary to bowel dilation when the overall bowel length is not limiting. Taping is often performed at the same time as an anastamotic revision as chronic dilation may be due to intermittent partial obstruction due to kinking at the anastamosis.

There are two commonly used techniques that combine bowel lengthening and tapering. The longitudinal intestinal lengthening and tailoring (LILT) procedure was first described by Adrian Bianchi in 1981.[35] In this procedure, the mesentery to a dilated loop of the remnant small bowel is dissected and split so that two leaves of mesentery are created to each side of the dilated bowel loop. The bowel segment is then divided longitudinally so that each side has its only separated mesenteric blood supply. This results in two segments of bowel that are the same length but half the original diameter. These segments can be anastamosed together to double the length of the small bowel remnant. The procedure has shown success in achieving enteral autonomy in the case series. However, the procedure is technically challenging, may put the small bowel mesentery at risk, and can only be performed in the setting of a significantly dilated small bowel. In addition, it is not feasible to perform the LILT procedure twice on the same segment of small bowel, so that re-dilation after the LILT remains problematic.

The serial transverse enteroplasty (STEP) procedure was first described in 2003.[36,37] The procedure incorporates consecutive applications of a tissue stapler across the antimesenteric border of the flattened, dilated small bowel remnant. The direction of the stapler is alternated from side to side and usually progresses from distal to proximal along the small bowel. The degree of tapering can be modified easily using the stapler so that the technique is quite versatile in children with IF and can be performed even in moderately dilated bowel. The procedure differs from the LILT in that it does not actually increase the mucosal surface area. Rather, it elongates the bowel and likely allows for improved absorption through increased transit time.[38,39] The procedure does not involve significant dissection of the mesenteric blood supply but does require multiple staple lines that can predispose to leak and long-term ulceration.[40]

There are no randomized studies that compare outcomes from the STEP and the LILT procedures. Many case series that have not controlled for patient selection have shown short- and long-term benefit for both the STEP and the LILT.[38,41–43] Both operative strategies have been shown to be effective in helping to decrease the percentage of calories required in PN and, in select children, to allow for enteral autonomy. There are some data to suggest a benefit from a second STEP procedure if the small bowel remnant re-dilates although this operative strategy remains controversial.[44,45] Complications exist including staple line and anastamotic leaks, bowel obstruction, redilation of the small bowel remnant, and long-term issues with staple line ulcers and dysmotility. Both procedures can be technically challenging as this patient cohort has undergone multiple prior abdominal operations and injury must be avoided at all costs to the short remnant small bowel.

At present, the timing and indications for autologous intestinal reconstruction in the child with IF continue to be debated.[46] It is important to remember that autologous intestinal reconstruction is one of many tools in the management of IF, and that not every child with short bowel syndrome and bowel dilation needs a bowel lengthening or tapering procedure. It is likely that only select patients benefit from this surgical strategy. In general, children with IF who benefit from autologous intestinal reconstruction have plateaued in their enteral advancement, have bowel that is significantly dilated, and have developed complications such as refractory bacterial overgrowth leading to bacterial translocation or bleeding small bowel ulcerations. It has been recently proposed that the decision to pursue bowel lengthening and the actual procedure itself should be conducted only at multidisciplinary IF centers and not by individual surgeons or gastroenterologists caring for these children outside of dedicated intestinal rehabilitation programs.[47]

Feeding Tube Access

The role for early placement of a feeding gastrostomy in pediatric IF remains controversial. Many of the young infants who undergo early bowel resection are premature and may experience oral feeding challenges. In addition, the feeding rate and specific diet for these patients may require significant alteration from those of a healthy child. Finally, placement of a gastrostomy after the index operation can be technically challenging in this cohort. At the same time, feeding access in the young infant can be associated with significant complication rates including leakage, infection, and erosion in the abdominal wall. There is no longer an urgent imperative to rapidly advance enteral feeds as the risk of liver disease from PN has been greatly reduced with alternative lipid strategies. Most importantly, many children with IF may not require a long-term gastrostomy if oral nutrition is prioritized from the early stages of intestinal rehabilitation.

A recent study found that the prevalence of feeding difficulty was associated with use of an enteral feeding tube early in life.[28] In current practice at our institution, we have a selective approach to which infants receive a surgical feeding access at the initial surgery, and we routinely close gastrostomies that are no longer needed after 1 year of age. If necessary, a redo percutaneous gastrotomy button can be placed in an interval fashion if the child develops a future need for enteral access.

PEDIATRIC INTESTINAL FAILURE FOR THE ADULT GENERAL SURGEON

With the improved survival recently observed in pediatric IF, children with this diagnosis are now surviving into late childhood and beyond. Ongoing research is evaluating this population's quality of life and neurocognitive function. But it is clear that these patients will continue to require ongoing surgical and medical care as they transition to young adulthood. This will require a necessary transition to adult care although the optimal timing and framework for this transition has yet to be studied.

When an adult surgeon encounters a child with IF, even in the teenage years, a referral to a regional pediatric IF center is strongly encouraged. A program that focuses on care of the IF patient likely has the experience necessary and access to the most recent medical and surgical advances to optimize short- and long-term outcomes. Even in the setting of geographic constraints, when the nearest intestinal rehabilitation program may be far away, this relationship is still preferred. In this way, the regional IF team can see the patient in the ambulatory setting every few months and provide recommendations for overarching care, whereas the primary management of the patient can be performed by the local adult or pediatric provider. Our program has implemented this framework for many patients in a wide multi-state geographic, and we have found it to be successful for the patient and family as well as the patient's local providers.

One of the most challenging issues in pediatric IF is how to transition young adults to the care of adult surgeons and gastroenterologists. From a medical standpoint, these patients will have ongoing needs for PN management, weight checks, electrolyte and micronutrient monitoring, and fluid and vitamin supplementation. They will need treatment for SIBO and aggressive management of CLABSI. In addition, they will remain at risk for complications that may require surgical intervention including intestinal ulceration, recurrent small bowel dilation, and bowel obstruction. They will also need expert care with difficult and long-term central venous access. In the future, specialization among adult general surgeons and gastroenterologists in IF care will be necessary to care for this growing population.

HOW TO MANAGE A CHILD WITH INTESTINAL FAILURE IN THE CONTEMPORARY ERA

Contemporary management of the infant and child with IF should emphasize early and aggressive rehabilitation of the remnant intestine. After early stoma closure, intestinal rehabilitation usually starts with the medical and nutritional strategies as outlined above. An alternative lipid strategy is initiated for the child on long-term PN. Aggressive treatment and prophylaxis of SIBO and CLABSI are prioritized. The patient is followed closely, usually weekly in the infant age group and monthly to quarterly in the older toddler and child. The goal is to allow the slow advancement of enteral nutrition as the bowel adapts, ideally prioritizing the oral route with consistent feeding therapy support to avoid oral aversion. Bowel lengthening and tapering are reserved for the child who is unable to attain enteral autonomy and who has reached a plateau in the wean from PN calories over time and is at risk for complications from IF. Even in this scenario, autologous intestinal reconstruction requires significant dilation of the small bowel.

It is important to note that intestinal rehabilitation in the child can be a chronic process, and it can take years to attain enteral autonomy. Data from the Pediatric IF Consortium (PIFCon) indicate that some children with IF are still able to wean off PN after 5 years of intestinal rehabilitation, and this finding was recently confirmed in a multinational study.[4,48] In addition, intestinal rehabilitation is safe with a long-term survival greater than 90% in multidisciplinary intestinal rehabilitation centers. Hence, intestinal rehabilitation is prioritized over early intestinal transplant in the young child with IF especially given the scarcity of available intestinal grafts that fit a small child and the long-term outcomes from transplantation. Recent data show the 1-year and 5-

year patient survival for intestinal transplant to be 73% and 57%, respectively.[49] Intestinal transplantation in the pediatric population has decreased over the past 10 to 15 years as intestinal rehabilitation as evolved.[50] Currently, intestinal transplantation is most commonly reserved for a child who has lost available sites for central venous access or who has developed late-stage IFALD although there is anecdotal evidence that some older teenagers may choose intestinal transplantation over ongoing intestinal rehabilitation.

The medical, nutritional, and surgical aspects of intestinal rehabilitation have evolved beyond the level of the general pediatric gastroenterologist and pediatric surgeon. Data have shown that multidisciplinary care of the child with IF in an intestinal rehabilitation program is associated with a reduction in mortality.[3] Moreover, multicenter data have confirmed that early referral of a child with IF and IFALD to an intestinal rehabilitation center is associated with improved survival.[51] Intestinal rehabilitation programs have dedicated providers in gastroenterology, surgery, and transplantation with advanced training in pediatric IF care. These programs likely also have better access to the most innovative and emerging therapies. Even when geography is a challenge, all children with IF should be enrolled in an intestinal rehabilitation program for the optimal long-term outcome.

CLINICS CARE POINTS

- Intestinal rehabilitation is a safe and successful strategy for children with intestinal failure.
- There is a survival benefit when children with intestinal failure are treated in dedicated, multidisciplinary intestinal rehabilitation programs.
- Early referral of children with intestinal failure to multidisciplinary intestinal rehabilitation programs has been associated with a decrease in mortality
- Alternative lipid strategies such as mixed lipid emulsions such be used early for children with intestinal failure who require long-term parenteral nutrition. These advances in intravenous lipid emulsions have been shown to decrease the risk of parenteral nutrition-associated liver disease.
- When patients are carefully selected, established bowel lengthening techniques have been shown to decrease the parenteral nutrition caloric requirement in children with intestinal failure
- In the infant with intestinal failure, intestinal rehabilitation is prioritized first before referral for intestinal transplantation based on the successful short- and long-term outcomes associated with intestinal rehabilitation.

DISCLOSURE

The authors have nothing to disclose.

REFERENCES

1. Javid PJ, Wendel DW, Horslen SP. Organization and outcomes of multidisciplinary intestinal failure teams. Semin Pediatr Surg 2018;27:218–22.
2. Javid PJ, Malone FR, Reyes J, et al. The experience of a regional pediatric intestinal failure program: successful outcomes from intestinal rehabilitation. Am J Surg 2010;199:676–9.
3. Modi BM, Langer M, Ching YA, et al. Improved survival in a multidisciplinary short bowel syndrome program. J Pediatr Surg 2008;43:20–4.

4. Daniela G, Roberts AJ, Wales PW, et al. Trends in pediatric intestinal failure: a multicenter, multinational study. J Pediatr 2021;237:16–23.

5. Modi BP, Galloway DP, Gura K, et al. ASPEN definitions in pediatric intestinal failure. J Parenter Enteral Nutr 2022;46:42–59.

6. Tappenden KA. Intestinal adaptation following resection. JPEN J Parenter Enteral Nutr 2014;38(1 Suppl):23S–31S.

7. Rodriguez D, Ryan P, Toro Monjaraz EM, et al. Small intestinal bacterial overgrowth in children: a state-of-the-art review. Front Pediatr 2019;7(1):1–19.

8. Rao SSC, Bhagatwala J. Small intestinal bacterial overgrowth: clinical features and therapeutic management. Clin Transl Gastroenterol 2019;10(10):e00078.

9. Dukowicz AC, Lacy BE, Levine GM. Small intestinal bacterial overgrowth: a comprehensive review. J Gastroenterol Hepatol 2007;3(2):112–22.

10. Bohm M, Siwiec RM, Wo JM. Diagnosis and management of small intestinal bacterial overgrowth. Nutr Clin Pract 2013;28(3):289–99.

11. Malik BA, Xie YY, Wine E, et al. Diagnosis and pharmacological management of small intestinal bacterial overgrowth in children with intestinal failure. Can J Gastroenterol 2011;25(1):41–5.

12. Reddy VS, Patole SK, Rao S. Role of probiotics in short bowel syndrome in infants and children–a systematic review. Nutrients 2013;5(3):679–99.

13. Pierret ACS, Wilkinson JT, Zilbauer M, et al. Clinical outcomes in pediatric intestinal failure: a meta-analysis and meta-regression. Am J Clin Nutr 2019;110(2):430–6.

14. Szydlowski EG, Rudolph JA, Vitale MA, et al. Bloodstream infections in patients with intestinal failure presenting to a pediatric emergency department with fever and a central line. Pediatr Emerg Care 2017;33(12):e140–5.

15. Bond A, Chadwick P, Smith TR, et al. Diagnosis and management of catheter-related bloodstream infections in patients on home parenteral nutrition. Frontline Gastroenterol 2020;11(1):48–54.

16. Robinson JL, Casey LM, Huynh HQ, et al. Prospective cohort study of the outcome of and risk factors for intravascular catheter-related bloodstream infections in children with intestinal failure. JPEN J Parenter Enteral Nutr 2014;38(5):625–30.

17. Rahhal R, Abu-El-Haija MA, Fei L, et al. Systematic review and meta-analysis of the utilization of ethanol locks in pediatric patients with intestinal failure. JPEN J Parenter Enteral Nutr 2018;42(4):690–701.

18. Quirt J, Belza C, Pai N, et al. Reduction of central line-associated bloodstream infections and line occlusions in pediatric intestinal failure patients receiving long-term parenteral nutrition using an alternative locking solution, 4% tetrasodium ethylenediaminetetraacetic acid. JPEN J Parenter Enteral Nutr 2021;45(6):1286–92.

19. Lambe C, Poisson C, Talbotec C, et al. Strategies to reduce catheter-related bloodstream infections in pediatric patients receiving home parenteral nutrition: the efficacy of taurolidine-citrate prophylactic-locking. JPEN J Parenter Enteral Nutr 2018;42(6):1017–25.

20. Drucker DJ. Gut adaptation and the glucagon-like peptides. Gut 2002;50(3):428–35.

21. Jeppesen PB, Gilroy R, Pertkiewicz M, et al. Randomised placebo-controlled trial of teduglutide in reducing parenteral nutrition and/or intravenous fluid requirements in patients with short bowel syndrome. Gut 2011;60(7):902–14.

22. Kocoshis SA, Merritt RJ, Hill S, et al. Safety and efficacy of teduglutide in pediatric patients with intestinal failure due to short bowel syndrome: a 24-week, phase III study. JPEN J Parenter Enteral Nutr 2020;44(4):621–31.

23. Wales PW, Allen N, Worthington P, et al. A.S.P.E.N. Clinical guidelines: support of pediatric patients with intestinal failure at risk of parenteral nutrition-associated liver disease. JPEN J Parenter Enteral Nutr 2014;38(5):538–57.

24. Nandivada P, Fell GL, Gura KM, et al. Lipid emulsions in the treatment and prevention of parenteral nutrition-associated liver disease in infants and children. Am J Clin Nutr 2016;103(2):629S–6234S.

25. Diamond IR, Grant RC, Pencharz PB, et al. Preventing the progression of intestinal failure-associated liver disease in infants using a composite lipid emulsion: a pilot randomized controlled trial of SMOFlipid. JPEN J Parenter Enteral Nutr 2017; 41(5):866–77.

26. Bines JE, Taylor RG, Justice F, et al. Influence of diet complexity on intestinal adaptation following massive small bowel resection in a preclinical model. J Gastroenterol Hepatol 2002;17(11):1170–9.

27. Kulkarni S, Mercado V, Rios M, et al. Breast milk is better than formula milk in preventing parenteral nutrition-associated liver disease in infants receiving prolonged parenteral nutrition. J Pediatr Gastroenterol Nutr 2013;57(3):383–8.

28. Boctor DL, Jutteau WH, Fenton TR, et al. The prevalence of feeding difficulties and potential risk factors in pediatric intestinal failure: Time to consider promoting oral feeds? Clin Nutr 2021;40(10):5399–406.

29. Ubesie AC, Kocoshis SA, Mezoff AG, et al. Multiple micronutrient deficiencies among patients with intestinal failure during and after transition to enteral nutrition. J Pediatr 2013;163(6):1692–6.

30. Laass MW, Straub S, Chainey S, et al. Effectiveness and safety of ferric carboxymaltose treatment in children and adolescents with inflammatory bowel disease and other gastrointestinal diseases. BMC Gastroenterol 2014;14:184.

31. Jeppesen PB, Høy CE, Mortensen PB. Deficiencies of essential fatty acids, vitamin A and E and changes in plasma lipoproteins in patients with reduced fat absorption or intestinal failure. Eur J Clin Nutr 2000;54(8):632–42.

32. Zemrani B, Bines JE. Monitoring of long-term parenteral nutrition in children with intestinal failure. JGH open 2019;3(2):163–72.

33. Stabler SP. Vitamin B12 deficiency. N Engl J Med 2013;368(21):2041–2.

34. Jimenez L, Stamm DA, Depaula B, et al. Is serum methylmalonic acid a reliable biomarker of vitamin b12 status in children with short bowel syndrome: a case series. J Pediatr Invalid date 2018;192:259–61.

35. Bianchi A. Intestinal loop lengthening–a technique for increasing small intestinal length. J Pediatr Surg 1980;15(2):145–51.

36. Kim HB, Fauza D, Garza J, et al. Serial transverse enteroplasty (STEP): a novel bowel lengthening procedure. J Pediatr Surg 2003;38:425–9.

37. Kim HB, Lee PW, Garza J, et al. Serial transverse enteroplasty (STEP) for short bowel syndrome: a case report. J Pediatr Surg 2003;38:881–5.

38. Jones BA, Hull MA, Potanos KM, et al. Report of 111 consecutive patients enrolled in the international serial transverse enteroplasty (STEP) data registry: a retrospective observational study. J Am Coll Surg 2013;216:438–46.

39. Chang RW, Javid PJ, Oh J-T, et al. Serial transverse enteroplasty enhances intestinal function in a model of short bowel syndrome. Ann Surg 2006;243:223–8.

40. Fisher JG, Stamm DA, Modi BP, et al. Gastrointestinal bleeding as a complication of serial transverse enteroplasty. J Pediatr Surg 2014;49:745–9.

41. Nagelkerke SCJ, van Poelgeest MY, Wessel LM, et al. Bowel lengthening procedures in children with short bowel syndrome: a systematic review. Eur J Pediatr Surg 2021. https://doi.org/10.1055/s-0041-1725187. Online ahead of print.

42. Reinshagen K, Kabs C, Wirth H, et al. Long-term outcome in patients with short bowel syndrome after longitudinal intestinal lengthening and tailoring. J Pediatr Gastroenterol Nutr 2008;47:573–8.

43. Sudan D, Thompson J, Botha J, et al. Comparison of intestinal lengthening procedures for patients with short bowel syndrome. Ann Surg 2007;246:593–604.

44. Lemoine C, Larkin K, Brennan K, et al. Repeat serial transverse enteroplasty procedure (reSTEP): is it worth it? J Pediatr Surg 2021;56:951–60.

45. Mercer DF, Burnett TR, Hobson BD, et al. Repeat serial transverse enteroplasty leads to reduction in parenteral nutrition in children with short bowel syndrome. J Pediatr Surg 2021;56:733–7.

46. Hukkinen M, Kivisaari R, Koivusalo A, et al. Risk factors and outcomes of tapering surgery for small intestinal dilatation in pediatric short bowel syndrome. J Pediatr Surg 2017;52:1121–7.

47. Fitzgerald K, Muto M, Belza C, et al. The evolution of the serial transverse enteroplasty for pediatric short bowel syndrome at a single institution. J Pediatr Surg 2019;54:993–8.

48. Squires RH, Duggan C, Teitelbaum DH, et al. Natural history of pediatric intestinal failure: initial report from the pediatric intestinal failure consortium. J Peds 2012; 161:723–8.

49. Raghu VK, Beaumont JL, Everly MJ, et al. Pediatric intestinal transplantation: analysis of the intestinal transplant registry. Pediatr Transplant 2019;23(8): e13580.

50. Horslen SP, Smith JM, Weaver T, et al. OPTN/SRTR 2020 annual data report: intestine. Am J Transplant 2022;22 S2:310–49.

51. Javid PJ, Oron AP, Duggan CP, et al. The extent of intestinal failure-associated liver disease in patients referred for intestinal rehabilitation is associated with increased mortality: an analysis of the pediatric intestinal failure consortium database. J Pediatr Surg 2018;53:1399–402.

Meconium Ileus, Distal Intestinal Obstruction Syndrome, and Other Gastrointestinal Pathology in the Cystic Fibrosis Patient

Joseph Tobias, MD[a], Mckinna Tillotson, BS[b], Lauren Maloney, BS[b], Elizabeth Fialkowski, MD[c],*

KEYWORDS

- Cystic fibrosis • Meconium ileus • Distal intestinal obstruction syndrome
- Exocrine pancreatic insufficiency • Constipation • Rectal prolapse
- Acute appendicitis

KEY POINTS

- Bilious emesis in the newborn is a surgical emergency until proven otherwise.
- Meconium ileus is often one of the first signs of cystic fibrosis.
- Water-soluble contrast enema may be diagnostic and therapeutic in simple meconium ileus.
- Complicated meconium ileus typically requires operative intervention.
- Distal intestinal obstruction syndrome is successfully managed nonoperatively in most cases.
- Meconium ileus in infancy is a strong risk factor for distal intestinal obstruction syndrome in childhood and adolescence.
- Constipation is a common gastrointestinal complaint in children with cystic fibrosis.
- Typical signs and symptoms of appendicitis may be masked or blunted by chronic antibiotic and steroid therapy.

INTRODUCTION
Cystic Fibrosis

Cystic fibrosis (CF) is an autosomal-recessive defect in the cystic fibrosis transmembrane conductance regulator (CFTR) gene located on chromosome 7 that affects 1 in 2500 live White births.[1] CFTR encodes a chloride channel that regulates electrolyte

[a] 3181 Southwest Sam Jackson Park Road, Portland, OR 97239, USA; [b] 2314 Northeast Multnomah Street, Portland, OR 97232, USA; [c] Pediatric General Surgery, Oregon Health and Science University, Portland, OR, USA
* Corresponding author.
E-mail address: fialkows@ohsu.edu

Surg Clin N Am 102 (2022) 873–882
https://doi.org/10.1016/j.suc.2022.07.016
0039-6109/22/© 2022 Elsevier Inc. All rights reserved.

surgical.theclinics.com

content at epithelial surfaces. Defects in the gene lead to decreased chloride secretion and increased sodium and water resorption. This results in abnormally thick secretions causing chronic obstruction in the respiratory and gastrointestinal tracts. Common gastrointestinal pathology in children with CF includes meconium ileus in infancy and distal intestinal obstruction syndrome (DIOS) in childhood and exocrine pancreatic insufficiency, constipation, and rectal prolapse.

Meconium Ileus

Meconium ileus is a condition of neonatal intestinal obstruction caused by thickened, so-called "inspissated" (from the Latin *spissus* meaning thick) meconium in the distal ileum. Meconium ileus may be the first sign of CF and occurs in 10% to 20% of neonates who have the disease.[2] Although highly suggestive of CF, meconium ileus also occurs in the setting of other pathology, such as Hirschsprung disease with total colonic aganglionosis. Meconium ileus is thought to be caused primarily by abnormal intestinal glandular secretions.

Distal Intestinal Obstruction Syndrome

DIOS is a fecal impaction of the distal ileum, which may be conceived as a chronic meconium ileus equivalent that occurs in children and adolescents who have CF. Meconium ileus is a strong risk factor for the development of DIOS later in life. Estimates of prevalence in children with CF range from 5 to 12 episodes per 1000 patients per year.[3] DIOS is thought to be caused by exocrine pancreatic insufficiency, abnormal intestinal glandular secretions, and intrinsic intestinal dysmotility.

Other Gastrointestinal Pathology

Children with CF are at a higher-than-normal risk for exocrine pancreatic insufficiency, constipation, and rectal prolapse. Additionally, acute appendicitis in the child with CF presents a special diagnostic dilemma.

MECONIUM ILEUS
Presentation and Differential Diagnosis

Meconium ileus is classified as either simple or complicated. Simple meconium ileus presents with failure to pass meconium within the first 24 to 48 hours of life, feeding intolerance, bilious emesis, and abdominal distention. Infants appear healthy for 1 to 2 days after birth. Complicated meconium ileus includes volvulus of the meconium-distended small bowel segment, accompanying intestinal atresias, ischemic necrosis of the bowel, intestinal perforation, meconium peritonitis, or meconium cyst formation. Complicated meconium ileus typically presents with a sicker infant, usually within the first 24 hours after birth. There may be abdominal wall edema and erythema, tenderness, a palpable abdominal mass, and hemodynamic instability. Roughly half of patients present with simple meconium ileus, whereas half present with complicated disease.[4] The differential diagnosis for neonatal intestinal obstruction must be kept broad because bilious emesis in the newborn is always a surgical emergency until proven otherwise. The differential diagnosis includes anorectal malformations, Hirschsprung disease, intestinal atresias, and malrotation with midgut volvulus. Of these causes, meconium ileus is estimated to account for 9% to 33% of cases of neonatal intestinal obstruction.[5]

Prenatal Diagnosis

Because thickened meconium forms in utero, meconium ileus may be diagnosed on prenatal ultrasound. Normal fetal meconium is hypoechoic or isoechoic, whereas inspissated meconium can present as a hyperechoic mass with or without the presence of calcifications and dilated bowel.[6] Hyperechoic bowel is also visualized in other conditions, however, and may be a normal variant.[7] The American College of Obstetrics and Gynecology recommends that all women of reproductive age undergo CF carrier screening.[8] If parents are carriers, fetal evaluation is performed with chorionic villus sampling or amniocentesis. When CF is suspected, monthly sonographic evaluation is performed, which may detect meconium ileus and its sequelae, such as intrauterine growth restriction and maternal polyhydramnios because of fetal intestinal obstruction.

Postnatal Imaging Studies

In simple meconium ileus, postnatal abdominal radiographs show dilated loops of small bowel with or without air-fluid levels. Air-fluid levels may be absent because of highly viscous meconium, which does not form an interface with air. Swallowed air bubbles can mix with meconium to give a "soap-bubble" or "ground-glass" appearance. Although one-third of cases of complicated meconium ileus have no additional radiographic findings, complicated disease may present with calcifications from in utero perforation.[9] Water-soluble contrast enema is performed under fluoroscopic guidance in neonates with suspected simple meconium ileus and shows a small-caliber, normally positioned colon (a so-called "unused" microcolon) and pellets of meconium (termed "scybala") in the distal ileum, with or without reflux of contrast into the dilated proximal small bowel (**Fig. 1**). Contrast enema should not be performed if peritonitis or perforation are present.

Laboratory Studies

If meconium ileus is suspected, standard laboratory analyses are performed to assess for sepsis and to correct electrolyte and coagulation abnormalities. The diagnosis of CF is made by biochemical analysis with a sweat chloride test, which is positive at

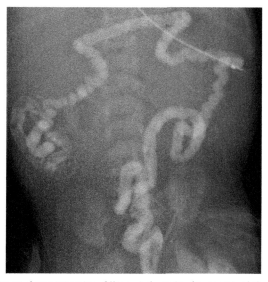

Fig. 1. Contrast enema demonstrating filling defects in the terminal ileum (scybala) and a microcolon.

a concentration of greater than 60 mmol in 100 mg of sweat.[10] This is typically a delayed diagnosis because sweat testing is optimally performed between 2 and 4 weeks of age, but may be performed as early as day-of-life 2. Genetic testing is concurrently performed to identify the specific CFTR mutation, which guides prognostication of disease severity. It is important to maintain a high index of suspicion for CF in infants who have meconium ileus because some infants may have had a falsely negative newborn screen.

Complicated Disease

When in utero perforation occurs, meconium is thought to cause a sterile chemical peritonitis. Dense adhesions form and a fibrous wall develops around the accumulated meconium, which may in turn develop into a cystic structure (technically a pseudocyst) (**Fig. 2**). If present for a longer duration, calcifications develop. Bacterial superinfection may then occur after birth leading to hemodynamic instability, sepsis, and peritonitis. Alternatively, the meconium-filled segment of small bowel may volvulize, leading to ischemic necrosis, or there may be associated atretic segments of small bowel. Notably, 12% to 17% of infants with jejunoileal atresias have CF.[4]

Nonoperative Management

Most neonates with simple meconium ileus are successfully managed nonoperatively. Management begins with gastric decompression, volume resuscitation, and empiric broad-spectrum antibiotic therapy. Water-soluble contrast enema under fluoroscopic guidance is diagnostic and potentially therapeutic of simple meconium ileus. Before instilling the enema, neonates must be adequately volume-resuscitated because there can be ensuing fluid shifts that lead to hypovolemia and end-organ damage, including necrotizing enterocolitis.[11] Under fluoroscopy, half-diluted hyperosmolar contrast (typically sodium meglumine diatrizoate or Gastrografin) is slowly instilled through a

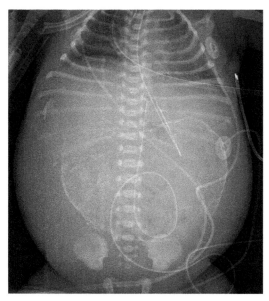

Fig. 2. Air-filled calcified mass consistent with perforation and meconium cyst formation.

catheter in the rectum, with the operator being careful to avoid catheter-balloon over-inflation or high pressures that could cause perforation. The hyperosmolar enema shifts fluid into the bowel lumen and acts as a direct solvent for the inspissated meconium. In successful cases, there is passage of meconium pellets and liquid meconium within the next 24 to 48 hours. Serial enemas should be attempted in cases of incomplete evacuation and ongoing obstruction. Progress is defined as contrast refluxing more and more proximally into dilated loops of small bowel under fluoroscopy. Success rates of contrast enemas are estimated at 30% to 50%.[2,12] Early or late perforation can occur as a complication. In cases where there is evidence of a meconium pseudocyst on imaging but intestinal continuity has been restored without evidence of ongoing perforation, operative exploration is not indicated because the cyst may resolve with time and not require intervention.

Operative Management

Operative management is indicated in simple meconium ileus when there is no passage of meconium after one or more trials of a contrast enema; when there is inadequate evacuation of meconium; or when a complication, such as perforation, occurs. Operative management is usually indicated in complicated meconium ileus except in cases of a sealed perforation with no ongoing obstruction. There are several approaches available to the operating surgeon (**Fig. 3**).

Enterotomy-irrigation
An enterotomy is made in the distal ileum proximal to the site of obstruction. An irrigating catheter is placed for instillation of a mucolytic agent, such as *N*-acetylcysteine (Mucomyst) solution to soften the inspissated meconium. Thereafter, meconium is gently milked distally into the colon or evacuated through the enterotomy, which is then closed primarily. Alternatively, the enterotomy may be made via the appendix as an appendicostomy.

Enterostomy-irrigation
Another approach is creation of a temporary enterostomy, which functions to relieve the obstruction and facilitate access for postoperative irrigation. There are several techniques available (see **Fig. 3**): the Mikulicz double-barreled enterostomy, the distal chimney enterostomy or Bishop-Koop procedure with an irrigation catheter passed through the chimney into the distal ileum, the proximal chimney enterostomy or Santulli procedure, and a simple tube enterostomy.

Resection of dilated, perforated, atretic, or necrotic bowel
At laparotomy for complicated disease, the operating surgeon must be prepared to find dense, adhesive disease, volvulus, atresia, ischemic intestine, and the possibility of purulent peritonitis. A conservative approach to lysis of adhesions and intestinal resection should be undertaken, although some neonates will unfortunately be left with short bowel syndrome. If a meconium pseudocyst is encountered, decortication of the pseudocyst should be performed as needed to mobilize the trapped intestine and control any contamination should be performed. Diversion enterostomy is preferable in cases of significant bowel size mismatch, purulent peritonitis, and hemodynamic instability.

Postoperative Care

Postoperatively, *N*-acetylcysteine solution is administered through an orogastric or nasogastric tube to liquefy gastrointestinal contents. If an irrigation catheter has been left in place, *N*-acetylcysteine solution may be instilled directly into the small

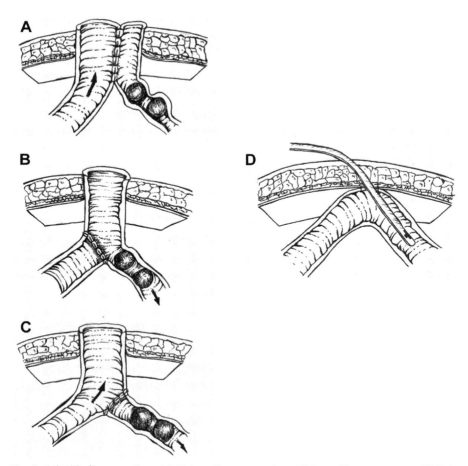

Fig. 3. (A) Mikulicz resection. (B) Bishop-Koop resection. (C) Santulli enterostomy. (D) Tube enterostomy.

bowel. Enteral nutrition is started as soon as possible, typically when there is confirmation of intestinal continuity and return of bowel function. Supplemental pancreatic enzymes should also be given. If there is a prolonged ileus, the neonate is supported with total parenteral nutrition. Antibiotic therapy is continued postoperatively, either for a short or long course depending on the clinical scenario. If an ileostomy is present, there must be meticulous repletion of electrolyte losses because patients with CF are at risk for sodium depletion. It remains important to confirm the diagnosis of CF and to establish a multidisciplinary team in the longitudinal care of the infant.

DISTAL INTESTINAL OBSTRUCTION SYNDROME
Presentation and Differential Diagnosis

DIOS presents as a partial to complete small bowel obstruction because of fecal impaction of the distal ileum in children, adolescents, and adults with CF, especially in patients with severe phenotypes. Signs and symptoms include crampy abdominal pain, often in the right lower quadrant; emesis; obstipation; abdominal distention; and a palpable right lower quadrant mass. DIOS may present with acute intestinal obstruction, but more commonly presents subacutely with partial obstruction causing episodic abdominal pain and distention. Meconium ileus in infancy is a strong predictor for DIOS later in life and may confer up to a 10-fold increase in risk.[13,14] A single previous episode of DIOS also confers enhanced risk for subsequent episodes.[15] The differential diagnosis includes constipation; appendicitis; ovarian pathology; intussusception; adhesive small bowel obstruction (particularly if the patient had a laparotomy in infancy for meconium ileus); inflammatory bowel disease; and fibrosing colonopathy, a rare stricturing condition of the colon that is associated with high-dose pancreatic enzyme supplementation.

Diagnostic Studies

The classic diagnostic triad for DIOS is abdominal pain, a right lower quadrant mass, and abdominal radiographs showing stool in the small bowel and right colon. DIOS may be differentiated from constipation, which is common in patents with CF, by a paucity of stool in the distal colon. Additionally, constipation may present with a more gradual onset. If obtained, computed tomography shows dilated small bowel with inspissated stool in the terminal ileum and may help to exclude other diagnoses, such as appendicitis. Laboratory analyses include a complete blood count, metabolic panel, liver enzymes, and lipase.

Management

DIOS can almost always be managed nonoperatively. Mainstays of treatment are volume resuscitation; correction of electrolyte abnormalities; and osmotic laxative therapy, either administered orally or via nasogastric tube. Current recommendations suggest the administration of polyethylene glycol (Golytely) in doses of 20 to 40 mL/kg per hour to a maximum of 1 L per hour for mild obstructive symptoms.[16] In cases of more severe obstruction with bilious emesis, nasogastric decompression and fluoroscopic hyperosmolar enemas, such as Gastrografin, are used. A standard enema preparation consists of 100 mL of Gastrografin diluted in 400 mL of water.[17] Rarely, patients fail to resolve nonoperatively. If operative intervention is indicated, the first strategy should be to milk impacted stool from the terminal ileum into the colon. Stool is softened with a retrograde enema of warm saline, Gastrografin, or N-acetylcysteine. If this is not feasible, appendicotomy or enterotomy proximal to the obstruction is fashioned for intestinal lavage. Last resort is ileocecectomy with primary anastomosis or temporary ileostomy in the case of an unstable patient. Although colonoscopy with lavage is possible, it is thought to confer an undue risk of perforation.[18] Postoperatively, maintenance daily laxative therapy should be instituted.

OTHER GASTROINTESTINAL PATHOLOGY
Exocrine Pancreatic Insufficiency

Up to 85% of patents with CF develop exocrine pancreatic insufficiency, many from the time they are born.[19] The cause is hypothesized to be ductal obstruction leading to destruction of acinar cells.[20] Signs and symptoms include dyspepsia; bloating; flatulence; steatorrhea; malnutrition; and growth failure because of malabsorption of fat-soluble vitamins A, D, E, and K. Pancreatic insufficient patents with CF are prescribed pancreatic enzyme replacement therapy.

Constipation

Constipation is one of the most common gastrointestinal complaints in patents with CF and occurs in up to one-half of children.[21] Patients may have regular bowel movements but still carry a significant intracolonic stool burden causing abdominal pain. Constipation may precede the development of DIOS or may be difficult to distinguish from DIOS. The current consensus definition is based on the presence of abdominal pain and/or abdominal distention, or a decrease in spontaneous bowel movement frequency, or an increase in stool consistency that is effectively relieved by laxative use.[15]

Rectal Prolapse

Rectal prolapse occurs in 3% of children with CF, most frequently in toddlers who are toilet training.[22] Before widespread newborn screening, rectal prolapse occurred in up to 23% of children with CF.[23] Rectal prolapse may be the initial symptom in some patents with CF, and CF should be considered in all pediatric patients presenting with rectal prolapse. Newborn screening has led to earlier diagnosis and earlier supplementation of pancreatic enzymes and laxative therapy, which are thought to be protective against prolapse. Prolapse may involve only the mucosa or may extend to all layers of the rectum. Management relies on manual reduction, which is almost always successful, followed by daily laxative and adherence to pancreatic enzyme replacement therapy.

Appendicitis in the Patient with Cystic Fibrosis

Appendicitis occurs less frequently in patents with CF than in the general pediatric population, but is more difficult to diagnose because it mimics symptoms of DIOS and constipation and is more frequently complicated by perforation.[24] Signs and symptoms of appendicitis may be masked by chronic antibiotic and steroid therapy. As such, a high index of suspicion for appendicitis is key in the child with CF. Additionally, the surgeon can consider performing incidental appendectomy during other abdominal operations.

SUMMARY

The general surgeon must be familiar with the significant, potentially life-threatening gastrointestinal manifestations of CF; chief among these, meconium ileus as a cause of intestinal obstruction in the newborn and DIOS as a cause of intestinal obstruction in children and adolescents. Most pediatric patients with CF also have exocrine pancreatic insufficiency and constipation, leading to abdominal pain, and these children are at a greater risk of rectal prolapse and of complicated appendicitis.

CLINICS CARE POINTS

- Meconium ileus can cause bilious emesis in the newborn and has different imaging characteristics than malrotation.
- Water-soluble contrast enema is diagnostic and is therapeutic for simple meconium ileus.
- Management of complicated meconium ileus focuses on controlling perforation or bowel obstruction if present and restoration of intestinal continuity.
- Distal intestinal obstruction syndrome can often be treated nonoperatively with hydration and bowel cleanout.
- Constipation is common in patients with cystic fibrosis and long-term bowel management is important.
- Rectal prolapse is a presenting sign of cystic fibrosis in pediatric patients.

DISCLOSURE

The authors have nothing to disclose.

REFERENCES

1. Kleven DT, McCudden CR, Willis MS. Cystic fibrosis: newborn screening in America. MLO Med Lab Obs 2008;40:16–8, 22, 4-18.
2. Sathe M, Houwen R. Meconium ileus in cystic fibrosis. J Cyst Fibros 2017; 16(Suppl 2):S32–9.
3. Colombo C, Ellemunter H, Houwen R, et al. Guidelines for the diagnosis and management of distal intestinal obstruction syndrome in cystic fibrosis patients. J Cyst Fibros 2011;10(Suppl 2):S24–8.
4. Escobar MA, Grosfeld JL, Burdick JJ, et al. Surgical considerations in cystic fibrosis: a 32-year evaluation of outcomes. Surgery 2005;138:560–71 [discussion: 71-2].
5. DeLorimier AA, Fonkalsrud EW, Hays DM. Congenital atresia and stenosis of the jejunum and ileum. Surgery 1969;65:819–27.
6. Dicke JM, Crane JP. Sonographically detected hyperechoic fetal bowel: significance and implications for pregnancy management. Obstet Gynecol 1992;80: 778–82.
7. Lince DM, Pretorius DH, Manco-Johnson ML, et al. The clinical significance of increased echogenicity in the fetal abdomen. AJR Am J Roentgenol 1985;145: 683–6.
8. Opinion No Committee. 691: Carrier screening for genetic conditions. Obstet Gynecol 2017;129:e41–55.
9. Ziegler MM. Meconium ileus. Curr Probl Surg 1994;31:731–77.
10. Farrell PM, White TB, Ren CL, et al. Diagnosis of cystic fibrosis: consensus guidelines from the cystic fibrosis foundation. J Pediatr 2017;181s:S4–15.e1.
11. Rowe MI, Furst AJ, Altman DH, et al. The neonatal response to gastrografin enema. Pediatrics 1971;48:29–35.
12. Carlyle BE, Borowitz DS, Glick PL. A review of pathophysiology and management of fetuses and neonates with meconium ileus for the pediatric surgeon. J Pediatr Surg 2012;47:772–81.
13. Jaffe BF, Graham WP 3rd, Goldman L. Postinfancy intestinal obstruction in children with cystic fibrosis. Arch Surg 1966;92:337–43.
14. Hort A, Hameed A, Middleton PG, et al. Distal intestinal obstruction syndrome: an important differential diagnosis for abdominal pain in patients with cystic fibrosis. ANZ J Surg 2020;90:681–6.
15. Houwen RH, van der Doef HP, Sermet I, et al. Defining DIOS and constipation in cystic fibrosis with a multicentre study on the incidence, characteristics, and treatment of DIOS. J Pediatr Gastroenterol Nutr 2010;50:38–42.
16. Littlewood JM. Cystic fibrosis: gastrointestinal complications. Br Med Bull 1992; 48:847–59.
17. Zahra M, Frederick C, Thomas R, et al. Gastrografin enemas for treatment of distal intestinal obstruction syndrome in children and adults with cystic fibrosis. J Pharm Nutr Sci 2014;4:76–80.
18. Shidrawi RG, Murugan N, Westaby D, et al. Emergency colonoscopy for distal intestinal obstruction syndrome in cystic fibrosis patients. Gut 2002;51:285–6.
19. Nousia-Arvanitakis S. Cystic fibrosis and the pancreas: recent scientific advances. J Clin Gastroenterol 1999;29:138–42.

20. Durie PR, Forstner GG. Pathophysiology of the exocrine pancreas in cystic fibrosis. J R Soc Med 1989;82(Suppl 16):2–10.
21. Stefano MA, Poderoso RE, Mainz JG, et al. Prevalence of constipation in cystic fibrosis patients: a systematic review of observational studies. J Pediatr (Rio J 2020;96:686–92.
22. El-Chammas KI, Rumman N, Goh VL, et al. Rectal prolapse and cystic fibrosis. J Pediatr Gastroenterol Nutr 2015;60:110–2.
23. Waldhausen JHT, Richards M. Meconium ileus. Clin Colon Rectal Surg 2018;31: 121–6.
24. Coughlin JP, Gauderer MW, Stern RC, et al. The spectrum of appendiceal disease in cystic fibrosis. J Pediatr Surg 1990;25:835–9.

Chest Wall Deformities and Congenital Lung Lesions
What the General/Thoracic Surgeon Should Know

J. Duncan Phillips, MD[a,b],*, John David Hoover, MD[c]

KEYWORDS

- Pectus excavatum • Pectus carinatum • Pectus arcuatum • Poland syndrome
- Congenital cystic adenomatoid malformation • Pulmonary sequestration
- Bronchogenic cyst

KEY POINTS

- Pectus excavatum, carinatum, and aruatum are relatively rare developmental malformations of the chest wall that may progressively compress the heart and lungs (and other mediastinal structures), causing various symptoms including shortness of breath with exertion and chest pain.
- Nonoperative and operative approaches to chest wall deformities have changed dramatically during the past several decades.
- Surgical approaches to treat chest wall deformities may result in various acute and long-term complications including deformity recurrence, chronic pain, floating sternum, and acquired asphyxiating thoracic dystrophy syndrome.
- In utero ultrasonography has increased the early detection of asymptomatic congenital lung lesions. Short-term follow-up studies, suggesting spontaneous regression/disappearance, may be inaccurate.
- Minimally invasive techniques, including thoracoscopy, may be successfully used in toddlers and infants for the treatment of congenital lung malformations.

INTRODUCTION

Formation of the sternum and anterior chest wall structures occurs during early human embryogenesis, with sternal fusion typically complete by week 10. Typically, ribs 1 to 5 are connected separately to the sternum by cartilage segments, beginning at roughly the midclavicular line and extending medially. In most patients, cartilages 6 to 10 fuse

[a] WakeMed Children's Hospital, WakeMed Chest Wall Deformity Center, 3024 New Bern Avenue, Suite 304, Raleigh, NC 27610, USA; [b] University of North Carolina at Chapel Hill; [c] WakeMed Chest Wall Deformity Center, 3024 New Bern Avenue, Suite 304, Raleigh, NC 27610, USA
* Corresponding author.
E-mail address: dphillips@wakemed.org

Surg Clin N Am 102 (2022) 883–911
https://doi.org/10.1016/j.suc.2022.07.017
0039-6109/22/© 2022 Elsevier Inc. All rights reserved.

surgical.theclinics.com

and form the costal margin and connect medially as a single unit. Ribs 11 and 12 have no costal cartilage and may be called false or floating ribs (**Fig. 1**).

PECTUS EX CAVATUM

In some patients, the sternum and attached costal cartilages may bow posteriorly, toward the mediastinum. This condition, known as pectus excavatum, or sunken chest syndrome or funnel chest, may be noted soon after birth, and therefore be considered congenital, or, more commonly, it may gradually develop during childhood, and therefore be considered developmental Although the entire sternum may be sunken, more commonly only the inferior one-third to one-half is involved, with cartilages 3 to 6 most commonly affected (**Fig. 2**).

The exact etiology of pectus excavatum is unknown, with various authors speculating about possible excessive growth of the involved ribs or weakness/deficiency in the involved cartilages and/or abnormalities in the congenital fusion of the bony segments that form the sternum.

The exact pathophysiology of excavatum remains somewhat controversial (and hotly debated). Current thinking is that pulmonary compression may not be the primary

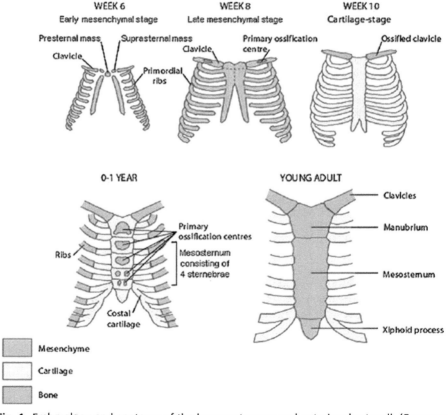

Fig. 1. Embryology and anatomy of the human sternum and anterior chest wall. (*From* van der Merwe AE, et al. A review of the embryological development and associated developmental abnormalities of the sternum in the light of a rare palaeopathological case of sternal clefting. Journal of Comparative Human Biology 2013;64(2):89-162.)

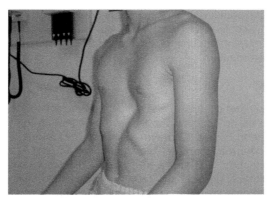

Fig. 2. Pectus excavatum. Typical adolescent boy with sternal indentation, primarily involving inferior one-third of the sternum.

factor causing symptoms. Recent studies suggest decreased right heart function (with diminished right ventricular outflow) and subsequent decreased pulmonary blood flow (especially during vigorous exercise) may be the mechanism.[1–7]

PECTUS CARINATUM

Also called pigeon or chicken chest, pectus carinatum is characterized by protrusion of the sternum and attached cartilages (**Fig. 3**). This is a distinctly different entity than excavatum, and is almost never seen in infancy or during early childhood. It is likely caused by overgrowth of the costal cartilages, with a relatively normal manubrium but progressive anterior angulation of the sternal body (and attached cartilages). Some authors term this chondrogladiolar prominence (or type 1 carinatum). Typical patients develop their deformities during early adolescent growth spurts.

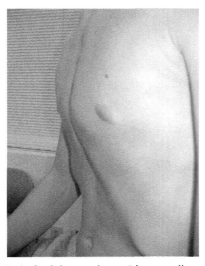

Fig. 3. Pectus carinatum. Typical adolescent boy with normally positioned manubrium and anterior angulation/protrusion of the sternal body.

Children and young adults with carinatum may present with anterior chest wall pain, exertional dyspnea, and exercise limitation.[8,9] Although the exact mechanism remains poorly understood, stretch/irritation of the intercostal nerves may be the cause. This is also true for pectus arcuatum.

PECTUS ARCUATUM

This is probably the most confusing and misunderstood anterior chest wall deformity and has also been called costomanubrial pectus carinatum (type 2), pouter pigeon breast, arcuate pigeon breast, Currarino-Silverman syndrome, and even the horns of the steer deformity. It is characterized by anterior angulation of the superior ribs and cartilages (especially 1–3) and a foreshortened unusual sternum with anterior angulation of the manubrium and, typically, a 90° angulation with posterior indentation[10] (**Fig. 4**). Some authors state the chest appears to be a type of carinatum superiorly and excavatum inferiorly.[11] Following the initial descriptions by Cincinnati pediatric radiologists Currarino and Silverman, pediatric cardiologists suggested this deformity is frequently associated with various types of structural heart disease,[12] but that is no longer felt to be true.

Most children with arcuatum are misdiagnosed with pectus carinatum, prior to presentation to an experienced chest wall surgeon.

POLAND SYNDROME

Poland syndrome,[13] initially described in 1841, is a more complex chest wall deformity of unilateral chest wall embryonic development, with a wide array of presentations. It may be relatively mild, with simple absence of the nipple/areola complex and/or breast, but most cases also have absence of most of the underlying pectoralis musculature. In some patients, the ipsilateral latissimus dorsi muscle may be absent, and in still others, there may be absence of underlying cartilages and/or ribs (most commonly 3–6) (**Fig. 5**). Affected individuals may have short webbed fingers on the ipsilateral side.

Patients with Poland syndrome may also progressively develop other abnormalities of the anterior chest wall with adolescent growth spurts, including significant indentation of the chest wall (pectus excavatum) or anterior protrusion of the sternum (carinatum).

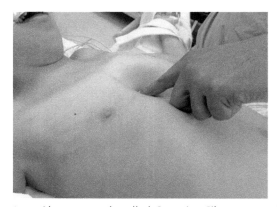

Fig. 4. Pectus arcuatum. Also commonly called Currarino-Silverman syndrome. Sternum is foreshortened (surgeon's left index finger is placed inferior to the xiphoid)—manubrium and superior sternum angulate anteriorly and inferior sternum angulates posteriorly.

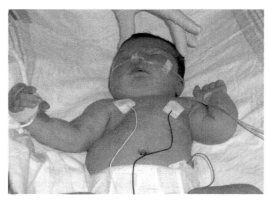

Fig. 5. Neonate with Poland syndrome. Note absence of right breast, pectoralis major, and multiple segments of the anterior rib cage.

PREVALENCE/INCIDENCE

The incidence of anterior chest wall deformities such as excavatum, carinatum, and arcuatum, is estimated to be between 1 in 300 people and 1 in 1000. Males are 4 to 5 times more often affected than females. In North America, excavatum may be 10 times more common than carinatum, but in some other parts of the globe, carinatum is reportedly more common. Poland syndrome affects roughly 1 in 20,000 newborns, with boys affected twice as often as girls.

SYMPTOMS

Patients with chest wall deformities may remain asymptomatic for many years, despite impressive changes in their external appearance. Children with relatively early onset of pectus excavatum may compensate and adapt to their condition and achieve acceptable exercise tolerance until midadolescence, or even early adulthood.[14] Symptoms typically begin gradually with progressive shortness of breath with exertion, exercise intolerance (early fatigue), and chest pain (typically brought on or worsened by exercise).[15] Dyspnea is frequently misdiagnosed as exercise-induced asthma or reactive airways disease. Still other patients develop recurrent respiratory tract infections, such as pneumonia and/or bronchitis. Although some patients may present with palpitations caused by cardiac arrhythmias, this is more commonly seen in adult patients than children.

Many adolescents and young adult describe psychological symptoms from their deformities, including shame, embarrassment, and fear of taking one's shirt off in public.[16,17] Rare patients may even develop major reactive depression.

EVALUATION/WORKUP

Thorough evaluation should begin with a complete history and physical examination, with emphasis on respiratory symptoms/previous illnesses/medications. Approximately 15% to 20% of pectus excavatum patients may have idiopathic scoliosis,[18,19] and many carinatum patients may have significant kyphosis. Roughly 5% of pectus patients have connective tissue disorders, such as Marfan or Ehlers-Danlos syndromes, and have usually been diagnosed earlier in life.[11] As stated previously, pectus arcuatum (also called Currarino-Silverman Syndrome) may be associated with structural congenital heart disease.[12] Any previous thoracic/chest wall surgery should be noted, as that may have a profound impact on treatment. A family history of chest wall deformities may be found in up to 43% of patients.[15]

Physical examination should note absence of any chest wall structures, such as the pectoralis muscles and breast and should also note sternal length, as some children with these deformities may have foreshortened sternums. A rough estimate of excavatum severity can be made by placing a wooden tongue blade transversely across the chest at the deepest portion of the concavity, with the patient lying supine and breathing normally, and measuring the distance from the tongue blade to the skin overlying the sternum. Auscultation of the heart may reveal murmurs, and inspection of the spine may reveal previously-undiagnosed curvature.

Evaluation of pectus severity typically begins with a chest radiograph followed by a chest computed tomography (CT) scan (without contrast, done at the end of full expiration). The Haller index (HI) (described in 1987) involves measuring the ratio of the transverse internal chest distance (measured at the deepest part of the concavity) and dividing that by the distance from the posterior periosteum of the sternum (at that deepest point) to the anterior periosteum of the associated underlying vertebral body[20] (**Fig. 6**). CT scans done in full inspiration (as is typically done at most institutions) may underestimate the HI (and pectus severity) by over 20%.[21] The authors have found that 3-dimensional reconstructions, using shaded surface display (SSD) technology is helpful[22] (**Fig. 7**).

Although the HI has never been subsequently validated as predictive of pectus severity, it has generally become accepted that a value of roughly 2.5 is normal. A value greater than 3.25 is significant and a possible indication for surgical repair of pectus excavatum, and a value of less than 2.0 is considered positive for carinatum.

Some authors prefer the correction index (CI); using an axial image at the deepest part of the pectus, a transverse line is drawn at the level of the anterior border of the underlying vertebral body. The distance between that line and the posterior sternum is measured, and the distance between that line and the most anterior aspect of the chest is measured. The distance between the two is divided by the latter (x100) to give the percentage of chest depth the defect represents.[23] In general, a 28% CI correlates with an approximate HI of 3.25.

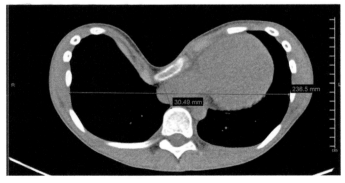

Fig. 6. Preoperative chest CT scan of 14-year-old boy with symptomatic pectus excavatum. At the deepest part of the concavity, transverse internal diameter divided by distance between posterior sternum and anterior aspect of the associated vertebral body yields an HI of 7.8. The scan also documents compression of the right atrium and displacement of the heart into the left hemithorax.

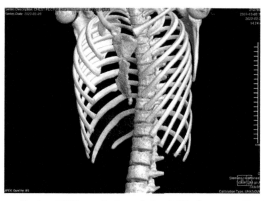

Fig. 7. Shaded surface display (SSD) rendering of chest CT of same patient as shown in **Fig. 7.**

MRI has been shown by several authors to be as accurate as CT scanning and offers the advantages of lack of ionizing radiation and the ability to more accurately assess compression of the right and left ventricles.[24]

Pulmonary function tests (PFTs) may be obtained and may or may not show significant impairment from excavatum.[25,26] Potential explanations for this include

They are typically done at rest and may not accurately reflect actual lung function during exercise.

Most pulmonologists consider forced expiratory volume in 1 second (FEV1) and forced vital capacity (FVC) values that are 80% or greater of predicted (based on patient age, height, weight) to be normal, and thus a symptomatic adolescent athlete, whose values are diminished by 19% (versus expected) would, in most pulmonary laboratories, be labeled as normal.

Most PFT studies were done prior to the use of the minimally invasive technique, and thus postoperative patients often had significant chest wall scarring, which caused a partial iatrogenic diminution in lung function.

For these, and other reasons, many investigators in the 1970s and 1980s concluded that repair of pectus excavatum was primarily a cosmetic procedure without true physiologic benefit. Fortunately, cardiorespiratory investigations done during exercise have helped correct this misunderstanding.

Echocardiography may be helpful by documenting right heart compression and showing valve distortion.[1,2,7] The most commonly affected valves are tricuspid (with subsequent regurgitation) and mitral (with regurgitation or prolapse). Unfortunately, because of anterior chest wall distortion from excavatum, it may be difficult for the echo technician or cardiologist to get adequate windows to view the cardiac chambers well. This can be overcome by using transesophageal echocardiography (TEE), but, because this typically requires conscious sedation or even general anesthesia, it is rarely done.[27]

Perhaps the most useful test for evaluation of excavatum patients is cardiopulmonary exercise testing (CPET), which is typically performed by a cardiologist.[1,2,4,5] Patients are placed on a treadmill (or exercise bicycle) with a metabolic cart, so that inhaled/exhaled air can be measured, and, with exercise, various measurements of cardiac function can be recorded. Perhaps the most useful is maximum oxygen consumption (VO_{2max}) (the maximum rate of oxygen consumption with exercise), typically

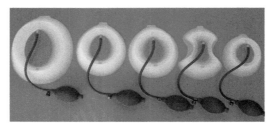

Fig. 8. Assorted sizes of the Klobe vacuum bell.

expressed in mL/(kg-min). In a well-organized laboratory, a pulmonologist may be able to simultaneously measure exercise PFTs.

NONOPERATIVE TREATMENT

Although exercises and physical therapy have been advocated for the treatment of chest wall deformities, there are currently no reliable reports of their proven success. A German engineer, Eckart Klobe, has developed a vacuum bell for the treatment of excavatum, requiring the patient to apply external suction to his or her anterior chest wall in order to gradually change shape of the anterior cartilages[28] (**Fig. 8**). Typical treatment regimens require use for at least 1 hour 2 times each day for up to 2 years. Although adverse effects, such as skin bruising, are rare and relatively mild, dropout rates are high, with successful treatment reported in only about 20% of treated patients. Retrospective reports suggest that the best candidates for the vacuum bell are patients 11 years of age or younger with relatively mild indentations (1.5 cm or less) with chest wall flexibility.[29]

The most extensive experience with nonoperative management of chest wall deformities has been described with carinatum. An external compression brace, popularized by Azizkhan, can be custom-made and worn either beneath or on top of clothing to compress the anterior chest wall during adolescent growth[30] (**Fig. 9**). Up

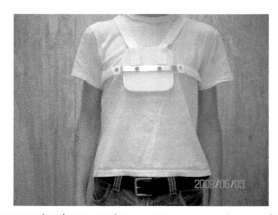

Fig. 9. External compression brace used to correct pectus carinatum during early adolescence. This particular child has chosen to wear the brace over his T-shirt, but most children prefer to wear the brace directly on the skin of the chest, with 1 or even 2 shirts worn over the brace to minimize its appearance while at school or at play with peers.

to 70% to 80% of appropriately chosen patients achieve good or excellent results with this technique. Typical treatment protocols require use for 22 to 23 hours per day for the first six months of treatment, followed by 18 months of maintenance, with brace use typically only when sleeping at night. A similar compression brace, developed in Argentina, allows for pressure measurements to be done and help guide patients (and parents) with the treatment.[31] Adverse effects of bracing are rare, but include bruising and skin changes (typically transient and reversible). Rarely, enthusiastic adolescents can overcorrect their carinatum deformities and develop excavatum, so periodic visits with a chest wall surgeon are typically required during treatment. Bracing is so effective that the American Pediatric Surgical Association (APSA) recommends a trial of bracing for most patients with carinatum before considering surgery.[32]

SURGICAL APPROACHES
Open

Although various techniques have been reported, the description of the open repair (with sternal osteotomy and resection of deformed anterior cartilages) by Ravitch in 1949[33] is considered by most pediatric surgeons to have established a gold standard by which all subsequent techniques should be compared. Because Ravitch did not initially use internal stabilization with a metal support bar or pin (or prosthetic mesh), recurrence was problematic. Many authors subsequently described minor changes to the operation, including the use of retrosternal support and more limited cartilage resections, and thus the term modified Ravitch has been extensively used. Large series with excellent results have been reported[34–40] (**Table 1**).

The operation is typically done through a vertical midline or transverse submammary incision with elevation of the pectoralis major and minor muscles off of the chest wall, subperichondrial resection of deformed/abnormal cartilages, transverse sternal osteotomy, placement of a retrosternal temporary support bar, and reapproximation of the pectoralis major muscles in the midline (**Fig. 10**). Modifications of the retrosternal (or trans-sternal) stabilization include use of a Steinman pin,[34] use of an Adkins strut,[40] use of prosthetic mesh,[37,38] and the addition of vertical stabilization bars.[39]

Until recently, most surgical repairs of pectus carinatum were done using the Ravitch technique (or one of its modifications). Most authors did not advocate placement of a support bar, anterior to the sternum, to prevent recurrence, but some did.[40,41] Transverse sternal osteotomies are now routinely stabilized with small titanium plates, adapted from those originally developed for sternotomy patients undergoing open heart surgery and patients requiring rib stabilization following traumatic injuries[42] (**Fig. 11**). Advantages of this new technique include decreased postoperative pain (because of decreased motion of the transected sternum during respiration) and avoidance of a subsequent second operation for bar removal (typically done roughly 6 months later in patients who have undergone open carinatum and excavatum surgery).

A modification of this operation is usually what is done for the treatment of pectus arcuatum (Currarino-Silverman syndrome).[43,44] However, because the cartilage protrusion is typically high (at the level of ribs 1–3), more inferior cartilages may not require removal. In order to achieve good correction, several sternal osteotomies may be required, including (on rare occasions) a transverse cut through the manubrium (Ravitch described the first successful surgical repair of Currarino-Silverman syndrome in 1952, 6 years before its radiographic description by Currarino and Silverman).

Surgery for Poland syndrome is typically delayed until the patient reaches skeletal maturity. This may be determined with plain radiographs of the hand bones, by a

Table 1
Large series of open repairs of pectus excavatum patients

Authors	Year Published	Institution	Patients	Follow-up	Complications	Recurrence
Shamberger, Welch	1988	Boston Children's Hospital	704	2 weeks – 27 years (mean 4.3 years)	4.4%	2.7% (major)
Haller, Scherer, Turner, et al	1989	Johns Hopkins University	664	1–40 years	<5%	5%
Lacquet, Morshuis, Folgering	1998	University Hospital St. Radboud, Netherlands	662 (390 pectus excavatum)	2.8–17.7 years (mean 8.1 years)	Unknown	4.6% (pectus excavatum repeat surgery rate)
Robicsek, Fokin	1999 (and 1974)	Carolinas Medical Center, Charlotte, North Carolina	"More than 850" (608 by 1974)	1–25 years	Unknown, with 1 serious complication (author's claim)	12% recurrence rate (1974 series) 7% reoperation rate (1974 series)
Saxena, Willital	2007	Muenster, Germany	1262 (1031 with pectus excavatum)	2–12 years (mean 5.4 years)	5.7%	5%
Fonkalsrud	2009	UCLA	912	Mean 7.6 years		

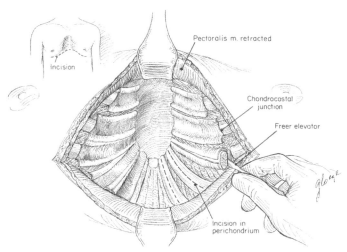

Fig. 10. Modified Ravitch procedure, as popularized by Fonkalsrud and others in the 1970s, 1980s, and 1990s. (*From* Fonkalsrud, et al. Repair of pectus deformities with sternal support. J Thorac Cardiovasc Surg 1994;107:37-42.)

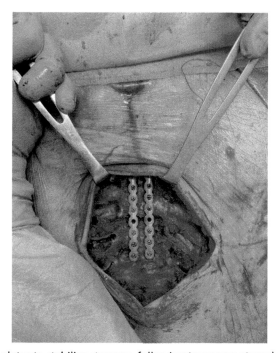

Fig. 11. Titanium plates to stabilize sternum, following transverse sternal osteotomy during open (Ravitch-type) repair of pectus carinatum. This typically allows avoidance of a temporary support bar (such as an Adkins strut or Nuss bar) during bone healing, obviating the need for a second operation for bar removal.

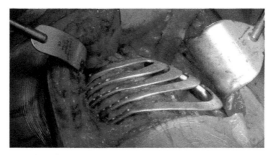

Fig. 12. Custom-designed and manufactured titanium implants for chest wall reconstruction for Poland syndrome in 15-year-old girl. This is the same child as shown in **Fig. 5** (as neonate). Additional reconstruction will require placement of an overlying saline-filled breast implant.

pediatric radiologist. For girls, this may be as young as age 15 to 16 years, but for boys it is typically age 17 to 18 years. If underlying bone/cartilage involvement is present, various chest wall reconstruction techniques have been developed, including the use of customized implants using 3-dimensional printer technology[45] (**Fig. 12**). For males, a latissimus dorsi muscle flap can be rotated anteriorly as a soft tissue substitute for a missing pectoralis muscle. For females, a breast prosthesis is often used,[45] but should not be placed over a bone/cartilage defect without first repairing that defect. Augmentation mammoplasty (for Poland syndrome or to treat simple breast hypoplasia) may be performed simultaneous with the Nuss procedure.[46]

Potential Risks/Complications of the Ravitch Approach

The modified Ravitch procedure, popular from the 1950s through the late 1990s, was advocated for the early correction of affected children with both excavatum and carinatum, often before the age of 5 or 6 years.[14,35] This was done for several reasons: to prevent the commonly seen progression of the deformity during adolescence, to decrease operative time (the procedure on a small child can be done much quicker and therefore require a much shorter duration of general anesthesia, than that on a teenager or adult), and to decrease the postoperative length of hospitalization and recovery (well-described in children following many different surgical procedures). As previously stated, large series suggested low short-term complication rates and recurrence risks. Unfortunately, long-term follow-up identified several potential life-altering consequences, including floating sternum syndrome (**Fig. 13**), acquired Jeune syndrome, breast deformities, and chronic chest wall pain.

Floating sternum syndrome

Floating sternum syndrome was initially described by Haller's group in 2001,[47] and is thought to occur when the cartilages resected during the modified Ravitch procedure fail to regrow, leaving the sternum essentially floating and connected to the ribs laterally by only thin bands of connective tissue and scar. The resultant deformity makes it appear that the heart is almost subcutaneous, with unsightly visible pulsations (and patient/parental concern regarding risks of cardiac trauma from minor blunt injuries).

Surgical repair of this condition should probably only be done by surgeons with extensive experience in complex chest wall repair. Evaluation typically includes all of the studies described previously, as well as a review of previous operative notes.[48]

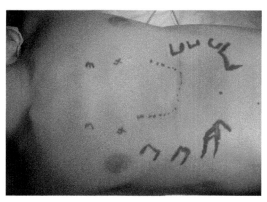

Fig. 13. Floating sternum syndrome, in patient who had undergone previous Ravitch-type open repair of pectus excavatum. Dotted line marks inferior edge of palpable sternum. This child underwent aggressive resection of cartilages 5 to 8 on each side, with failure of regrowth.

If not available, every effort should be made to obtain them and/or speak with the original operating surgeon. Most patients require extensive mobilization of anterior chest wall soft tissue, with retrosternal placement of permanent prosthetic mesh, attached to the tips of adjacent mesh, to act as a hammock to support the sternum. This is a modification of the technique popularized by Robicsek in the 1980s and 1990s for the treatment of pectus excavatum.[37,38] Cadaveric ribs and/or iliac bone grafts may be used to bridge the anterior aspects of the defect and recreate a costal margin (**Fig. 14**).

Acquired Jeune syndrome
Also initially described by Haller,[48] in 1996, acquired Jeune syndrome (also called asphyxiating thoracic dystrophy, or acquired restrictive thoracic dystrophy) (**Fig. 15**), is perhaps the most devastating consequence of early aggressive resection of the affected cartilages and may result from damage to the physis (growth plate) of

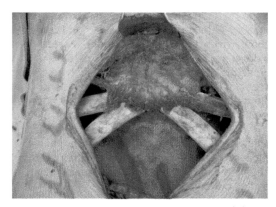

Fig. 14. Floating sternum reconstruction, involving extensive mobilization of chest wall soft tissue, retrosternal placement of permanent prosthetic mesh, and the use of multiple cadaveric rib grafts, as well as iliac bone crest as a graft.

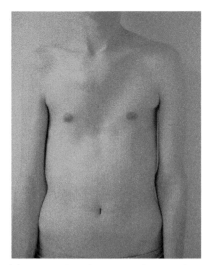

Fig. 15. 14-year-old boy with acquired asphyxiating thoracic dystrophy (acquired Jeune syndrome), 11 years after modified Ravitch procedure for pectus excavatum. Although size and shape of the manubrium are normal, the midthorax is unusually slender and constricted.

the adjacent ribs. Affected patients may develop failure of subsequent rib growth, with a resultant small tubular chest.[49] A common feature of almost all of these patients is that they were operated on at age 6 years or younger. They may present years or even decades later, in late adolescence or early adulthood (most do not have recurrence of their sternal indentation). Patients complain of severe progressive dyspnea with exertion. PFTs reveal severe restrictive disease, with FEV1 and FVC values as low as 25% to 50% of predicted.

Repair of this deformity was initially described by Haller, using modified Rehbein splints in an attempt to elevate the sternum and expand the chest volume.[48] Although subjective exercise tolerance improved in operated patients, splint failure occurred in almost half of the patients, and objective improvement in pulmonary function could not be documented.[50]

Weber described a technique to divide the sternum vertically and use transversely oriented bone grafts to hold the 2 halves of the sternum permanently apart, allowing lung tissue to essentially herniate anteriorly.[51] He documented slight improvement in pulmonary function, which took up to 24 months after surgery.[52] The authors have previously reported a similar experience[49] (**Fig. 16**).

More recent approaches to this devastating condition have been described. These typically involve release of the sternum and remaining anterior chest wall from fibrous scar tissue, multiple osteotomies of adjacent ribs/scar/cartilage, and some sort of sternal stabilization with a metallic bar,[53] some combination of retrosternal bar support and anterior plating,[54] or even the use of absorbable biomaterials.[55] Common features of all of these operations appear to be lengthy operative times and a significant risk of perioperative morbidity and major complications. Although many patients report a subjective improvement in exercise tolerance and quality of life, objective documentation of improvement is currently lacking.

Breast deformities

Although typically not reported in males, female patients may have devascularization injuries to their mammary buds during early childhood chest wall surgery and, as a

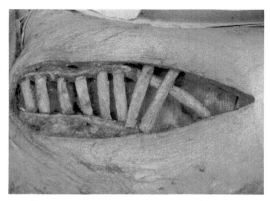

Fig. 16. Intraoperative photograph of 15-year-old boy undergoing sternal split with autologous rib graft interposition procedure, as initially described by Weber. Multiple grafts interposed between the 2 sternal halves and secured in place with stainless steel wires. Note mesh used to bridge defect between rectus abdominus muscles.

result, may develop tuberous breasts or breast hypoplasia as they go through adolescence.[56]

Plastic surgery intervention may be required during early adulthood, with the placement of prosthetic breast implants. The assistance of a general/thoracic surgeon may be helpful, as extensive mobilization of the pectoralis major muscles is typically done during the modified Ravitch procedure, and as a result, there may be fairly extensive scar tissue present. If the chest wall is still flexible and the ribs have not completely calcified yet, these girls are at high risk for recurrent pectus excavatum if large implants are used, especially if placed in a subpectoral position (**Fig. 17**).

Chronic chest wall pain
Although rare, some patients may have chronic irritation of their intercostal nerves, often exacerbated by movement/exercise. Multiple techniques have been described

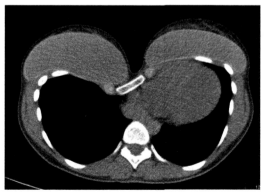

Fig. 17. Chest CT scan of 23-year-old woman with uncorrected pectus excavatum. Large saline-filled breast implants had been placed previously, by a plastic surgeon, to improve her appearance, resulting in significant worsening of her skeletal deformity. HI was 8.0. Implant removal was required prior to performing minimally invasive repair of her deformity.

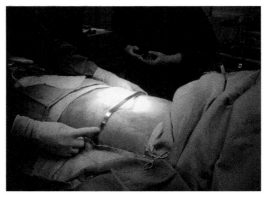

Fig. 18. Nuss procedure. A stainless steel bar is custom bent to conform to the chest wall of the patient during the operation. Bars are typically between 10 and 13 inches long.

to treat this including multi-level intercostal nerve blocks (typically with the addition of corticosteroid) and even cryoanalgesia.

Thoracoscopic

In 1998, Nuss and colleagues[57] reported their 10-year review with a minimally invasive approach for the correction of pectus excavatum. Via small lateral chest wall incisions, a curved stainless steel retrosternal support bar is passed behind the sternum (concave side forward) and then flipped over to elevate the sternum (**Fig. 18**). The bar sits on 2 to 4 ribs laterally for support. The bar acts like orthodontic braces on a teenager's teeth, applying forces to the chest to bend and remodel the ribcage. Small transverse fractures, which slowly heal, may also occur at the congenital fusion points of the sternum.[58] Bars are typically removed as an outpatient procedure 2 to 3 years later.

Although Nuss did not initially utilize intraoperative thoracoscopy, this quickly became routine in order to decrease the risk of intraoperative injury to the lungs and mediastinal structures (**Fig. 19**). Most authors call this operation the Nuss procedure or the minimally invasive repair of pectus excavatum (MIRPE).

Few operations have undergone such extensive modifications in the 20 years since its introduction. These have included

1. The addition of lateral stability bars, which slide over the ends of the transverse bars, to diminish the risk of bar shift or movement[59]
2. Anchoring sutures or wires, to secure the bars to the underlying ribs or cartilages[60]
3. The use of multiple[2,3] bars in older/stiffer patients, including adults[61]
4. Asymmetric bar bending to compensate for sternal angulation/tilt, found in many pectus excavatum patients[62]
5. The use of 2 crossed bars, in patients with significant sternal shortening[63] (**Fig. 20**)
6. The development of bars made of alternative metals (such as titanium) for patients with allergies to components of stainless steel[64]
7. Intraoperative use of sterilized vacuum bells to temporarily assist with sternal elevation before bars are flipped over[65]
8. Subxiphoid incisions to allow introduction of blunt retractors, attached to a Rul-tract retractor, for intraoperative sternal elevation[66]

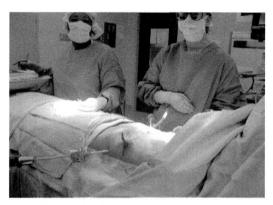

Fig. 19. Nuss procedure. Curved stainless steel bar (concave side oriented anteriorly) has been passed beneath the sternum (between the sternum and pericardium) with thoracoscopic guidance and will be flipped to elevate the sternum.

9. Enhanced recovery after surgery (ERAS) protocols to streamline perioperative management[67]
10. Improvements in perioperative pain management including the use of thoracic epidural catheters[68] and intraoperative thoracoscopic-directed multilevel intercostal nerve blocks[69] and/or cryoanalgesia[70]

the Reverse Nuss for treatment of pectus carinatum

Following the original description by Nuss in 1998 of anterior chest wall remodeling to treat pectus excavatum, various investigators have tried to utilize these same principles to treat pectus carinatum by placing a Nuss bar subcutaneously (anterior to the sternum), pushing down on the sternum, and then securing the bar laterally to the ribcage, typically with wires, cables, and/or screws. The most well-known of these is

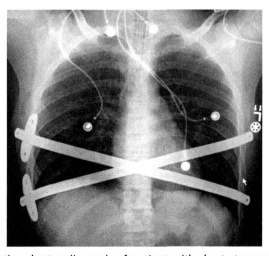

Fig. 20. Intraoperative chest radiograph of patient with short sternum undergoing Nuss procedure with the placement of 2 retrosternal crossed bars. Note lateral stability bars have been slipped over each bar on patient's right side, to improve stability and reduce chance of slippage/movement.

probably Abramson, from Buenos Aires, Argentina, who reported his 5-year experience with 40 patients in 2009[71] (**Fig. 21**). Indeed, most chest wall surgeons now call this the Abramson technique or the Abramson repair. Follow up was available on only half of these patients, with excellent results reported in only 50% and a high rate of complications, including wire breakage. Other investigators have experienced similar frustrations, with the most common technical problem being wire/cable breakage or gradual erosion of wires/cables through the ribs, with resultant loss of correction.[72] The patients who were felt to be the best candidates for this operation (young children with flexible, symmetric protrusions) are those who typically respond best to external compression bracing.

Magnetic Treatment (the Minimover)

Based on the success of the Nuss procedure in the late 1990s and early 2000s, with remodeling of the anterior chest wall achieved by applying pressure to the sternum (rather than the more traditional approach of sternal osteotomy and cartilage removal), Harrison proposed a technique to gradually remodel the sternum by implanting a retrosternal magnet (roughly the size of a hockey puck) and then having patients wear vests with external magnets to essentially pull the sternum forward and correct pectus excavatum[73] (**Fig. 22**). After demonstrating safety and obtaining US Food and Drug Administration sponsorship,[74,75] the investigators received 540 inquiries regarding study participation. Out of these 540, 15 patients underwent implantation.[76] Children were young (ages 8 to 14 years) with flexible chests. Despite this, implant cables broke in 7 of the 15 patients (47%). Pretreatment and post-treatment HIs (used as an objective measurement of chest wall improvement) were not significantly different. Although most chest wall surgeons consider this a very small trial and, technically, a treatment failure, it caught the eye of the US mainstream media[77] and was widely discussed on various Internet chat rooms. It remains one of the most asked about treatment modalities for parents seeking surgical opinions regarding pectus excavatum.

Long-Term Follow-Up

As mentioned previously, several large series of open pectus repair surgeries have now been reported (see **Table 1**) with excellent long-term success. Most patients perceive their corrections as either excellent or good with a low risk of recurrence

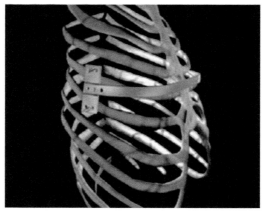

Fig. 21. The Abramson technique (or reverse Nuss technique) with subcutaneous tunneling and placement of an antesternal compression bar for the correction of pectus carinatum.

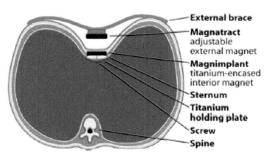

External brace

Magnatract
adjustable
external magnet

Magnimplant
titanium-encased
interior magnet

Sternum

**Titanium
holding plate**

Screw

Spine

Fig. 22. The magnetic minimover procedure. (*From* Harrison MR, et al. Magnetic mini-mover procedure for pectus excavatum II: initial findings of a Food and Drug Administration-sponsored trial. J Pediatr Surg 2010;45:185-192.)

(typically 5% to 10%). Similarly, large series of patients having undergone the Nuss procedure have now been reported, including a series of 2037 patients from Dr. Nuss' group.[66]

The Nuss procedure has been used successfully for the treatment of recurrent pectus excavatum (either after previous open repair or after a previous Nuss procedure).[78] In general, complication rates are somewhat higher than they would be for primary repair, with results that are acceptable but, subjectively, not as good. Jaroszewski's group has described a hybrid approach to adult patients with recurrent pectus excavatum (following previous repair) with the placement of 2 to 3 retrosternal bars and, in many patients, anterior sternal and/or parasternal osteotomies with titanium plating.[79] Intrathoracic adhesions are commonly encountered, with adhesiolysis required in 85% of patients. These operations typically require the surgeon to use all of his or her technical tricks, including bilateral thoracoscopy, intraoperative transesophageal echocardiography, and sternal elevation.

CONGENITAL LUNG LESIONS (OR CONGENITAL LUNG MALFORMATIONS)
Introduction

Congenital lung lesions are rare entities. The most common are congenital pulmonary airway malformations (CPAM), pulmonary sequestrations (PS), congenital lobar emphysema (CLE), and bronchogenic cysts (BC).[80,81]

Congenital Cystic Adenomatoid Malformations

Formation of the lung begins in the first weeks of in utero development and does not stop until at least 8 years of age. CPAMs usually develop during the pseudoglandular stage (seventh to sixteenth week). They are the most frequent abnormal lung lesions of the newborn. Because of improved prenatal screening, they are estimated at 1 in 7200 pregnancies. Ninety-five percent are now found on prenatal ultrasounds[82] (**Fig. 23**).

Pulmonary Sequestrations

PS is thought to occur due the formation of an accessory supernumerary lung bud, either inferior to (extralobar) or within (intralobar) the normal lung bud.[83] They are rare and account for approximately 5% of all congenital lung lesions. They frequently have a systemic blood supply with a feeding vessel from the descending thoracic aorta, typically traversing the inferior pulmonary ligament.

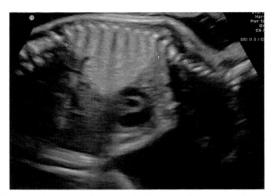

Fig. 23. In utero ultrasound image of congenital cystic adenomatoid malformation (congenital pulmonary airway malformation). Fetal spine is superior, head is to the right, liver is noted to the left, and heart is noted inferiorly. Because the fetus does not breath air, cystic structures are not air-filled, and the malformation often appears as a large solid intrathoracic mass.

Congenital Lobar Emphysema

CLE is defined as the hyperinflation of one or more pulmonary lobes caused by the partial obstruction of its bronchus, causing compression of adjacent organs[84] (**Fig. 25**). The incidence is around 1 case in 30,000 births.

Congenital pediatric airway malformations, until recently known as congenital cystic adenomatoid malformations, are rare birth defects of the pulmonary tree resulting in a mass that encompasses abnormal lung tissue (**Fig. 24**).

Pulmonary sequestration is a congenital lung defect that occurs from the abnormal formation of lung without any bronchial tree or pulmonary artery connections.

Bronchogenic Cysts

BCs are yet another distinct clinical entity. These cystic structures are typically adherent to mainstem bronchi and may enlarge dramatically during childhood as they fill with mucous secreted by respiratory epithelial cells (**Fig. 26**). They can cause a CLE-like picture because of the pressure effect on the adjacent bronchial tree.

Congenital Pulmonary Airway Malformations

CPAMs, formerly called congenital cystic adenomatoid malformations (CCAM), are the most common congenital lung lesion of the pediatric patient and account for nearly 90% of all lung lesions. Up to 95%[82] are diagnosed prenatally. In the early 1980s, postnatal chest radiographs suggested that many would actually disappear during prenatal development. Unfortunately, this misconception was propagated in obstetric, pediatric, and surgical textbooks for several decades. Recent studies with more sophisticated radiographic imaging have found this not to be true.

Prenatal diagnosis enables risk stratification based on the size of the lesion by comparing the calculated volume of the lesion to the circumference of the neonates head. The CPAM volume ratio (CVR) is calculated by dividing the CPAM volume by the head circumference of the fetus. A CVR greater than 1.6 has an increased risk of hydrops fetalis developing and therefore requires close follow-up and potentially intrauterine therapy and/or corticosteroids; CVR less than 1.2 suggests a low risk of complications and does not, in general, require as frequent follow-up. CVR between

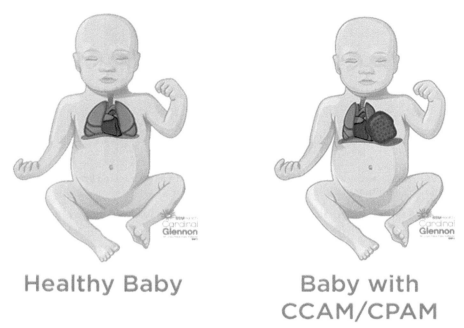

Healthy Baby

Baby with CCAM/CPAM

Fig. 24. Congenital cystic adenomatoid malformation (also called congenital pulmonary airway malformation)—note mediastinal displacement toward the right, and compression of normal lung tissue. (*From* the Fetal Care Institute of the Cardinal Glennon Children's Hospital, St. Louis, Mo.)

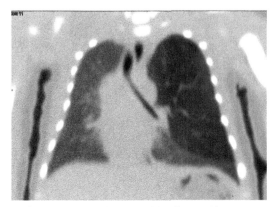

Fig. 25. Preoperative chest CT scan of 2-day-old infant with respiratory distress demonstrating hyperexpansion of the left upper lobe and mediastinal shift to the right, consistent with congenital lobar emphysema. Histologic examination reveals dilated alveoli and alveolar ducts scattered throughout the lobe.

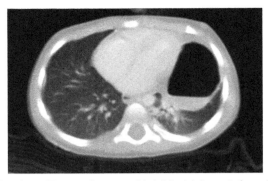

Fig. 26. Preoperative chest CT scan of 1-year-old child with large infected bronchogenic cyst within left hemithorax. Note air/fluid level.

1.2 and 1.6 is classified as intermediate and needs to be followed closely for complications. It is unusual for the CRV to increase during the last trimester.

Asymptomatic Management

When should one image?
Prenatal screening has increased the awareness and diagnosis of CPAMs, PS, and BC but not CLE. Most infants born with a prenatal diagnosis of a CLM are asymptomatic at birth and do require any immediate intervention. It is common to perform a chest radiograph after delivery and if there is no abnormality noted, follow-up with cross-sectional imaging in the first few months of postnatal life is indicated. The type of cross-sectional imaging in debatable. Some surgeons prefer CT scan, because sedation or general anesthesia can be avoided; others use MRI to avoid radiation exposure. A recent consensus statement from the American Pediatric Surgical Association (APSA) does recommend a CT scan but does not comment on timing.[85]

Why should one operate?
The indications for asymptomatic lesions are at least three-fold[86–88]:

1. Avoiding the eventual complication of the CLM becoming infected. These infections may be life-threatening, with systemic sepsis. Additionally, the inflammatory

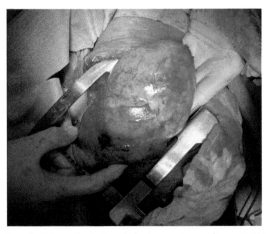

Fig. 27. Intraoperative photograph during left thoracotomy for resection of large infected congenital pulmonary airway malformation of the left lower lobe. Patient is 8 years old.

reaction that is induced, and the subsequent adhesions and scarring, may significantly increase the risks of subsequent surgical resection (**Fig. 27**).
2. Avoiding malignant transformation. Rhabdomyosarcoma, pleuropulmonary blastoma, and bronchioalveolar carcinoma are known to have developed within CPAMs. Malignancy has been reported in specimens resected during infancy, but the incidence is low (less than 1%). The incidence and timing of malignant transformation are unknown but most likely underappreciated.
3. Enabling optimal lung function after resection. Because alveolar formation continues during the first 7 to 8 years of life, the remaining lobes (following lobectomy) have their optimal chance to expand and form functional lung tissue the earlier the planned resection is completed.

When should one operate?

Most surgeons recommend resection during the first year of life to avoid complications from infection and allow residual lung tissue growth to accommodate for loss of volume. One study found that resection prior to 4 months of age had similar complications and less operative time compared with later resections.[89] Komori showed that patients operated on when they were less than 1 year of age had better pulmonary functions than those who were older at the time of operation, and demonstrated that alveolar multiplication mainly occurs in patients younger than 1 year as opposed to overinflation that occurs after the age of on year.[90]

How should one operate?

Thoracoscopy versus thoracotomy. Thoracoscopy has become the preferred modality for resection of CPAMs, BC and PS (**Fig. 28**). It remains challenging for CLE because of the overinflation and loss of domain; therefore most CLE cases require a thoracotomy for resection. Rothenberg reported his experience with over 20 years of thoracoscopic resection in nearly 350 patients with complication rate less than 2% and average operative time less of 160 minutes.[91]

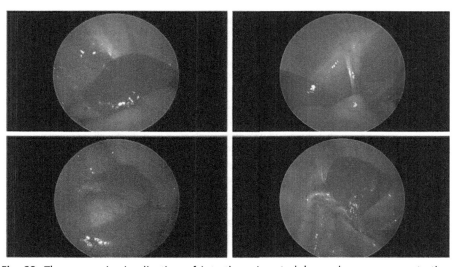

Fig. 28. Thoracoscopic visualization of intrathoracic extralobar pulmonary sequestration. Patient is 10 months old and weighs 9.6 kg. Note arterial blood supply directly from descending thoracic aorta.

Symptomatic. CLMs that are symptomatic at birth should be resected prior to discharge from the hospital. The symptoms may be related to a space-occupying lesion resulting in compression of normal tissue and high-flow cardiac output failure. Space-occupying lesions (CPAM, BC, and CLE) can cause compression of the normal surrounding lung parenchyma, decreasing normal pulmonary functions. PS because of their systemic blood flow, can cause a high output failure from recirculation.

Typically, infants will have an increased work of breathing and may require supplemental oxygen and have poor oral intake. It is not unusual for the symptoms to resolve over the first few days of life; therefore, it is appropriate to monitor in the neonatal intensive care unit with frequent chest radiographs to make sure there is resolution of any compression or mediastinal shift.

If increased work of breathing does not normalize despite medical intervention or there is a significant mediastinal shift on subsequent imaging, then lobectomy prior to discharge is indicated.

CLINICS CARE POINTS

- Most chest wall deformities are not present at birth but develop and worsen during childhood and are therefore considered "developmental" rather than "congenital."
- With pectus excavatum, most studies suggest that right heart compression, with subsequent decreased pulmonary blood flow during exercise (rather than actual lung compression) is the primary mechanism for decreased exercise tolerance in these patients.
- Most children with pectus arcuatum (Currarino-Silverman syndrome) are misdiagnosed before referral to a chest wall surgical specialist.
- Dyspnea in children with pectus excavatum may be misdiagnosed as "asthma" since children typically stop activity to utilize inhalers and therefore the brief break from activity may actually be what relieves their symptoms.
- The Haller index, calculated from a chest CT scan, is often done incorrectly (in full inspiration, rather than expiration), and therefore may significantly underestimate the severity of the deformity. A value greater than 3.25 is considered significant.
- Although some patients with pectus excavatum may respond to nonoperative vacuum bell therapy, overall published success rates are relatively low, at about 20%.
- External compression bracing is considered "treatment of choice" for compressible, flexible young patients with symmetric pectus carinatum.
- Since one of many different effective surgical approaches may be appropriate for an individual patient with a chest wall deformity, evaluation by a chest wall specialist with expertise in multiple different approaches may be beneficial.
- Multiple large series of patients undergoing chest wall reconstruction for pectus excavatum have shown relatively low complication rates and high rates of long-term success.
- The Modified Ravitch procedure, or "open repair" of pectus excavatum and carinatum has been associated with significant chest wall constriction and diminished lung function, if done at an early age. These include floating sternum syndrome, acquired Jeune syndrome, breast deformities, chronic chest wall pain, and recurrent pectus.
- The Nuss procedure (Minimally Invasive Repair of Pectus Excavatum) has undergone multiple revisions and modifications since its original description in 1998.
- Congenital lung anomalies are often discovered as "incidental findings" during routine in-utero ultrasound evaluations.

- Congenital Pulmonary Airway Malformations may enlarge, causing compression of adjacent lung tissue and mediastinal structures. If not resected, they may become infected or eventually undergo malignant transformation.
- Although somewhat controversial, most pediatric surgeons recommend prophylactic resection of many asymptomatic lung anomalies to prevent complications.
- Thoracoscopic instrumentation and techniques now allow for minimally-invasive approaches to many congenital lung anomalies.

DISCLOSURE

Authors have nothing to disclose.

REFERENCES

1. Neviere R, Montaigne D, Benhamed L, et al. Cardiopulmonary response following surgical repair of pectus excavatum in adult patients. Eur J Cardio-thoracic Surg 2011;40:e77–82.
2. Tand M, Nielsen HHM, Lesbo M, et al. Improved cardiopulmonary exercise function after modified Nuss operation for pectus excavatum. Eur J Cardio-thoracic Surg 2012;41:1063–7.
3. Neviere R, Benhamed L, Pentiah AD, et al. Pectus excavatum repair improves respiratory pump efficacy and cardiovascular function at exercise. J Thorac Cardiovasc Surg 2013;145:605–6.
4. Tardy MM, Filaire M, Patoir A, et al. Exercise cardiac output limitation in pectus excavatum. J Am Coll Cardiol 2015;66:976–7.
5. Jayaramakrishnan K, Wotton R, Bradley A, et al. Does repair of pectus excavatum improve cardiopulmonary function? Interactive CardioVascular Thorac Surg 2013;16:865–71.
6. Malek MH, Berger DE, Housh TJ, et al. Cardiovascular function following surgical repair of pectus excavatum: a metaanalysis. Chest 2006;130:506–16.
7. Coln E, Carrasco J, Coln D. Demonstrating relief of cardiac compression with the Nuss minimally invasive repair for pectus excavatum. J Pediatr Surg 2006;41:683–6.
8. Fonkalsrud EW, Beanes S. Surgical management of pectus carinatum: 30 years' experience. World J Surg 2001;25:898–903.
9. Fonkalsrud EW, Anselmo DM. Less extensive techniques for repair of pectus carinatum: the undertreated chest deformity. J Am Coll Surg 2004;198:898–905.
10. Currarino G, Silverman FN. Premature obliteration of the sternal sutures and pigeon-breast deformity. Radiology 1958;70:532–40.
11. Kelly RE Jr, Quinn A, Varela P, et al. Dysmorphology of chest wall deformities: frequency distribution of subtypes of typical pectus excavatum and rare subtypes. Arch Bronconeumol 2013;49:196–200.
12. Chidambaram B, Mehta AV. Currarino-Silverman syndrome (pectus carinatum type 2 deformity) and mitral valve disease. Chest 1992;102:780–2.
13. Fox JP, Seyfer AE. Setting the record straight: the real history of Poland's syndrome. Bull Am Coll Surg 2012;97:27–9.
14. Humphreys GH, Jaretzki A. Pectus excavatum: late results with and without operation. J Thorac Cardiovasc Surg 1980;80:686–95.
15. Kelly RE Jr, Shamberger RC, Mellins RB, et al. Prospective multicenter study of surgical correction of pectus excavatum: design, perioperative complications,

pain, and baseline pulmonary function facilitated by internet-based data collection. J Am Coll Surg 2007;205:205–16.

16. Kelly RE Jr, Cash TF, Shamberger RC, et al. Surgical repair of pectus excavatum markedly improves body image and perceived ability for physical activity: a multicenter study. Pediatrics 2008;122:1218–22.

17. Lawson ML, Cash TF, Akers R, et al. A pilot study of the impact of surgical repair on disease-specific quality of life among patients with pectus excavatum. J Pediatr Surg 2003;38:916–8.

18. Waters P, Welch K, Micheli LJ, et al. Scoliosis in children with pectus excavatum and pectus carinatum. J Pediatr Orthop 1989;9:551–6.

19. Ghionzoli M, Martin A, Bongini M, et al. Scoliosis and pectus excavatum in adolescents: does the Nuss procedure affect the scoliotic curvature? J Laparoendosc Adv Surg Tech A 2016;26:734–9.

20. Haller JA Jr, Kramer SS, Lietman SA. Use of CT scans in selection of patients for pectus excavatum surgery: a preliminary report. J Pediatr Surg 1987;22:904–6.

21. Birkemeier KL, Podberesky DJ, Salisbury S, et al. Breathe in… breathe out… stop breathing: does phase of respiration affect the Haller index in patients with pectus excavatum? AJR Am J Roentgenol 2011;197:W934–9.

22. Calloway EH, Chhotani AN, Lee YZ, et al. Three-dimensional computed tomography for evaluation and management of children with complex chest wall anomalies: useful information of just pretty pictures? J Pediatr Surg 2011;46:640–7.

23. Poston PM, McHugh MA, Rossi NO, et al. The case for using the correction index obtained from chest radiography for evaluation of pectus excavatum. J Pediatr Surg 2015;50:1940–4.

24. Birkemeier KL, Podberesky DJ, Salisbury S, et al. Limited, fast magnetic resonance imaging as an alternative for preoperative evaluation of pectus excavatum: a feasibility study. J Thorac Imaging 2012;27:393–7.

25. Cahill JL, Lees GM, Robertson HT. A summary of preoperative and postoperative cardiorespiratory performance in patients undergoing pectus excavatum and carinatum repair. J Pediatr Surg 1984;19:430–3.

26. Lawson ML, Mellins RB, Tabangin M, et al. Impact of pectus excavatum on pulmonary function before and after repair with the Nuss procedure. J Pediatr Surg 2005;40:174–80.

27. Xu B, Xu T, Wang S, et al. The use of nonthoracoscopic Nuss procedure for the correction of pectus excavatum by trans-esophageal echocardiography monitoring. Medicine 2019;98:1–4.

28. Haecker FM. The vacuum bell for conservative treatment of pectus excavatum: the Basle experience. Pediatr Surg Int 2011;27:623–7.

29. Obermeyer RJ, Cohen NS, Kelly RE Jr, et al. Nonoperative management of pectus excavatum with vacuum bell therapy: a single center study. J Pediatr Surg 2018;53:1221–5.

30. Frey AS, Garcia VF, Brown RL, et al. Nonoperative management of pectus carinatum. J Pediatr Surg 2006;41:40–5.

31. Martinez-Ferro M, Fraire C, Bernard S. Dynamic compression system for the correction of pectus carinatum. Semin Pediatr Surg 2008;17:194–200.

32. APSA Practice Committee, Shaul DB, Phillips JD, et al. American pediatric surgical association pectus carinatum guideline, Available at: www.eapsa.org 2012. Accessed August 8, 2022

33. Ravitch MM. The operative treatment of pectus excavatum. Ann Surg 1949;129:429–44.

34. Shamberger RC, Welch KJ. Surgical repair of pectus excavatum. J Pediatr Surg 1988;23:615–22.
35. Haller JA Jr, Scherer LR, Turner CS, et al. Evolving management of pectus excavatum based on a single institutional experience of 664 patients. Ann Surg 1989; 209:578–83.
36. Lacquet LK, Morshuis WJ, Folgering HT. Long-term results after correction of anterior chest wall deformities. J Cardiovasc Surg 1998;39:683–8.
37. Robicsek F, Fokin A. Surgical correction of pectus excavatum and carinatum. J Cardiovasc Surg 1999;40:725–31.
38. Robicsek F, Daugherty HK, Mullen DC, et al. Technical considerations in the surgical management of pectus excavatum and carinatum. Ann Thorac Surg 1974; 18:549–64.
39. Saxena AK, Willital GH. Valuable lessons from two decades of pectus repair with the Willital-Hegemann procedure. J Thorac Cardiovasc Surg 2007;134:871–6.
40. Fonkalsrud EW. 912 open pectus excavatum repairs: changing trends, lessons learned: one surgeon's experience. World J Surg 2009;33:180–90.
41. Saxena AK, Willital GH. Surgical repair of pectus carinatum. Int Surg 1999;84: 326–30.
42. Young S, Lau ST, Shaul DB, et al. A new technique in complex chest wall reconstruction: open reduction and internal fixation. J Pediatr Surg 2018;53:2488–90.
43. Shamberger RC, Welch KJ. Surgical correction of chondromanubrial deformity (Currarino Silverman syndrome). J Pediatr Surg 1988;23:319–22.
44. Gritsiuta AI, Bracken A, Beebe K, et al. Currarino-Silverman syndrome: diagnosis and treatment of rare chest wall deformity, a case series. J Thorac Dis 2021;13: 2968–78.
45. Rodriguez IE, Heare T, Bruny J, et al. Customized titanium implant for chest wall reconstruction in complex Poland syndrome. Plast Reconstr Surg Glob Open 2014;2:3112.
46. Park HJ, Gu JH, Jang JC, et al. Correction of pectus excavatum with breast hypoplasia using simultaneous pectus bar procedure and augmentation mammoplasty. Ann Plast Surg 2014;73:190–5.
47. Prabhakaran K, Paidas CN, Haller JA, et al. Management of a floating sternum after repair of pectus excavatum. J Pediatr Surg 2001;36:159–64.
48. Haller JA Jr, Colombani PM, Humphries CT, et al. Chest wall constriction after too extensive and too early operations for pectus excavatum. Ann Thorac Surg 1996; 61:1618–25.
49. Phillips JD, van Aalst JA. Jeune's syndrome (asphyxiating thoracic dystrophy): congenital and acquired. Semin Pediatr Surg 2008;17:167–72.
50. Pretorius ES, Haller JA, Fishman EK. Spiral CT with 3D reconstruction in children requiring reoperation for failure of chest wall growth after pectus excavatum surgery: preliminary observations. Clin Imaging 1998;22:108–16.
51. Weber TR, Kurkchubasche AG. Operative management of asphyxiating thoracic dystrophy after pectus repair. J Pediatr Surg 1998;33:262–5.
52. Weber TR. Further experience with the operative management of asphyxiating thoracic dystrophy after pectus repair. J Pediatr Surg 2005;40:170–3.
53. Casamassima MGS, Goldstein SD, Salazar JH, et al. Operative management of acquired Jeune's syndrome. J Pediatr Surg 2014;49:55–60.
54. Jaroszewski DE, Notrica DM, McMahon LE, et al. Operative management of acquired thoracic dystrophy in adults after open pectus excavatum repair. Ann Thorac Surg 2014;97:1764–70.

55. Miller DL. Reoperative pectus repair using biomaterials. Ann Thorac Surg 2020; 110:383–9.
56. Van Aalst JA, Phillips JD, Sadove AM. Pediatric chest wall and breast deformities. Plast Reconstr Surg 2009;124:38e–49e.
57. Nuss D, Kelly RE Jr, Croitoru DP, et al. A 10-year review of a minimally invasive technique for the correction of pectus excavatum. J Pediatr Surg 1998;33:545–52.
58. Ohno K, Morotomi Y, Harumoto K, et al. Prelimary study on the effects of bar placement on the thorax after the Nuss procedure for pectus excavatum using bone scintigraphy. Eur J Pediatr Surg 2006;16:155–9.
59. Karakus OZ, Ulusoy O, Hakguder G, et al. Nuss procedure: technical modifications to ease bending of the support bar and lateral stabilizer placement. Ann Thorac Med 2016;11:214–8.
60. McMahon LE, Johnson KN, Jaroszewski DE, et al. Experience with FiberWire for pectus bar attachment. J Pediatr Surg 2014;49:1259–63.
61. Lo P-C, Tzeng I-S, Hsieh M-S, et al. The Nuss procedure for pectus excavatum: an effective and safe approach using bilateral thoracoscopy and a selective approach to use of multiple bars in 296 adolescent and adult patients. PLoS One 2020;15:e0233547.
62. Park HJ, Lee SY, Lee CS, et al. The Nuss procedure for pectus excavatum: evolution of techniques and early results on 322 patients. Ann Thorac Surg 2004;77: 289–95.
63. Pilegaard HK. Nuss technique in pectus excavatum: a mono-institutional experience. J Thorac Dis 2015;7:S172–6.
64. Obermeyer RJ, Gaffar S, Kelly RE Jr, et al. Selective versus routine patch metal allergy testing to select bar material for the Nuss procedure in 932 patients over 10 years. J Pediatr Surg 2018;53:260–4.
65. Haecker F-M, Krebs T, Kocher GJ, et al. Sternal elevation techniques during the minimally invasive repair of pectus excavatum. Interact Cardiovasc Thorac Surg 2019;29:497–502.
66. Obermeyer RJ, Goretsky MJ, Kelly RE Jr, et al. Selective use of sternal elevation before substernal dissection in more than 2000 Nuss repairs at a single institution. J Pediatr Surg 2021;56:649–54.
67. Yu P, Wang G, Zhang C, et al. Clinical application of enhanced recovery after surgery (ERAS) in pectus excavatum patients following Nuss procedure. J Thorac Dis 2020;12:3035–42.
68. Heo MH, Kim JY, Kim JH, et al. Epidural analgesia versus intravenous analgesia fter minimally invasive repair of pectus excavatum in pediatric patients: a systematic review and meta-analysis. Korean J Anesthesiol 2021;74:449–58.
69. Lukosiene L, Rugyte DC, Macas A, et al. Postoperative pain management in pediatric patients undergoing minimally invasive repair of pectus excavatum: the role of intercostal block. J Pediatr Surg 2013;48:2425–30.
70. Graves CE, Moyer J, Zobel MJ, et al. Intraoperative intercostal nerve cryoablation during the Nuss procedure reduces length of stay and opioid requirement: a randomized clinical trial. J Pediatr Surg 2019;54:2250–6.
71. Abramson H, D'Agostino J, Wuscovi S. A 5-year experience with a minimally invasive technique for pectus carinatum repair. J Pediatr Surg 2009;44:118–24.
72. Cohee AS, Lin JR, Frantz FW, et al. Staged management of pectus carinatum. J Pediatr Surg 2013;48:315–20.
73. Harrison MR, Estefan-Ventura D, Fechter R, et al. Magnetic Mini-Mover Procedure for pectus excavatum: I. development, design, and simulations for feasibility and safety. J Pediatr Surg 2007;42:81–5.

74. Harrison MR, Curran PF, Jamshidi R, et al. Magnetic mini-mover procedure for pectus excavtum II: initial findings of a Food and Drug Administration-sponsored trial. J Pediatr Surg 2010;45:185–91.

75. Harrison MR, Gonzales KG, Bratton BJ, et al. Magnetic mini-mover procedure for pectus excavatum III: safety and efficacy in a Food and Drug Administration-sponsored clinical trial. J Pediatr Surg 2012;47:154–9.

76. Graves CE, Hirose S, Raff GW, et al. Magnetic mini-mover procedure for pectus excavatum IV. FDA sponsored multicenter trial 2017;52:913–9.

77. Standen A. Magnets may pull kids with sunken chests out of operating room. NPR. 2012. Available at: https://www.npr.org/section/health-shots/2012/07/30/157441675/magents-may-pull-kids-with-sunken-chests-out-of-operating-room. Accessed August 8, 2022.

78. Croitoru DP, Kelly RE Jr, Goretsky MJ, et al. The minimally invasive Nuss technique for recurrent or failed pectus excavatum repair in 50 patients. J Pediatr Surg 2005;40:181–6.

79. Ashfaq A, Beamer S, Ewais MM, et al. Revision of failed prior Nuss in adult patients with pectus excavatum. Ann Thorac Surg 2018;105:371–8.

80. Cass DL, Crombleholme TM, Howell LJ, et al. Cystic lung lesions with systemic arte- rial blood supply: a hybrid of congenital cystic adenomatoid malformation and bronchopulmonary sequestration. J Pediatr Surg 1997;32(7):986–90.

81. Fowler DJ, Gould SJ. The pathology of congenital lung lesions. Semin Pediatr Surg 2015;24(4):176–82.

82. Azizkhan RG, Crombleholme TM. Congenital cystic lung disease: contemporary antenatal and postnatal management. Pediatr Surg Int 2008;24(6):643–57.

83. SadeRM, Clouse M, Ellis FH. The Spectrum of pulmonary sequestration. Ann Thorac Surg 1974;18(6):644–58.

84. Olutoye OO, Coleman BG, Hubbard AM, Adzick NS. Prenatal diagnosis and management of congenital lobar emphysema. J Pediatr Surg 2000;35(5):792–5.

85. Downard CD, Calkins CM, Williams RF, et al. Treatment of congenital pulmonary air- way malformations: a systematic review from the APSA outcomes and evidence based practice committee. Pediatr Surg Int 2017. https://doi.org/10.1007/s00383-017-4098-z.

86. Chetcuti PA, Crabbe DC. CAM lungs: the conservative approach. Arch Dis Child Fetal Neonatal Ed 2006;91(6):F463–4.

87. Aziz D, Langer JC, Tuuha SE, et al. Perinatally diagnosed asymptomatic congenital cystic adenomatoid malformation: to resect or not? J Pediatr Surg 2004;39(3):329–34 [discussion: 34].

88. Pelizzo G, Barbi E, Codrich D, et al. Chronic inflammation in congenital cystic adenomatoid malformations. An underestimated risk factor? J Pediatr Surg 2009;44(3):616–9.

89. Style CC, Cass DL, Olutoye OO, et al. Early vs late resection of asymptomatic congenital lung malformations. J Pediatr Surg 2019;54:70–4.

90. Komori K, Kamagata S, Hirobe S, et al. Radionuclide imaging study of long-term pulmonary function after lobectomy in children with congenital cystic lung disease. J Pediatr Surg 2009;44(11):2096–100.

91. Rothenberg SS, Middlesworth W, Kadennhe-Chiweshe A, et al. Two decades of experience with thoracoscopic lobectomy in infants and children: standardizing techniques for advanced thoracoscopic surgery. J Laparoendosc Adv Surg Tech 2015;25(5):423–8.

Pediatric Inflammatory Bowel Disease for General Surgeons

Michael R. Phillips, MD, MSCR, FACS[a,b,*], Erica Brenner, MD, MSCR[c],
Laura N. Purcell, MD, MPH[a], Ajay S. Gulati, MD[c]

KEYWORDS

- Inflammatory bowel disease • Ulcerative colitis • Crohn disease
- Inflammatory bowel disease-unclassified • Ileal pouch anal anastomosis

KEY POINTS

- Pediatric inflammatory bowel disease (IBD) presents with more severe symptoms, frequently requiring surgical intervention. Severe disease may manifest as failure to meet growth and developmental milestones and requires a multidisciplinary approach.
- Perianal Crohn disease requires a combination of medical and surgical interventions to improve symptom management, which should be considered in patients with any complex perianal infections.
- Severe and refractory ulcerative colitis can be effectively managed with proctocolectomy with ileal pouch anal anastomosis.
- Patients with IBD may require emergency intestinal resection due to disease severity or instability. For Crohn disease, this should be performed with the intent to minimize the length of intestinal resection, and for ulcerative colitis, an abdominal colectomy with end ileostomy should be performed.
- For patients with stable disease requiring surgery, referral to multidisciplinary care teams specializing in IBD is recommended to ensure medical, nutritional, and psychological needs are met in addition to surgical.

KEY/ESSENTIAL HEADINGS

Introduction and Definitions: Inflammatory bowel disease (IBD) is caused by a dysregulation of the patient's immune system causing inflammation of the gastrointestinal

[a] Department of Surgery, The University of North Carolina School of Medicine, 170 Manning Drive, CB #7223, Chapel Hill, NC 27599-7223, USA; [b] Department of Pediatrics, The University of North Carolina School of Medicine, 260 MacNider Hall, CB# 7220333 South Columbia St Chapel Hill, NC 27599-7220; [c] Department of Pediatrics, Division of Gastroenterology, The University of North Carolina School of Medicine, 230 MacNider, CB #7229, Chapel Hill, NC 27599, USA
* Corresponding author.
E-mail address: miphilli@med.unc.edu

Surg Clin N Am 102 (2022) 913–927
https://doi.org/10.1016/j.suc.2022.07.018
0039-6109/22/© 2022 Elsevier Inc. All rights reserved.

surgical.theclinics.com

Table 1
Comparison of phenotypes of inflammatory bowel disease (CD, UC, IBD-U)

	Crohn Disease	Ulcerative Colitis	Inflammatory Bowel Disease-Unclassified[b]
Location	Any area in the GI tract	Colon[a]	Colon
Layers of intestine affected	Transmural	Mucosa	Mucosa
Phenotypes	Inflammatory Stricturing Penetrating Peri-anal Combination	Colitis	Colitis
Histologic features	Active and chronic inflammation Noncaseating granulomas (~60% of patients)	Active and chronic inflammation	Active and chronic inflammation

Abbreviation: GI, Gastrointestinal tract.
[a] Patients with severe ulcerative colitis may develop backwash ileitis or gastritis, may not be contraindication to IPAA.
[b] Reserved for patients who cannot be defined as CD or UC.

tract.[1,2] The incidence of IBD in children in the United States is increasing from 33.0/100,000 in 2007 to 77.0/100,000 in 2016.[1] This means that approximately 25% of patients with IBD present before 20-years of life, with peak onset in pediatric patients occurring in adolescence.[1,2] IBD is classified in 3 phenotypes: (1) Crohn disease (CD), (2) ulcerative colitis (UC), and (3) Inflammatory bowel disease-unclassified (IBD-U; **Table 1**).

Pediatric Crohn Disease

CD causes full thickness inflammation that can affect the intestinal tract in any location from mouth to anus. CD may also affect areas that are not contiguous (ie, skip lesions). It is classified by the location affected and the phenotypic behavior it exhibits.[3–5] (**Table 2**) Pediatric CD is often more extensive and more severe than in adults. Specifically, Goodhand and colleagues found higher rates of ileocolonic (L3) disease compared with adults, 67% vs 22%, respectively. They also demonstrated higher rates of upper GI (L4) disease (28% vs 0%) at the time of diagnosis.[5] The rate of ileocolonic disease at diagnosis was similar in studies performed by Vernier-Masouille and Van Limbergent.[3,4] Goodhand demonstrated an 18% incidence of surgery in adolescent patients with CD compared with 9% in adult patients with CD propensity matched by disease duration with a mean follow-up of 4.7 years in both groups.[5] Van Limbergent performed an observational study of adolescent and adult patients with CD, and noted that while fewer children underwent surgery at the time of diagnosis, the percentages of adolescent patients undergoing surgery compared with adult-onset CD were 34.5% and 55.5%, respectively. Vernier-Masouille demonstrated a cumulative incidence of intestinal resection in a cohort of 394 pediatric patients with CD to be 44%.[3] The extensive nature of CD and the frequent need for surgery in pediatric patients highlight the need for clear indications for surgery.

Indications for surgery

A summary of indications for surgery and potential surgical options is located in **Table 3** and may apply to adult patients as well.[6] (see **Table 3**) Risk factors for surgery

Table 2
Classification schema for Crohn disease

Category	Definition
Location (L)	
L1	Terminal ileum
L2	Colon
L3	Ileum and colon (ileocolon)
L4	Upper gastrointestinal tract
Behavior (B)	
B1	Nonstricturing/inflammatory
B2	Stricturing
B3	Penetrating
P	Perianal

in pediatric CD include diagnosis in adolescence compared with younger ages, growth impairment at diagnosis, and stricturing or internal penetrating phenotype.[7] In contrast, CD located only within the colon seems to be protective from the need for surgery compared with other locations.[7]

Stricturing Crohn disease. Intestinal narrowing or obstruction is frequently associated with a stricturing phenotype. Select cases can be treated with medical therapy first, particularly if the stricture is inflammatory. The timing of surgical intervention depends on the degree of obstruction from the strictured segment, specifically waves of peristaltic abdominal pain, weight lows, proximal dilation, and distal decompression are all signs of a more severe luminal narrowing.

A recent systematic review of pediatric patients with stricturing CD demonstrated complete response in only 8% of patients treated with medical therapy alone.[8] For fibrotic strictures, intestinal resection, strictureplasty, or endoscopic balloon dilation are potential therapies.[6,8] The pooled recurrence rate for all types of procedural interventions was 22% at 1.9 years. Individual recurrence rates for resection, strictureplasty, and endoscopic balloon dilation were 9%, 38%, and 47%, respectively.[8] Acute intestinal obstruction due to stricturing disease that fails medical management requires intestinal

Table 3
Indications for surgery in pediatric Crohn disease

Indication	Surgery
Intestinal stricture or obstruction	Resection or stricturoplasty
Penetrating disease	
Phlegmonous changes	Medical therapy
Intra-abdominal abscess	Percutaneous drainage or resection
Enteric fistula	Fistula closure ± intestinal resection
Perforation	Intestinal resection
Fulminant of hemorrhagic disease refractory to medical therapy	Intestinal resection
Neoplastic changes	Intestinal resection
Complex perianal fistula or abscess	Incision and drainage ± Seton placement
Growth or pubertal delay	

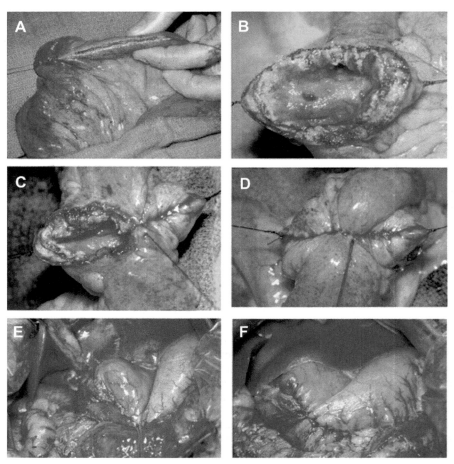

Fig. 1. Surgical images from Heineke-Mikulicz strictureplasty (*A–D*), and Finney (Jaboulay) strictureplasty (*E, F*).[9]

resection. Strictureplasty can be performed in 1 of 3 methods: (1) Heineke-Mikulicz strictureplasty (<10 cm), (2) Finney (Jaboulay) strictureplasty (10–20 cm), or (3) side-to-side isoperistaltic strictureplasty (>25 cm).[9] Strictureplasty should not be used in localized perforation, fistula, multiple strictures in a short segment, stricture near a planned resection, radiation strictures, colonic strictures, or in patients with malnutrition.[9]

Heineke-Mikulicz strictureplasty is performed by a longitudinal incision in the anti-mesenteric border along the length of the stricture. This is followed by transverse closure of the stricture as in **Fig. 1**A–D. For strictures ~20 to 25 cm, a Finney or Jaboulay strictureplasty can be performed by creating a U-shape or a V-shape with the midpoint of the stricture at the apex of the V. The stricture is then opened on the mesenteric side along its length, and the lateral borders are sutured in a running fashion as in **Fig. 1**E and F.[9] The side-to-side isoperistaltic strictureplasty is performed for strictures greater than 25 cm. The bowel is divided at the midpoint of the stricture, and then the proximal and distal portions are placed next to each other in an isoperistaltic configuration. The antimesenteric border is opened in either direction to normal appearing bowel extending at least 2 cm onto the normal bowel.

The opened bowel is then sutured together.[9] The side-to-side strictureplasty is rarely required in children.

Nonperianal penetrating Crohn disease. Penetrating CD may present as phlegmonous changes, intra-abdominal abscesses, an enteric fistula, or free perforation.[6,10] For penetrating disease, which presents as phlegmonous changes, treatment with intravenous broad-spectrum antibiotics is the first step in treatment. Following resolution of infection, initiation of anti-inflammatory therapy is associated improvement in many small series.[10] For patients who experience an intra-abdominal abscess secondary to penetrating CD, Hirten and colleagues recommend a strategy, which involves intravenous antibiotics followed by percutaneous or endoscopic drainage for abscesses greater than 3 cm. If patients worsen or fail to improve, then reimaging to ensure complete drainage followed by consideration for surgery is indicated. If the abscess is completely treated and infection has resolved, immunosuppressive therapy may be initiated.[10] For patients who fail medical management, intestinal resection with or without ostomy creation should be considered.

Enteric fistulas. These require complex multidisciplinary management, and referral to a tertiary care center of pediatric IBD specialization should be considered. Patients with enteric fistulas represent advanced penetrating disease, and, following control of localized infection or inflammation, nutritional optimization should be prioritized.[10] Surgical excision of the diseased area of bowel should be considered, and care taken to avoid recurrent fistulas.[10]

Fulminant or hemorrhagic Crohn disease. For fulminant or hemorrhagic disease that is not responsive to medical management, stabilization of the patient when possible should be performed. For fulminant disease, this includes fluid resuscitation and antibiotics as well as vigilance to rule our perforation or abscess (to ensure adequate source control). For hemorrhage, identification of the intestinal location responsible the bleeding is critical, and surgical exploration without identification of the bleeding site may result in injury to normal bowel or friable diseased bowel. In either case, if patients do not respond to medical therapy, intestinal resection is indicated.

Approach to intestinal resection in pediatric Crohn disease. For patients with complicated or medically refractory CD, intestinal resection of the affected segment should be performed. The risk of resection increases with time from diagnosis, with rates of 16.3%, 33.3%, and 46.6% at 1 year, 5 years, and 10 years from diagnosis, respectively.[11] In pediatric CD, the annual incidence of surgical resection increased by 3.8% from 1997 to 2009, with a corresponding increase in hospital charges.[12]

Patients who require intestinal resection for CD should undergo preoperative medical optimization to decrease the risk of postoperative complications when possible. Intestinal resection should be performed by surgeons with experience in IBD, with a goal of preservation of intestinal length. This can be done laparoscopically or through an open approach or a combination of the two. In the combination approach, laparoscopy is used to identify the affected area, and then the diseased intestine is withdrawn from the abdomen for excision with or without anastomosis. This can be done with suture or stapled techniques. Patients who are at high risk for anastomotic complications (malnourished, immunocompromised, actively infected, smokers, diabetics, or others) may benefit from ostomy creation at the time of resection. After a period of stabilization and better disease control, this ostomy could be reversed.

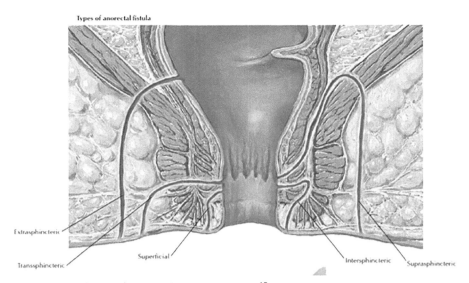

Fig. 2. Anatomic classification of perianal fistulas.[15]

Management of pediatric perianal Crohn disease. Perianal CD is a heterogenous manifestation of CD in children, with rates varying from 10% to 62% of children with CD.[13,14] The management of perianal CD has evolved from primarily surgical management to a combination of surgery and antibiotics to relieve infection and medical therapy to assist with wound healing and disease control.[13] De Zoeten and colleagues proposed guidelines for evaluation and treatment of perianal fistulae and abscesses in pediatric CD. Comprehensive management includes diagnosis and classification using imaging and an examination under anesthesia, followed by medical therapy with agents such as antibiotics, immunomodulators and/or biologic therapy in conjunction with surgical intervention.[14] Data from a systematic review supports this multidisciplinary approach to therapy using combination of surgery and medical therapy, and as such should be performed in centers capable of providing this coordinated care.[13]

Fistulas are classified by their location and pathway, including extrasphincteric, transphincteric, superficial, intersphincteric, and suprasphincteric (**Fig. 2**).[15] Due to the path of the fistula and associated CD activity, a fistula may present with an associated abscess. Before the initiation of medical therapy, complete drainage of the abscess should be performed, and frequently a Seton will be placed to prevent recurrent infection while on medical therapy. Setons are inert foreign material (vessel loop, rubber drain, silk suture) that are attached to themselves and remain in place until the area has healed. This allows maximal medical therapy to occur uninterrupted due to recurrent infection without injury to the sphincter complex.[13] Systematic review of pediatric patients with perianal disease demonstrate recurrence rates between 1 and 2 years of 35.7%, 23.4%, and 4.3% for Seton placement alone, infliximab therapy alone, and combination therapy, respectively.[13]

Ulcerative Colitis

UC is chronic superficial inflammation of the colon and is common than CD children aged under 6 years (31%–47%).[16] Pediatric patients present with more extensive and severe colitis than adults with UC, with some studies reporting 61% to 90% of

Table 4
Surgical approaches to total proctocolectomy with ileal pouch anal anastomosis

Stages	Approach	Patient Population
One-stage	Total proctocolectomy with ileal pouch anal anastomosis	Stable patients without risk factors anastomotic leak
Two-stage	1. Total proctocolectomy with ileal pouch anal anastomosis and diverting ileostomy 2. Ileostomy closure	Stable patients with risk factors for anastomotic leak
Modified 2-stage	1. Total abdominal colectomy with end ileostomy 2. Ileal pouch anal anastomosis without diverting ileostomy	Unstable patients requiring urgent surgery who improve following surgery and undergo ileal pouch procedure without risk of anastomotic leak
Three-stage	1. Total abdominal colectomy with end ileostomy 2. Ileal pouch anal anastomosis without diverting ileostomy 3. Ileostomy closure	Unstable patients who later undergo ileal pouch procedure with risk of anastomotic leak

children presenting with pancolitis, nearly double the rates of extensive disease in adults.[5,16] However, the increased use of infliximab has resulted in reduced rates of surgical intervention for UC.[17] Surgical management of UC includes total proctocolectomy with ileal pouch–anal anastomosis (TPC-IPAA).[17–19] Surgery can be accomplished as a single stage or in multiple stages.[18,20,21] (**Table 4**) Indications for surgery in UC are summarized in **Table 5**. Before surgery for UC, CD and other causes of colitis should be ruled out (**Box 1**).[22]

Surgical approach
TPC-IPAA has similar long-term outcomes whether performed open or laparoscopic. However, as minimally invasive surgery has become more common, there is increasing utilization of laparoscopy for the procedure. Regardless of technique, the removal of the colon with ileal pouch reconstruction is considered the standard of care for patients with UC that require surgery. Although various options for ileal pouch reconstruction are available (S-pouch, W-pouch, J-pouch), the most commonly used technique is the J-pouch.[23] When comparing postoperative function and patient satisfaction with TPC-IPAA, laparoscopic versus open surgical approaches have produced similar outcomes with high rates of patient satisfaction.[23]

Total proctocolectomy can be performed by dividing the colonic mesentery and controlling the arterial blood supply to the colon (**Fig. 3**), taking care to avoid injury

Table 5
Indications for surgery in pediatric ulcerative colitis

Indication	Surgery
Life-threatening complications of colitis (ie, hemorrhage or perforation)	Staged total proctocolectomy with ileal pouch anal anastomosis
Uncontrolled disease refractory to medical therapy	Staged total proctocolectomy with ileal pouch anal anastomosis
Neoplastic changes	Total proctocolectomy with ileal pouch anal anastomosis
Growth/pubertal delay	

to the adjacent structures.[23] Following mobilization and removal of the colon, attention is turned to the rectum. The lateral peritoneum along the length of the rectum is opened adjacent to the rectum while carefully avoiding the nervi erigentes on the lateral wall (**Fig. 4**).[23] The rectum is dissected from the sacral promontory to the pelvic floor posteriorly, and then dissection is continued close to the distal rectal wall, avoiding the pelvic plexus anteriorly (see **Fig. 4**).[23] At the pelvic floor, the rectum is divided 1 to 2 cm above the dentate line. This anatomic area corresponds to the anal transition zone, the most innervated area of the colon and rectum.[23] This innervated area is responsible for sensing pressure, liquid, solid, and gas, which plays a critical role in continence following IPAA.[23] After TPC, an ileal pouch is constructed using the terminal ileum. The apex of the pouch is identified at the area of the terminal ileum, which most easily reaches the pelvic floor. The terminal ileum is then folded at that point and measured to approximately 15 cm in length (**Fig. 5A, B**). An enterotomy is created and the 2 lumens of small intestine are then connected on their antimesenteric border to create a pouch using 2 fires of a 10-cm stapler. The apex can then be attached to the rectal cuff using a circular stapler or by absorbable sutures, with similar outcomes. In some patients, a diverting loop ileostomy may be created proximal to the pouch to decrease pouch leaks.

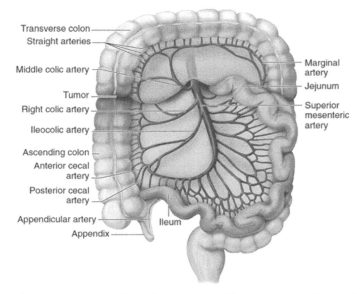

Fig. 3. Superior mesentery artery branches to the small intestine, ascending, and transverse colon.[9]

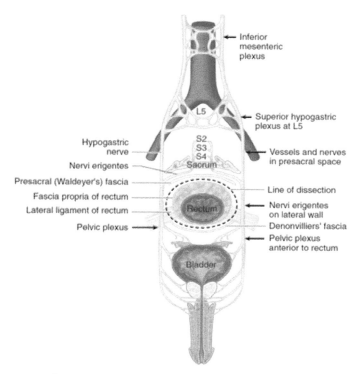

Fig. 4. Anatomy of pelvic nerves, which should be identified and preserved during proctocolectomy-ileal pouch anal anastomosis.[9]

Straight ileal pull-through

The performance of a TPC with straight ileal pull-through is unique to pediatric surgery and used most commonly for congenital agangliosis of the colon and rectum.[24] The ileoanal pull-through (IPT; without pouch reconstruction) is well documented in the pediatric surgical literature but little data exist in patient outcomes in UC. The largest study examined 250 total children and 168 with UC from multiple institutions. The study examined stooling frequency as the primary outcome and pouchitis as the secondary outcome.[24] These data demonstrated more frequent stooling in the IPT groups at 1-year and 2-years postop but similar stooling patters compared with IPAA at 3-year follow-up.[24] The frequency of pouchitis in the IPAA was 49% compared with 26% in the IPT group.[24] This unique approach should be noted on assumption of care by adult surgeons in patients who present with complications following IPAA.

Staging ileal reconstruction

The frequency of diverting ileostomy after ileal reconstruction in pediatric patients is controversial.[21,25] Specifically, in patients with well-controlled disease without risk factors for anastomotic leak the benefit to diverting ileostomy is less clear than in adult patients.[21,25] Although, diverting ileostomy is thought to decrease fecal peritonitis in adult patients with an anastomotic leak, it has been shown to be associated with increased cost, pouch failure, rectovaginal fistula, and bleeding.[26] As such efforts to safely avoid ileostomy are important to improving care, retrospective data in children demonstrate similar outcomes between patients with and without diverting ileostomy after ileal pouch reconstruction.[21,25]

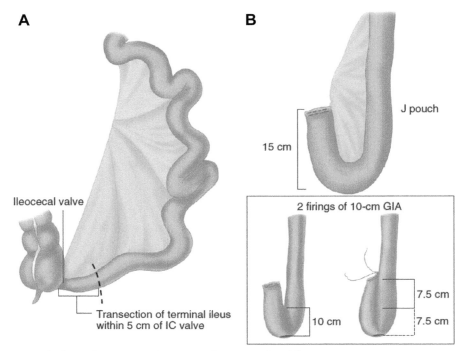

A

B

J pouch

15 cm

Ileocecal valve

Transection of terminal ileus
within 5 cm of IC valve

2 firings of 10-cm GIA

7.5 cm

10 cm   7.5 cm

Fig. 5. Ileal pouch creation using a J-configuration (A, B).[9]

Surgical Outcomes

A recent systematic review of outcomes after surgery for pediatric UC demonstrated high rates of postoperative complications, with acute pouchitis affecting just more than 40% of patients.[18] Small bowel obstruction, stricture or stenosis, and fistula were frequently reported as well.[18] Chronic pouchitis (13.2% [39/295, 3 studies]), anastomotic leak or pelvic abscess (10.7% [29/270, 7 studies]), and wound infections (8.9% [29/326, 4 studies]) occurred less commonly.[18] There are few well-controlled studies examining the quality of life for pediatric patients following TPC-IPAA.[18] At long-term follow-up, 79% of adolescent and young adult patients were very satisfied with their surgery.[27] In adult patients, satisfaction was not affected by laparoscopic or open approaches.[23]

Special considerations

Referral to pediatric surgical care. Due to the chronic-relapsing nature of IBD and its associated psychosocial impacts, establishing connections to multidisciplinary care teams that include pediatric gastroenterologists, surgeons, dieticians, psychologists, and social workers are paramount.[28] Formation of a comprehensive care team allows for screening and management of nonsurgical conditions as well as coordination of care.[28] This also facilitates the performance of surgical and endoscopic interventions in coordination with the patient and family goals.[28] This can be done in nonemergent settings for patients who present to general surgical care. In emergency settings, early follow-up with multidisciplinary care to address nutritional and psychosocial needs following surgery is recommended.

Emergency surgery. For pediatric patients with emergent or life-threatening conditions (perforation, hemorrhage, hemodynamic instability), damage control surgery may be necessary outside of their typical care team and environment. For IBD patients who require intestinal resection in an emergency, care should be taken to minimize the length of intestinal resection in CD, especially if the surgical emergency is their presenting symptom and they have not been exposed to medical therapy. This typically involves resection of the gross abnormal intestine, which may include a perforated segment or short stricture that has associated segment of bowel with creeping fat or thickened mesentery. For patients with UC who present with severe life-threatening sepsis related to colitis refractory to medical management or perforation subtotal colectomy with end ileostomy and rectal closure is the preferred approach. This allows time for pathology to be finalized and clinical optimization before definitive pelvic surgery. After emergency surgery a referral to a specialized center for ileal-pouch reconstruction and psychosocial and nutritional optimization can be performed.

Inflammatory bowel disease-unclassified. Patients with IBD-U have inflammation confined to the colon without features specific to UC or CD.[16] This could be a presentation of UC with the presence of transmural inflammation, significant growth delay, ileitis or duodenitis, rectal sparing, or reversal of the gradient of mucosal inflammation.[16] IBD-U is more common in children than in adult patients with IBD[29]; however, most patients with IBD-U can ultimately be assigned to either CD or UC phenotypes.[1] When examining outcomes after IPAA for IBD-U, Delaney and colleagues[30] reported similar outcomes, quality of life, and pouch failure compared with patients with UC. Patients with IBD-U were more likely to have their diagnosis change to CD than patients with UC but reported very high levels of satisfaction and likelihood of recommending surgery to other patients (>90%).[30]

Growth delay. Patients with pediatric IBD may experience growth and developmental deficits.[16,31,32] Growth failure is defined as consistent height less than third percentile or z-score for height −2 standard deviations (SD).[32] This occurs more commonly in patients with CD than UC and is variably present in IBD-U.[16] This leads to patients with CD having a decrease in height of 0.50 SD and a final deficit of 0.29 SD of final height.[31] Unfortunately, even with therapy, Sawczenko and colleagues[31] identified 19% of patients with greater than 8 cm deficit in final height, although notably this study was performed before biologics were used in pediatric IBD treatment. As such, growth delay represents a unique and subtle indication for surgical intervention in pediatric IBD and should be included in multidisciplinary discussions of treatment efficacy and surgical candidacy.

Pubertal delay. In addition to growth delay, pediatric patients with IBD may develop delays in pubertal development. This is more common in female patients with CD and presents as an absence of breast development.[32] In male patients, this presents as testicular enlargement of z-score−2.5 SD below the mean.[32] The underlying mechanisms, which were initially thought to be primarily related to malnutrition, are unclear but may be associated with nutritional deficiency and proinflammatory cytokines found in active disease.[32,33] As such, this may represent a more subtle finding of treatment failure, and the patient's candidacy for surgery should be reviewed in a multidisciplinary fashion.

Transitional clinic. Due to the chronic nature of pediatric IBD, the transition from pediatric care teams to adult care teams is critical for providing continuity of care. Previous studies have demonstrated poorer health outcomes during these transition periods.[34] Although resources exist to improve transitional care, data are based on descriptive analysis rather than prospective studies.[34] A recent review suggested assessing transition readiness, planning and documenting goals of transition, and implementing changes with continual reassessment of progress.[34] This requires collaboration and communication between adult and pediatric care teams. To facilitate this transition, operative notes with pathology results from the pediatric care team should be given to the adult care team to allow for a thorough understanding of the patient's anatomy.

SUMMARY

IBD is a chronic, relapsing-remitting condition in children, and frequently requires multidisciplinary care. Important to patient care is identifying the phenotype of IBD, which includes distinguishing between CD, UC, and IBD-U, understanding that this may change over time. The type of IBD changes the approach to surgery; however, surgical indications are similar between groups and generally include severe or life-threatening disease or disease refractory to medical therapy. In CD, attention should be paid to preservation of bowel length and intestinal resection should be followed with close medical follow-up to prevent disease recurrence. UC and IBD-U can be effectively treated with TPC-IPAA but many patients experience complications following surgery, including pouchitis in nearly 40% of patients. However, patients who do undergo surgery demonstrate high rates of satisfaction and quality of life in spite of this morbidity. IBD-unclassified may progress to CD and should be discussed with patients and families before surgical intervention. Special considerations for pediatric patients with IBD include growth delays, delayed onset or progression of puberty, and the transition period from pediatric teams to adult care teams being associated with poorer outcomes.

CLINICS CARE POINTS

- Pediatric inflammatory bowel disease frequently requires surgery.

- Crohn disease may require intestinal resection for severe stricturing or penetrating disease. Efforts should be made to minimize the length of resection and restart medical therapy postoperatively to prevent recurrence.

- Peri-anal Crohn disease may present as a perirectal abscess with associated fistula; patients have lowest recurrence rates with a combination of Seton placement and immune suppression.

- Ulcerative colitis in children with life-threatening disease or who fail medical management may require total proctocolectomy with ileal pouch anal anastomosis. Although patients experience early postoperative complications (including pouchitis), the majority are satisfied with their surgical outcomes.

- A thorough understanding of the patients' operative and pathologic history is critical on assuming care of pediatric patients transitioning to adult care teams.

- Delays in growth, pubertal onset, and pubertal progression are manifestations of IBD, which are specific to pediatric patients, and should be considered when evaluating therapeutic success or failure.

- Multidisciplinary care is critical to optimizing care for pediatric patients with IBD, including expertise in pediatric gastroenterology, surgery, social work, nutrition, and psychology.

- When the patient condition permits, transfer to a multidisciplinary team should be considered. In emergencies (perforation, instability), intestinal resection may be required with the goal of stabilization with limited bowel resection in Crohn disease and abdominal colectomy with end ileostomy in ulcerative colitis.

- Transitioning of care from pediatric to adult providers represents a vulnerable time in the care of children with IBD, and a standardized approach to care transitions, which involve pediatric and adult care teams are critical.

DISCLOSURE

The authors have nothing to disclose.

REFERENCES

1. Ye Y, Manne S, Treem WR, et al. Prevalence of inflammatory bowel disease in pediatric and adult populations: recent estimates from large national databases in the united states, 2007-2016. Inflamm Bowel Dis 2020;26(4):619–25.
2. Rosen MJ, Dhawan A, Saeed SA. Inflammatory bowel disease in children and adolescents. JAMA Pediatr 2015;169(11):1053–60.
3. Vernier-Massouille G, Balde M, Salleron J, et al. Natural history of pediatric Crohn's disease: a population-based cohort study. Gastroenterology 2008; 135(4):1106–13.
4. Van Limbergent J, Russell RK, Drummond HE, et al. Definition of phenotypic characteristics of childhood-onset inflammatory bowel disease. Gastroenterology 2008;135(4):1114–22.
5. Goodhand J, Dawson R, Hefferon M, et al. Inflammatory bowel disease in young people: the case for transitional clinics. Inflamm Bowel Dis 2010;16(6): 947–52.
6. Kim S. Surgery in pediatric crohn's disease: indications, timing and postoperative management. Pediatr Gastroenterol Hepatol Nutr 2017;20(1):14–21.
7. Ricciuto A, Aardoom M, Orlanski-Meyer E, et al. Predicting outcomes in pediatric crohn's disease for management optimization: systematic review and consensus statements from the pediatric inflammatory bowel disease-ahead program. Gastroenterology 2021;160(1):403–436 e426.
8. Neville JJ, Macdonald A, Fell J, et al. Therapeutic strategies for stricturing Crohn's disease in childhood: a systematic review. Pediatr Surg Int 2021;37(5): 569–77.
9. James W, Fleshman JMDF, Birnbaum EH, Hunt SR, et al. Atlas of surgical techniques for colon, rectum and anus: (A volume in the surgical techniques atlas series) (expert consult - online and print). Philadelphia: Elsevier Health Sciences; 2012.
10. Hirten RP, Shah S, Sachar DB, et al. The management of intestinal penetrating crohn's disease. Inflamm Bowel Dis 2018;24(4):752–65.
11. Frolkis AD, Dykeman J, Negron ME, et al. Risk of surgery for inflammatory bowel diseases has decreased over time: a systematic review and meta-analysis of population-based studies. Gastroenterology 2013;145(5):996–1006.
12. Debruyn JC, Soon IS, Hubbard J, et al. Nationwide temporal trends in incidence of hospitalization and surgical intestinal resection in pediatric inflammatory bowel diseases in the United States from 1997 to 2009. Inflamm Bowel Dis 2013;19(11): 2423–32.

13. Forsdick VK, Tan Tanny SP, King SK. Medical and surgical management of pediatric perianal crohn's disease: A systematic review. J Pediatr Surg 2019;54(12): 2554–8.
14. de Zoeten EF, Pasternak BA, Mattei P, et al. Diagnosis and treatment of perianal Crohn disease: NASPGHAN clinical report and consensus statement. J Pediatr Gastroenterol Nutr 2013;57(3):401–12.
15. Delaney CP. Netter's surgical anatomy and approaches. Saint Louis, UNITED STATES: Elsevier; 2013.
16. Yu YR, Rodriguez JR. Clinical presentation of Crohn's, ulcerative colitis, and indeterminate colitis: symptoms, extraintestinal manifestations, and disease phenotypes. Semin Pediatr Surg 2017;26(6):349–55.
17. Bolia R, Rajanayagam J, Hardikar W, et al. Impact of changing treatment strategies on outcomes in pediatric ulcerative colitis. Inflamm Bowel Dis 2019;25(11): 1838–44.
18. Tan Tanny SP, Yoo M, Hutson JM, et al. Current surgical practice in pediatric ulcerative colitis: a systematic review. J Pediatr Surg 2019;54(7):1324–30.
19. Orlanski-Meyer E, Aardoom M, Ricciuto A, et al. Predicting outcomes in pediatric ulcerative colitis for management optimization: systematic review and consensus statements from the pediatric inflammatory bowel disease-ahead program. Gastroenterology 2021;160(1):378–402 e322.
20. Rubalcava NS, Moreno NA, Adler J, et al. Does the timing of pouch creation in 2-stage operations for pediatric patients with ulcerative colitis matter? J Pediatr Surg 2021;56(6):1203–7.
21. Marulanda K, Purcell LN, Egberg MD, et al. Analysis of a modified two-stage approach to ileal pouch-anal anastomosis without fecal diversion in pediatric patients. Am Surg 2022;88(1):103–8.
22. Turner D, Levine A, Escher JC, et al. Management of pediatric ulcerative colitis: joint ECCO and ESPGHAN evidence-based consensus guidelines. J Pediatr Gastroenterol Nutr 2012;55(3):340–61.
23. Lavryk OA, Stocchi L, Ashburn JH, et al. Case-matched comparison of long-term functional and quality of life outcomes following laparoscopic versus open ileal pouch-anal anastomosis. World J Surg 2018;42(11):3746–54.
24. Seetharamaiah R, West BT, Ignash SJ, et al. Outcomes in pediatric patients undergoing straight vs J pouch ileoanal anastomosis: a multicenter analysis. J Pediatr Surg 2009;44(7):1410–7.
25. Rubalcava NS, Gadepalli SK, Criss CN, et al. Single-stage restorative proctocolectomy for ulcerative colitis in pediatric patients: a safe alternative. Pediatr Surg Int 2021;37(10):1453–9.
26. Samples J, Evans K, Chaumont N, et al. Variant two-stage ileal pouch-anal anastomosis: an innovative and effective alternative to standard resection in ulcerative colitis. J Am Coll Surg 2017;224(4):557–63.
27. Shannon A, Eng K, Kay M, et al. Long-term follow up of ileal pouch anal anastomosis in a large cohort of pediatric and young adult patients with ulcerative colitis. J Pediatr Surg 2016;51(7):1181–6.
28. Wren AA, Maddux MH. Integrated multidisciplinary treatment for pediatric inflammatory bowel disease. Children (Basel) 2021;8(2):1–4.
29. Prenzel F, Uhlig HH. Frequency of indeterminate colitis in children and adults with IBD - a metaanalysis. J Crohns Colitis 2009;3(4):277–81.
30. Delaney CP, Remzi FH, Gramlich T, et al. Equivalent function, quality of life and pouch survival rates after ileal pouch-anal anastomosis for indeterminate and ulcerative colitis. Ann Surg 2002;236(1):43–8.

31. Sawczenko A, Ballinger AB, Savage MO, et al. Clinical features affecting final adult height in patients with pediatric-onset Crohn's disease. Pediatrics 2006; 118(1):124–9.
32. Amaro F, Chiarelli F. Growth and Puberty in Children with Inflammatory Bowel Diseases. Biomedicines 2020;8(11):1–17.
33. Ballinger AB, Savage MO, Sanderson IR. Delayed puberty associated with inflammatory bowel disease. Pediatr Res 2003;53(2):205–10.
34. Menon T, Afzali A. Inflammatory bowel disease: a practical path to transitioning from pediatric to adult care. Am J Gastroenterol 2019;114(9):1432–40.

UNITED STATES POSTAL SERVICE ®

Statement of Ownership, Management, and Circulation
(All Periodicals Publications Except Requester Publications)

1. Publication Title	2. Publication Number	3. Filing Date
SURGICAL CLINICS	529 – 800	9/18/2022

4. Issue Frequency	5. Number of Issues Published Annually	6. Annual Subscription Price
FEB, APR, JUN, AUG, OCT, DEC	6	$456.00

7. Complete Mailing Address of Known Office of Publication *(Not printer)* *(Street, city, county, state, and ZIP+4®)*

ELSEVIER INC.
230 Park Avenue, Suite 800
New York, NY 10169

Contact Person
Malathi Samayan

Telephone *(Include area code)*
91-44-4299-4507

8. Complete Mailing Address of Headquarters or General Business Office of Publisher *(Not printer)*

ELSEVIER INC.
230 Park Avenue, Suite 800
New York, NY 10169

9. Full Names and Complete Mailing Addresses of Publisher, Editor, and Managing Editor *(Do not leave blank)*

Publisher *(Name and complete mailing address)*

DOLORES MELONI, ELSEVIER INC.
1600 JOHN F KENNEDY BLVD. SUITE 1800
PHILADELPHIA, PA 19103-2899

Editor *(Name and complete mailing address)*

JOHN VASSALLO, ELSEVIER INC.
1600 JOHN F KENNEDY BLVD. SUITE 1800
PHILADELPHIA, PA 19103-2899

Managing Editor *(Name and complete mailing address)*

PATRICK MANLEY, ELSEVIER INC.
1600 JOHN F KENNEDY BLVD. SUITE 1800
PHILADELPHIA, PA 19103-2899

10. Owner *(Do not leave blank. If the publication is owned by a corporation, give the name and address of the corporation immediately followed by the names and addresses of all stockholders owning or holding 1 percent or more of the total amount of stock. If not owned by a corporation, give the names and addresses of the individual owners. If owned by a partnership or other unincorporated firm, give its name and address as well as those of each individual owner. If the publication is published by a nonprofit organization, give its name and address.)*

Full Name	Complete Mailing Address
WHOLLY OWNED SUBSIDIARY OF REED/ELSEVIER, US HOLDINGS	1600 JOHN F KENNEDY BLVD. SUITE 1800 PHILADELPHIA, PA 19103-2899

11. Known Bondholders, Mortgagees, and Other Security Holders Owning or Holding 1 Percent or More of Total Amount of Bonds, Mortgages, or Other Securities. If none, check box ▶ ☐ None

Full Name	Complete Mailing Address
N/A	

12. Tax Status *(For completion by nonprofit organizations authorized to mail at nonprofit rates)* *(Check one)*
The purpose, function, and nonprofit status of this organization and the exempt status for federal income tax purposes:
☒ Has Not Changed During Preceding 12 Months
☐ Has Changed During Preceding 12 Months *(Publisher must submit explanation of change with this statement)*

PS Form **3526**, July 2014 *(Page 1 of 4 (see instructions page 4))*   PSN: 7530-01-000-9931   PRIVACY NOTICE: See our privacy policy on www.usps.com.

---

13. Publication Title	14. Issue Date for Circulation Data Below
SURGICAL CLINICS	JUNE 2022

15. Extent and Nature of Circulation

			Average No. Copies Each Issue During Preceding 12 Months	No. Copies of Single Issue Published Nearest to Filing Date
a. Total Number of Copies *(Net press run)*			399	332
b. Paid Circulation *(By Mail and Outside the Mail)*	(1)	Mailed Outside-County Paid Subscriptions Stated on PS Form 3541 *(Include paid distribution above nominal rate, advertiser's proof copies, and exchange copies)*	186	156
	(2)	Mailed In-County Paid Subscriptions Stated on PS Form 3541 *(Include paid distribution above nominal rate, advertiser's proof copies, and exchange copies)*	0	0
	(3)	Paid Distribution Outside the Mails Including Sales Through Dealers and Carriers, Street Vendors, Counter Sales, and Other Paid Distribution Outside USPS®	169	136
	(4)	Paid Distribution by Other Classes of Mail Through the USPS *(e.g., First-Class Mail®)*	0	0
c. Total Paid Distribution *(Sum of 15b (1), (2), (3), and (4))*		▶	355	292
d. Free or Nominal Rate Distribution *(By Mail and Outside the Mail)*	(1)	Free or Nominal Rate Outside-County Copies included on PS Form 3541	24	19
	(2)	Free or Nominal Rate In-County Copies Included on PS Form 3541	0	0
	(3)	Free or Nominal Rate Copies Mailed at Other Classes Through the USPS *(e.g. First-Class Mail)*	0	0
	(4)	Free or Nominal Rate Distribution Outside the Mail *(Carriers or other means)*	24	19
e. Total Free or Nominal Rate Distribution *(Sum of 15d (1), (2), (3) and (4))*		▶	24	19
f. Total Distribution *(Sum of 15c and 15e)*		▶	379	311
g. Copies not Distributed *(See Instructions to Publishers #4 (page #3))*		▶	20	21
h. Total *(Sum of 15f and g)*		▶	399	332
i. Percent Paid *(15c divided by 15f times 100)*			93.66%	93.89%

* If you are claiming electronic copies, go to line 16 on page 3. If you are not claiming electronic copies, skip to line 17 on page 3.

16. Electronic Copy Circulation

	Average No. Copies Each Issue During Preceding 12 Months	No. Copies of Single Issue Published Nearest to Filing Date
a. Paid Electronic Copies	▶	
b. Total Paid Print Copies (Line 15c) + Paid Electronic Copies (Line 16a)	▶	
c. Total Print Distribution (Line 15f) + Paid Electronic Copies (Line 16a)	▶	
d. Percent Paid (Both Print & Electronic Copies) (16b divided by 16c × 100)	▶	

☒ I certify that 50% of all my distributed copies (electronic and print) are paid above a nominal price.

17. Publication of Statement of Ownership

☒ If the publication is a general publication, publication of this statement is required. Will be printed ☐ Publication not required.

in the OCTOBER 2022 issue of this publication.

18. Signature and Title of Editor, Publisher, Business Manager, or Owner

Malathi Samayan - Distribution Controller

Malathi Samayan

Date 9/18/2022

I certify that all information furnished on this form is true and complete. I understand that anyone who furnishes false or misleading information on this form or who omits material or information requested on the form may be subject to criminal sanctions (including fines and imprisonment) and/or civil sanctions (including civil penalties).

PS Form **3526**, July 2014 *(Page 3 of 4)*   PRIVACY NOTICE: See our privacy policy on www.usps.com.

Moving?

Make sure your subscription moves with you!

To notify us of your new address, find your **Clinics Account Number** (located on your mailing label above your name), and contact customer service at:

Email: journalscustomerservice-usa@elsevier.com

800-654-2452 (subscribers in the U.S. & Canada)
314-447-8871 (subscribers outside of the U.S. & Canada)

Fax number: 314-447-8029

Elsevier Health Sciences Division
Subscription Customer Service
3251 Riverport Lane
Maryland Heights, MO 63043

*To ensure uninterrupted delivery of your subscription, please notify us at least 4 weeks in advance of move.